Mary M. Mckay, PhD
Roberta L. Paikoff, PhD
Editors

W9-BWN-137

Community Collaborative Partnerships: The Foundation for HIV Prevention Research Efforts

Community Collaborative Partnerships: The Foundation for HIV Prevention Research Efforts has been co-published simultaneously as *Social Work in Mental Health*, Volume 5, Numbers 1/2 and 3/4 2007.

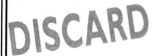

Pre-publication REVIEWS, COMMENTARIES, EVALUATIONS . . .

"This book will be a foundational resource for anyone interested in: (a) urban African-American communities (b) factors impacting on initiation of sexual behaviors, (c) how a research study (CHAMP) can influence clinical practice, (d) establishing long-term and meaningful partnerships between university-based researchers and community members, (e) transferring externally funded research programs into community-based organizations in order to ensure the sustainability of effective programs, and (f) diffusing innovations nationally and internationally."

Kathleen M. Nokes, PhD, RN, FAAN
Professor
Hunter-Bellevue
School of Nursing
Hunter College
City University of New York

Community Collaborative Partnerships: The Foundation for HIV Prevention Research Efforts

Community Collaborative Partnerships: The Foundation for HIV Prevention Research Efforts has been co-published simultaneously as *Social Work in Mental Health*, Volume 5, Numbers 1/2 and 3/4 2007.

Monographic Separates from the *Social Work in Mental Health*

For additional information on these and other Haworth Press titles, including descriptions, tables of contents, reviews, and prices, use the QuickSearch catalog at http://www.HaworthPress.com.

Community Collaborative Partnerships: The Foundation for HIV Prevention Research Efforts, edited by Mary M. McKay, PhD, and Roberta L. Paikoff, PhD (Vol. 5, Nos. 1/2 and 3/4, 2007). *Exploration of ways to develop, design, and evaluate strong community partnerships to support youth health prevention efforts in the United States and around the world.*

Clinical and Research Uses of an Adolescent Mental Health Intake Questionnaire: What Kids Need to Talk About, edited by Ken Peake, DSW, Irwin Epstein, PhD, and Daniel Mederios, MD (Vol. 3, Nos. 1/2, 2004, and Vol. 3, No. 3, 2005). *"Clinical and Research Uses of an Adolescent Mental Health Intake Questionnaire: What Kids Need to Talk About" explores the research on adolescent behavior culled from the answers to a clinician-designed intake questionnaire given to adolescent clients asking how they view their own risks, what they worry about, and what they wish to talk about. Respected authorities discuss the enlightening findings and present ways to reshape services, taking into account customer preference, risk and worry, and youth development (YD) perspectives while presenting practical clinical strategies to engage at-risk adolescents in mental health treatment.*

Social Work Approaches in Health and Mental Health from Around the Globe, edited by Anna Metteri, MSocSc, Teppo Kröger, PhD, Anneli Pohjola, PhD, and Pirkko-Liisa Rauhala, PhD (Vol. 2, No. 2/3, 2004). *"BROAD-BASED AND UNIQUE . . . . A much-needed publication for training and practice." (Charlene Laurence Carbonatto, DPhil, Senior Lecturer, Department of Social Work, University of Prestoria, South Africa)*

Psychiatric Medication Issues for Social Workers, Counselors, and Psychiatrists, edited by Kia J. Bentley, PhD, LCSW (Vol. 1, No. 4, 2003). *"OUTSTANDING . . . . All social workers, counselors, and psychologists working in the mental health field would benefit from reading this outstanding book." (Deborah P. Valentine, PhD, MSSW, Professor and Director, School of Social Work, Colorado State University)*

Community Collaborative Partnerships: The Foundation for HIV Prevention Research Efforts

Mary M. McKay, PhD
Roberta L. Paikoff, PhD
Editors

Gary Rosenberg, PhD
Andrew Weissman, PhD
Series Editors

Community Collaborative Partnerships: The Foundation for HIV Prevention Research Efforts has been co-published simultaneously as *Social Work in Mental Health*, Volume 5, Numbers 1/2 and 3/4 2007.

The Haworth Press, Inc.

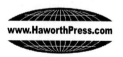

www.HaworthPress.com

Published by

The Haworth Press, Inc., 10 Alice Street, Binghamton, NY 13904-1580 USA.

Community Collaborative Partnerships: The Foundation for HIV Prevention Research Efforts has been co-published simultaneously as *Journal of Social Work in Mental Health* Volume 5, Numbers 1/2 and 3/4 2007.

The development, preparation, and publication of this work has been undertaken with great care. However, the publisher, employees, editors, and agents of The Haworth Press and all imprints of The Haworth Press, Inc., including The Haworth Medical Press® and The Pharmaceutical Products Press®, are not responsible for any errors contained herein or for consequences that may ensue from use of materials or information contained in this work. Opinions expressed by the author(s) are not necessarily those of The Haworth Press, Inc. With regard to case studies, identities and circumstances of individuals discussed herein have been changed to protect confidentialty. Any resemblance to actual persons, living or dead, is entirely coincidental.

The Haworth Press is committed to the dissemination of ideas and information according to the highest standards of intellectual freedom and the free exchange of ideas. Statements made and opinions expressed in this publication do not necessarily reflect the views of the Publisher, Directors, management, or staff of The Haworth Press, Inc., or an endorsement by them.

Library of Congress Cataloging-in-Publication Data

Community Collaborative Partnerships: The Foundation for HIV Prevention Research Efforts/ Mary M. McKay, Roberta L. Paikoff, editors.
　　p. cm.
　　"Co-published simultaneously as social work in mental health, vol. 5, no. 1-4 2007."
　　Includes bibliographical references and index.
　　ISBN 13: 978-0-7890-3253-9 (hard cover : alk. paper)
　　ISBN 10: 0-7890-3253-8 (hard cover : alk. paper)
　　ISBN 13: 978-0-7890-3254-6 (soft cover : alk. paper)
　　ISBN 10: 0-7890-3254-6 (soft cover : alk. paper)
　　1. AIDS (Disease) in adolescence–United States–Prevention. 2. HIV infections–United States–Prevention. 3. HIV viruses–United States–Prevention. 4. African American youth–Sexual behavior–United States. 5. African American youth--Services for–United States. 6. Minority youth–Services for–United States. 7. Urban youth–Services for–United States. 8. Community health services–United States. 9. Social work with youth–United States. I. McKay, Mary M. II. Paikoff, Roberta Lynn.
　　[DNLM: 1. HIV Infections–prevention & control–United States. 2. Adolescent–United States. 3. African Americans–United States. 4. Community Health Services–organization & administration–United States. 5. Consumer Participation–United States. 6. Minority Groups–United States. 7. Urban Health–United States. W1 SO135Q v.3 no.1-4 2007 / WC 503.6 C7347 2007]
　　RJ387.A25C63 2007
　　362.196'979200835–dc22　　　　　　　　　　　　　　　　　　　　　　　　2007000986

The HAWORTH PRESS _Inc._

Abstracting, Indexing & Outward Linking

PRINT _and_ ELECTRONIC BOOKS & JOURNALS

This section provides you with a list of major indexing & abstracting services and other tools for bibliographic access. That is to say, each service began covering this periodical during the the year noted in the right column. Most Websites which are listed below have indicated that they will either post, disseminate, compile, archive, cite or alert their own Website users with research-based content from this work. (This list is as current as the copyright date of this publication.)

Abstracting, Website/Indexing Coverage . . . . Year When Coverage Began

- *(CAB ABSTRACTS, CABI) <http://www.cabi.org>* 2003

- *(IBR) International Bibliography of Book Reviews on the Humanities and Social Sciences (Thomson) <http://www.saur.de>* 2006

- *(IBZ) International Bibliography of Periodical Literature on the Humanities and Social Sciences (Thomson) <http://www.saur.de>* 2002

- ***Academic Search Premier (EBSCO)** <http://search.ebscohost.com>* 2006

- ***CINAHL (Cumulative Index to Nursing & Allied Health Literature) (EBSCO)** <http://www.cinahl.com>* 2003

- ***CINAHL Plus (EBSCO)** <http://search.ebscohost.com>* 2006

- ***MasterFILE Premier (EBSCO)** <http://search.ebscohost.com>* . . 2006

- ***Psychological Abstracts (PsycINFO)** <http://www.apa.org>* . . . 2003

- ***Social Services Abstracts (Cambridge Scientific Abstracts)** <http://www.csa.com>* 2003

- ***Social Work Abstracts (NASW)** <http://www.silverplatter.com/catalog/swab.htm>* 2006

- *Abstracts on Hygiene and Communicable Diseases (CAB ABSTRACTS, CABI) <http://www.cabi.org>* 2006

- *Academic Source Premier (EBSCO) <http://search.ebscohost.com>* . . . 2007

(continued)

(continued)

(continued)

Bibliographic Access

- **Cabell's Directory of Publishing Opportunities in Psychology** *<http://www.cabells.com>*

- **MediaFinder** *<http://www.mediafinder.com>*

- **Ulrich's Periodicals Directory: The Global Source for Periodicals Information Since 1932** *<http://www. bowkerlink.com>*

Special Bibliographic Notes related to special journal issues (separates) and indexing/abstracting:

- indexing/abstracting services in this list will also cover material in any "separate" that is co-published simultaneously with Haworth's special thematic journal issue or DocuSerial. Indexing/abstracting usually covers material at the article/chapter level.
- monographic co-editions are intended for either non-subscribers or libraries which intend to purchase a second copy for their circulating collections.
- monographic co-editions are reported to all jobbers/wholesalers/approval plans. The source journal is listed as the "series" to assist the prevention of duplicate purchasing in the same manner utilized for books-in-series.
- to facilitate user/access services all indexing/abstracting services are encouraged to utilize the co-indexing entry note indicated at the bottom of the first page of each article/chapter/contribution.
- this is intended to assist a library user of any reference tool (whether print, electronic, online, or CD-ROM) to locate the monographic version if the library has purchased this version but not a subscription to the source journal.
- individual articles/chapters in any Haworth publication are also available through the Haworth Document Delivery Service (HDDS).

As part of Haworth's continuing committment to better serve our library patrons, we are proud to be working with the following electronic services:

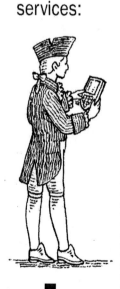

AGGREGATOR SERVICES

EBSCOhost

Ingenta

J-Gate

Minerva

OCLC FirstSearch

Oxmill

SwetsWise

MINERVA

FirstSearch

Oxmill Publishing

SwetsWise

LINK RESOLVER SERVICES

1Cate (Openly Informatics)

CrossRef

Gold Rush (Coalliance)

LinkOut (PubMed)

LINKplus (Atypon)

LinkSolver (Ovid)

LinkSource with A-to-Z (EBSCO)

Resource Linker (Ulrich)

SerialsSolutions (ProQuest)

SFX (Ex Libris)

Sirsi Resolver (SirsiDynix)

Tour (TDnet)

Vlink (Extensity, *formerly Geac*)

WebBridge (Innovative Interfaces)

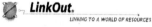

LinkOut.
LINKING TO A WORLD OF RESOURCES

atypon

A to Z

LinkSolver

ULRICH'S RESOURCE LINKER

S·F·X

SerialsSolutions

SirsiDynix

TOUR

(extensity)

WebBridge

ABOUT THE EDITORS

Mary M. McKay, PhD, has received substantial federal funding for research focused on meeting the mental health and prevention needs of inner-city youth and families. Currently, she is Professor of Psychiatry and Community Medicine at the Mount Sinai School of Medicine in New York. She has held professorships at Columbia University and University of Illinois at Chicago. One of her most sucessful research projects is the CHAMP (Collaborative HIV Prevention and Adolescent Mental Health Project) Family Program which is a collaborative effort between university and community members to provide HIV prevention and mental health promtion services in urban, low income communities. This project began in Chicago with Dr. Roberta Paikoff as the Principal Investigator and is now being replicated in New York City, South Africa (Dr. Carl Bell, Principal Investigator), and Trinidad (Dr. Donna Baptiste, Principal Investigator). She is embarking on a new project where the same collaborative model will be used to provide HIV prevention and mental health promotion services in family homeless shelters.

Additionally, Dr. McKay has developed a substantial body of research findings around engagement pratices to improve engagement with mental health services in urban areas. She has worked closely with New York State Office of Mental Health, New York City Department of Health and Mental Hygiene and the National Institute of Mental Health to create evidence-based engagement interventions and test models of dissemination and training of mental health professionals in engagement best practices.

Dr. McKay holds a PhD in Social Work and has a strong clinical background as a family therapist. She has published over 50 peer-reviewed publications on the topics of HIV/AIDS, mental health, and urban health issues.

Roberta L. Paikoff, PhD, is Associate Professor of Psychology, Department of Psychiatry, Institute for Juvenile Research, University of Illinois, Chicago. She received her BS in Human Development and Family Studies from Cornell University and her PhD in Child Psychology from the Institute of Child Development, University of Minnesota. She has conducted numerous studies on the transition to adolescence among urban, African American youth, focusing on both basic developmental research and preventive interventions. Currently, she is interested in developmental transitions among children and adolescents with special needs.

Community Collaborative Partnerships: The Foundation for HIV Prevention Research Efforts

CONTENTS

PART II

PART I

Overview of Community Collaborative Partnerships and Empirical Findings: The Foundation for Youth HIV Prevention

Roberta L. Paikoff
Dorian E. Traube
Mary M. McKay

SUMMARY. This article presents a summary history and context of the CHAMP Family Program. Primarily, CHAMP was created and developed in response to rising levels of HIV and AIDS in inner-city commu-

Roberta L. Paikoff, PhD, is affiliated with the University of Illinois at Chicago. Dorian E. Traube, LCSW, is affiliated with the Columbia University School of Social Work. Mary M. McKay, PhD, is affiliated with the Mount Sinai School of Medicine.

This body of work is the result of the dedication of CHAMP Co-Investigators: Roberta Paikoff, PhD, Mary M. McKay, PhD, Carl C. Bell, MD, Donna Baptiste, PhD and Sybil Madison-Boyd, PhD. In addition, the significant contributions of CHAMP Project Directors (D. Coleman, McKinney, I. Coleman, Hibbert, Leachman, Lawrence and Miranda), CHAMP staff and participants is significant. Finally, CHAMP Collaborative Board members have worked tirelessly over the last decade to ensure the success of this work.

Funding from the National Institute of Mental Health (R01 MH55701; P. I. Paikoff; R01 MH63622; P. I. McKay; R01 MH58566; P. I. McKay; R01 MH64872; P. I. Bell) and the W. T. Grant Foundation is gratefully acknowledged. Dorian Traube is currently a pre-doctoral fellow at the Columbia University School of Social Work supported by a training grant from the National Institutes of Mental Health (5T32MH014623-24).

[Haworth co-indexing entry note]: "Overview of Community Collaborative Partnerships and Empirical Findings: The Foundation for Youth HIV Prevention." Paikoff, Roberta L., Dorian E. Traube, and Mary M. M. McKay. Co-published simultaneously in *Social Work in Mental Health* (The Haworth Press, Inc.) Vol. 5, No. 1/2, 2007, pp. 3-26; and: *Community Collaborative Partnerships: The Foundation for HIV Prevention Research Efforts* (ed: Mary M. McKay, and Roberta L. Paikoff) The Haworth Press, Inc., 2007, pp. 3-26. Single or multiple copies of this article are available for a fee from The Haworth Document Delivery Service [1-800-HAWORTH, 9:00 a.m. - 5:00 p.m. (EST). E-mail address: docdelivery@haworthpress.com].

nities of color. Concurrently, major changes in the field of psychology were underway during the late 1980s and early 1990s including new perceptions of the effect of culture and context on development; the birth of development psychopathology as a field; and increasing interest in–and recognition of–adolescent psychology. It is within the context of these transformations that this article places the design and implementation of CHAMP. The evolution of the CHAMP Family Program a relatively small, cyclical study in Chicago, to a major, multi-site project is discussed, with particular emphasis on the role of community collaboration in the transitions that CHAMP has experienced thus far. doi:10.1300/J200v05n02_01

[Article copies available for a fee from The Haworth Document Delivery Service: 1-800-HAWORTH. E-mail address: <docdelivery@haworthpress.com> Website: <http://www.HaworthPress.com> © 2007 by The Haworth Press, Inc. All rights reserved.]

KEYWORDS. Community collaborative partnerships, culture, context, adolescent psychology, family-based intervention, HIV-prevention

OVERVIEW

Adolescents are among the fastest growing population at risk for HIV/AIDS (Centers for Disease Control, 2003; 2000; 1998). Females and minority youth are disproportionately affected by STDs and the AIDS epidemic (Centers for Disease Control, 2001; 2003; DiLorenzo & Hein, 1993; Jemmott & Jemmott, 1992; 1998). Over the last decade, the incidence of HIV and AIDS infection has risen dramatically in low income, minority neighborhoods. African American and Latino youth are over represented among those living in poor neighborhoods with increased likelihood of exposure to HIV due to higher overall rates of neighborhood prevalence, along with poorer access to preventive health care, early detection and treatment services (Rotheram-Borus, Mahler & Rosario, 1995).

Prevention scientists have developed and tested a number of sexual risk reduction and STD or HIV prevention programs targeting urban minority youth. However, efforts to transport empirically supported prevention programs have encountered numerous obstacles, including insufficient school-based resources, poor community participation or tensions and suspicions between community residents and outside researchers (Dalton, 1989; Galbraith, Stanton, Feigelman, Ricardo, Black & Kalijee,

1996; Thomas & Quinn, 1991). As a result, it is becoming clear that community-based prevention programs targeting urban minority youth are likely to fail if they attempt to provide interventions in a non-collaborative manner (Aponte, 1988; Boyd-Franklin, 1993; Fullilove & Fullilove, 1993) or neglect to design and implement programs which do not appreciate stressors, scarce contextual resources or target groups' core values (Boyd-Franklin, 1993). Therefore, two steps are necessary to increase chances of success of HIV prevention efforts focused on urban youth. First, the establishment of strong community partnerships to support youth health prevention efforts is critical so that effective adolescent sexual risk prevention programs will be well received within urban communities. Second, any preventatively oriented program has increased chances for effectiveness if it is devised based upon empirical findings drawn directly from youth living in targeted communities.

Thus, the CHAMP (Collaborative HIV prevention and Adolescent Mental health Project; Paikoff, McKay & Bell, 1994; McKay, Paikoff, Bell, Madison & Baptiste, 2000) Family Program has been designed with these two steps as its foundation across national and international sites. More specifically, community collaborative research principles have guided the design, delivery and testing of the family-based HIV preventative intervention. In addition, the program has been continually informed by empirical findings derived directly from inner-city youth and their families living within target CHAMP communities. CHAMP focuses on building the capacities of community members to deliver a family-based HIV prevention program targeting preadolescent youth and their families living within inner-city U.S. communities and within countries hardest hit by the HIV/AIDS epidemic. The CHAMP Collaborative Board, consisting of urban parents, school staff, representatives from community-based organization and university-based researchers ensures that key stakeholders in the community are involved in every step of the research process, thereby, building further capacity for future prevention research oriented collaborations and community-level leadership. The CHAMP Collaborative Board oversees all aspects of the research project, including design and implementation of the intervention and evaluation of outcomes.

Further, the CHAMP Family Program is also informed by a developmentally grounded theoretical model of youth sexual risk taking that incorporates an understanding of multiple influences at the level of the child, peer group, family and community that impact initiation of youth sexual activity and risk behavior. Empirical findings identifying salient risk and protective factors related to youth sexual health protective behaviors and sexual risk taking informed the content, format and evaluation of the CHAMP Family Program. In this volume, seventeen articles overview the CHAMP program of research. The current chapter, written by Dr. Roberta Paikoff sets the stage for understanding the CHAMP program by providing a "History of Us: CHAMP, Moving from Chicago to Collaborative." It is the intention of the authors to provide an overview of the transition of the program over the years of its development. Next, Drs. Tolou-Shams, Piakoff, McKirnan and Holbeck report on key findings from basic research that inform some of the targets of the CHAMP Family Program. Findings related to mental health, youth sexual activity, racial socialization parenting practices, family communication about sensitive topics and social support are summarized by the next four articles. In the next three articles we describe mechanisms, motivators, and challenges to involving urban parents as collaborators in university based HIV prevention research efforts. The volume concludes with five articles addressing the translation of the CHAMP Family Program into a community operated intervention. The first of these five articles details the specific challenges and benefits that CHAMP experienced in the process of its move from a university lab to a community mental health agency. Secondly, Dr. Kerkorian contextualizes community experiences and perceptions of HIV prevention efforts, drawing on a study entitled Knowledge of the African American Research Experience (KAARE). The authors of "Voices from the Community" distill the ten most essential ingredients necessary for successful community collaboration. Dr. Baptiste follows with a discussion of an international Family-Based HIV/AIDS prevention intervention, working with teens in Trinidad and Tobago. Finally, Dr. McKay and her co-authors conclude with a discussion of the adaptation of family-based HIV Prevention programs for HIV pre-adolescents and their families. Dr. Kerkorian follows with an article about parent's experiences and motivation for allowing their children to participate in research studies like CHAMP. The volume concludes with three articles addressing the translation of the CHAMP Family Program into a community operated intervention, an intervention that can be used internationally, and an intervention that can be used with HIV+ youth. In the next article, Dr. Bell provides a commentary on using the Triadic Theory of Influence as a guide for adapting collaborative HIV prevention programs for new contexts and populations.

    In order to interpret the findings of the CHAMP Family Program and to understand the mechanisms of collaboration and translation, it is necessary to provide the reader with a description of how the program came into existence, why it was developed, key intervention variables and essential modes of service delivery. The history of CHAMP (Collaborative HIV prevention and Adolescent Mental health Project) had its humble beginnings in three tiny cramped offices on the third floor of the old (now defunct) Institute for Juvenile Research, and a one bedroom apartment in the Lincoln Park neighborhood of Chicago. From these two venues, many dedicated collaborators, students and staff worked to bring together the ideas which shaped two parallel lines of study: A basic longitudinal study focused on developmental process, and a family-based preventative intervention based on findings from the longitudinal study. These lines of inquiry were influenced by the authors training and experiences, as well as some of the scientific trends in the late 1980s and early 1990s. Changes in prevailing views of three areas in developmental psychology were of particular importance to the design and early approaches of CHAMP: (1) the role of culture/context in development, the importance of within sub-group variation, and the study of mechanisms toward adaptation within a subculture; (2) the promise of the newly developing fields of applied developmental psychology and developmental psychopathology; and (3) the growth in recognition of adolescent developmental psychology.

ROLE OF CULTURE AND CONTEXT

The recognition of the importance of culture within development had been recognized for some time, but was just beginning to be applied to diverse cultures within the United States. While prior applications of diversity in development had focused on evaluation of development relative to a particular standard (for the most part, white, male, middle class, and, two parent nuclear family structures), newer approaches emphasized the importance of looking within a particular subgroup for the important variations and predictive value of differences in development. A number of influential scientists (Spencer & Dornbusch, 1990; McLloyd, 1990) had written extensively about the importance of evaluating minority and other diverse subgroups separately as subpopulations in order to determine the relative importance of particular developmental processes and factors in determining adaptive outcomes.

In order to study developmental processes within the context of particular subgroups, additional theoretical models were needed and derived. In particular, numerous theoretical models focused on the perspective of risk and protective factors (Garmezy 1993a; 1993b; Cicchetti & Garmezy 1993;

Masten 2003; 2000). From this perspective, examinations of subgroups of children and adolescents could be undertaken with particular hypotheses about the effects of social, cognitive, biological, or mental health aspects of development that might yield different links between process and outcome, allowing for the possibility that factors which would affect some subgroups of youth negatively, might, in fact, have positive effects on other youth. Perhaps the most well-known of these studies is the Steinberg and colleagues (1992) study examining parenting styles among diverse groups of youth, and finding that authoritarian parenting, while less effective than authoritative parenting for White youth, was actually more effective in contributing to achievement levels among other youth (Asians and African Americans). The difference between these studies was primarily along the lines of interpretation: whereas prior studies might have focused on the important differences between groups in terms of pathology or health, these studies focused on important links within subgroups, allowing for the possibility of health across all cultures, thus changing the nature of the links to adaptation without assuming that any one culture is more or less adaptive than any another.

APPLIED DEVELOPMENTAL PSYCHOLOGY AND DEVELOPMENTAL PSYCHOPATHOLOGY

The field of developmental psychopathology (a term coined by Alan Sroufe and Sir Michael Rutter in their collected volume of *Child Development* in 1984) was at its very beginning, with key principles that were somewhat comparable to issues of cultural context above. Rather than examining discrete subgroups of children, with assumptions regarding separateness, developmental psychopathologists argued persuasively that adaptation should be considered on a continuum; that behavior that was diagnosed as "abnormal" or "dysfunctional" seldom represented a discrete break from normative development, but rather helped to elucidate principles of development. This theory raised an idea that continues to be popular today, that development should be thought of in sync with functionality, and that cases where development is less functional have much to tell us about the nature of development itself, just as normative development may help us to further understand the meanings and causes of functionality. Similar to the cultural context discussion above, theoretical models of developmental psychopathology often emphasize variation within groups of children, or conceiving of a range of development rather than discrete groupings, though they may also involve direct comparisons of particular groups of children, based on more applied characteristics (e.g., comparing children who have received different diagnoses with each other and with children considered to be typically developing, to discern where and whether these diagnoses and groupings have implications for functional development).

The potential importance of basic developmental studies for their promise of informing clinical and preventive interventions, as well as for influencing public policies, was just beginning to take shape (Brooks-Gunn et al., 1991; Chase-Lansdale et al., 1991). The study of prevention science was also becoming popular, primarily through its links with mental health and community psychology (Tolan & Gorman-Smith, 2002; Tolan, 2001; Tolan et al., 2000). A number of scholars in community psychology, in particular, became interested in cyclical models of prevention research, with basic studies being derived from applied questions in conjunction with theoretical models. Once basic studies were completed, the goal was to use targeted data to assist in developing and implementing prevention and intervention studies. These studies, in turn, were expected to raise new questions, and to inform further basic research, as well as assist in developing progressively more refined and definitive intervention and prevention programs to implement and ascertain effectiveness. Ironically, given the history of CHAMP that follows, I was very interested in these theoretical and pragmatic models, but did not pay particular attention to the other aspects of community psychology models that stress the importance of collaboration with a community. Rather, my collaborative interests stemmed from my more traditional developmental psychology training, which emphasized the importance of considering community and context from the perspective of getting reliable and accurate data on development.

ADOLESCENT PSYCHOLOGY

In addition, the field of adolescent development had begun to take on an importance of its own, with the increasing recognition of developmental psychologists that important changes continue to take place after childhood (Hill, 1987; Steinberg, 1987). The initial meeting of the Society for Research on Adolescence was held in 1986, and the Society grew extremely rapidly, providing many opportunities for those who were interested in development during the second decade of life, both from basic and applied perspectives, and encompassing a wide range of disciplines.

What these changes in the landscape of developmental psychology meant for young faculty members, such as myself, was that the academic world was split wide open, with huge new areas of potential study. It was certainly the case at that time that few studies had been conducted examining large subgroups of gender or minority groupings in order to determine appropriate links between developmental process and adaptive outcome within particular groups of children and adolescents. It was also the case that, although much was known about normative developmental process, very little of this basic science had been undertaken using methodologies that could be of help for more applied uses. Very little discussion or interplay took place between basic research scientists and more clinical or applied faculty (e.g., educators, psychologists, social workers, or program developers/intervention specialists).

Although many would agree that the level of interdisciplinary communication between basic and applied scientists (and, perhaps, more critically, between academics in general and those who are actually developing and implementing programs) still leaves much to be desired, it is important to recall that it was not so long ago when such communications essentially did not occur. Thus, while there is much room for improvement, one of the most stunning changes in the academic landscape of today is the need for all basic scientists to justify their social and behavioral science work, not just in terms of rationale, but also in terms of basic use in applied settings.

There was substantial work to be done, and many of us eager to do it. For myself, a number of critical experiences shaped my particular interests, and the methods by which I went about designing the initial CHAMP basic longitudinal study. First and foremost, was my personal belief that there was much that developmental psychology, and a developmental approach more generally, had to offer to fields that actually attempted to promote development (particular prevention and intervention programs aimed at significant public health issues for children and adolescents). My belief stemmed from my excellent undergraduate and graduate training, and my mentors, Andy Collins, Megan Gunnar, and Ritch Savin-Williams. It was fortified and nurtured through my post-doctoral experiences at Educational Testing Service with Jeanne Brooks-Gunn.

During my time at Educational Testing Service, I had several experiences that proved pivotal in my design of future work. First, I conducted a literature review on the effectiveness on programs aimed at preventing initial and repeat teenage pregnancies. In addition, I served as a consultant to the NYC Mayor's Committee on Teenage Pregnancy Prevention. Through these two experiences, I was able to understand and document, first-hand, how very little the domains of developmental psychology, program development and evaluation, and program design and implementation, had spoken to one another, and how potentially problematic that was for all disciplines. Those of us in developmental psychology had not yet learned to conduct our studies or discuss our findings in ways that could be straightforwardly helpful to program developers and implementers. Those developing programs at that time, had, for the most part, very little experience or consultation from people who could discuss their developmental relevance or rigorously evaluate their effects.

In addition to my work on teenage pregnancy prevention, other work aimed at adolescent development within a private parochial boys' school in Harlem affected me in other ways. I found an incredible disconnect between what I would see in my travels within Harlem and what I would watch on the news in my New Jersey living room. The depiction of urban teenage boys on the evening news was one of pathology and despair, and served largely to make them appear different and pathological relative to other cultural subgroups (stories on gang violence, urban destruction, etc.). In my travels in Harlem, I met young boys and their families, and found them more similar to than different from suburban families I knew, both in their values and in their hopes and dreams for their children and their family as a whole. I became very interested in doing the kind of research that would inform other cultures about the more normative aspects of inner city family life, and that would, at the same time, take a perspective of enhancing family strengths rather than focusing on documenting weakness or pathology. Given my interest in teenage pregnancy prevention, the growing concerns regarding HIV infection among teenagers, I chose to focus my work prospectively, on prevention of HIV risk and delay of initial sexual activity.

Another factor that highly influenced the development of the theoretical models of CHAMP, was an interest of mine of mapping out the role of context in contributing to youth sexual behavior. I was interested in two different aspects of context: one, the demographics of a context, and two, the specific social situations that children were exposed to. For the first, I became interested in locating my work in communities and neighborhoods of highest contextual risk, (e.g., where highest HIV seroprevalence rates were found). With regard to the second, I was concerned in my reading of the literature on early sexual experience that we did not have a sense of the actual contexts in which early sexual risk taking occurs, that is, what do these experiences "look like"? What is their meaning for youth? I began developing a theoretical model that would describe the progression through different social contexts that would influence sexual risk taking and sexual debut.

When the opportunity arose to consider a position at the Institute for Juvenile Research (IJR) at University of Illinois at Chicago, I was particularly excited given the work of Patrick Tolan and colleagues (in particular, Deborah Gorman-Smith) in the area of antisocial behavior and adolescent violence. The approach they took in working on the Chicago Youth Development Study (CYDS) and the Metropolitan Area Community Study (MACS) was a direct application of the community psychology prevention and intervention model, and served as an excellent example for me, a young faculty member with interests in this model as relevant to early sexuality and HIV/AIDS prevention.

Both at ETS and at IJR, I worked persistently over several years to get funding. Over the course of 3 years, I wrote 7 different proposals (9 if you include amended applications), and received a couple of small, seed grants that allowed me to formulate ideas and working plans, until one of the larger grants was funded. Within one year, I was funded by two granting agencies, the NIMH Office on AIDS and the William T. Grant Foundation. I was able to begin the first of the CHAMP studies, a basic study of approximately 300 families, examining associations between family process, social, cognitive, and biological (pubertal) development, as well as mental health of caregiver and child, in their contribution healthy relationship and heterosexual development during the transition to adolescence.

All the CHAMP studies have focused on a specific age range: the transition to adolescence, ages 10-15. We have done this for a specific reason: in many prior studies of teenage pregnancy and sexual risk taking, studies were begun after youth were already pregnant or had reported being sexually active. In order to study the development of sexual risk taking or sexual health, we needed to begin our studies earlier, prior to initial sexual activity. However, we also needed to begin them at an age that most families would find acceptable, and within a time frame where we could reasonably expect some change in sexual activity. Therefore, we aimed our studies at this initial period of pre/ early adolescence, where we expected some changes in behavior that could presumably be linked to health or to risk taking, but we also expected that the majority of youth would NOT be sexually active in the initial years of the study. This has allowed us to look prospectively at the development of heterosocial and heterosexual behaviors related to sexual health and sexual risk taking.

Early on, we learned several important lessons that would shape our basic study and our methods of beginning prevention and intervention work. One important and empowering lesson was, if you build it WELL, they will come! Over and over senior people told me, early in my career that good ideas paired with persistence will meet with success. It's hard to believe it, though, until you see it for yourself. The literal and figurative change in fortune that funding permits allows one to create a program and truly see one's ideas unfold before one's very eyes. The beauty of the NIMH system is that thoughtful peer review serves to improve and refine good ideas so they are doable.

A second key lesson was, NEVER work alone! One of the most important things I did in the years while I was working on small seed grants was to involve students, colleagues, community members and stakeholders in the development of research ideas and implementation plans. Doing so was not merely a gesture of good will (as I had thought initially it would be), but ended up being a critical factor in decision making regarding methodological issues, such as where particular aspects of the study would take place, and how different measures would be administered. For example, at the time we were preparing to examine HIV risk behavior in 10-12 year olds, a measure called the "secret ballot" was highly regarded in academic circles. This method recommended the administration of sexual behavior measures with a series of "yes-no" questions, each contained in a separate sealed envelope. Items were sequenced in what was assumed to be the logical progression of sexual behaviors up to and including sexual intercourse. Children were to open items only until they answered "no" to a question. In this way, we would not be exposing children to questions about sensitive behavior any more than was necessary (e.g., only up to the next behavior in a presumed sequence).

The parent and school-community liaison who worked with me at one of our schools, were both against this procedure. They felt strongly that it was our staff's responsibility to "protect" the children from items that were inappropriate based on their experiences, and should not be left to the children themselves. They gave several persuasive reasons, chief among them that for some children, reading items by themselves would not be possible based on literacy levels, and, for those children who could read the items, it would be too much of a temptation to continue the process and "uncover" all the information presented in the envelopes. Based on this, we developed our interview on Sexual Possibility Situations, which required trained interviewers to present to youth with a variety of detailed skip patterns aimed at keeping less sexually involved youth from answering more detailed and sensitive questions. The lessons learned here served us very well in our later community collaborative intervention work. In the following sections, I will provide a brief overview of the CHAMP projects, primarily to assist readers in understanding the background in which the studies contained in this issue were undertaken.

CHAMP I:
BASIC RESEARCH ON FAMILIES,
MENTAL HEALTH FACTORS, AND HIV RISK

In this initial, basic research study, the goal was to develop knowledge regarding key intervenable variables for HIV risk prevention programs. To that end, a sample of 315 urban, African American families with pre-adolescent children was recruited from the South and West side of Chicago. All families were recruited via their child's attendance at a school on or near a major public housing project in Chicago, an area with higher than average citywide rates of HIV infection that is primarily African American and poor (with high rates of joblessness, as well as other major health and social welfare concerns). This sample has now been interviewed three times; ages 10-12, 12-14, and 17-19 (refer to McBride, Paikoff & Holmbeck, 2003; Paikoff, 1997; Paikoff et al., 1997; Sagrestano et al., 1999; or Delucia, Paikoff & Holmbeck, and Tolou-Shams, Paikoff et al., in this volume, this volume for more information about sample recruitment and retention rates). At each data wave, age appropriate questions related to the theoretical model below were addressed (see Figure 1).

These data has been used to address a variety of research questions in numerous areas:

- *Family Demographics*: Both parent education (HS/GED vs. No HS/GED) and parent employment (work since the child's birth vs. no work since the child's birth) were associated with youth participating in sexual possibility situations. Children least likely to have participated in these situations were more likely to have parents who reported an education through high school completion or GED and who had worked since the child's birth (Paikoff, Parfenoff, Williams, McCormick, Greenwood, & Holmbeck, 1997). In addition, females were slightly more likely (p < .10) than males to be in these situations (Paikoff et al., 1997).

- *Family Relationships*: Four aspects of family relationships were associated with pre-adolescent participation in sexual possibility situations: (1) family interactions; (2) children's reports of parental control in decision making; (3) family support for children of teenaged mothers; and (4) parental communication and knowledge regarding HIV/AIDS.

    1. Family Interactions: Videotaped interactions of family problem solving were rated by two coders, both African American, and one from the target community (e.g., a parent without children in the sample). Family interaction scales that focused on family emotions (e.g., parent and child warmth and humor) as well as the overall health of the family have been associated with exposure to sexual possibility situations, with more healthy and more positive emotional interactions associated with lack of exposure to sexual possibility situations (Paikoff et al., 1997).

    2. Parental Control: In addition to family interaction, parent and child reports about family conflict, decision making, discipline and supervision were assessed at pre and early adolescence: Most parent and child reports about the family were uncorrelated with one another, and the only association with exposure to sexual possibility situations at preadolescence was the child report of family decision making. Children who reported that their parents had more control over family decision making also reported less exposure to sexual possibility situations (Paikoff et al., 1997). Parent reports of control were unassociated with children's exposure to sexual possibility situations (Paikoff et al., 1997, 1997).

    3. Family Support and Teenage Motherhood: For pre-adolescents whose mothers were teenagers at their first childbirth, greater family support was associated with lack of exposure to sexual possibility situations. For those preadolescents whose mothers were not teenagers at the time of their first childbirth, however, greater family support was associated with increased exposure to sexual possibility situations (Paikoff et al., 1997).

    4. Family Communication: Parents also were asked to rate whether or not they had discussed a variety of risk behavior

topics with their child, and their comfort in doing so. Parents completed a 28 question measure regarding their own AIDS knowledge. Children who had not experienced sexual possibility situations had parents with more HIV/AIDS knowledge than children who had experienced sexual possibility situations (Parfenoff & McCormick, 1997). In addition, children who had been in sexual possibility situations were more likely to have parents who reported having discussed abstinence (staying away from sex) with them than those who had not been in these situations. Overall, parents were less likely to have discussed sexuality and related topics (including HIV/AIDS) with their children than other risk topics (e.g., alcohol or drug use, cigarette smoking; Parfenoff & McCormick, 1997).

• *Friendship Relationships*: Relationship maintenance (i.e., extent to which child will tolerate risk behavior to maintain relationship) and likelihood of peer pressure in children's friendships were linked to exposure to sexual possibility situations. Youth who had not been in sexual possibility situations reported prioritizing resisting peer pressure over maintaining friendships and less likelihood of pressure from their friends; however, they also reported lower levels of friendship support overall (Paikoff, Holmbeck, Parfenoff, Bhorade, & Gillming, 1997). This finding regarding peer pressure and relationship maintenance is highly robust and is of particular interest, as it suggests that those pre-adolescents who experience sexual possibility situations are likely to perceive themselves as less motivated to resist pressure to engage in risk behaviors, and more like to experience such pressure.

• *Child Individual Processes*: Within our model, 3 individual child processes were examined: pubertal maturation, social problem solving, and mental health. We are just beginning to examine data with regard to child mental health and social problem solving; pubertal maturation has not been associated with exposure to sexual possibility situations in our analyses to date (Sagrestano, McCormick, Paikoff, & Holmbeck, 1999). This is not particularly surprising as participants were in pre-to early puberty at the pre-adolescent data wave. With regard to mental health, children with Oppositional Defiant Disorder (ODD), and particularly girls, were more likely to be in sexual possibility situations (Donahue, Parfenoff, & Holmbeck, 1998). Depressive affect is not linked to exposure to sexual possibility situations; other aspects of child mental health have not been examined to date (Sagrestano, Paikoff, Fendrich, Parfenoff, & Holmbeck, 1997).

In addition to our early adolescent, a number of longitudinal studies have been conducted.

First, a longitudinal study of youth's sexual debut and links to individual and family factors was completed and published in the *Journal of Consulting and Clinical Psychology* (McBride, Paikoff, & Holmbeck, 2003). In this study, pre-adolescent family and individual factors, such as family conflict, positive affect, and pubertal development, were studied longitudinally as linked to early sexual debut among urban African American young adolescents. Results indicated that girls were more likely to delay sexual debut past early adolescence than boys, and that more developed preadolescents with greater family conflict and less positive affect were least likely to delay sexual debut.

Second, a longitudinal study of family factors in contributing to depression among urban adolescents has appeared in the *Journal of Family Psychology* (Sagrestano, Paikoff, Holmbeck, & Fendrich, 2003). In this study, parent and adolescent levels of depression were examined in association with changes in family functioning, finding that increases in conflict and decreases in parental monitoring were associated with in-

FIGURE 1. Conceptual Model of Family Influences on HIV Risk Exposure

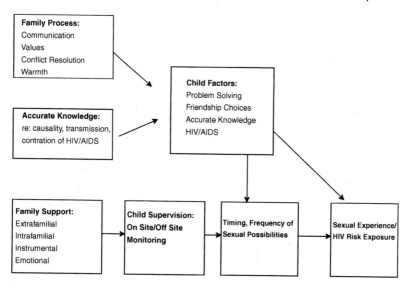

creases in child depressive symptomatology, and increases in conflict and decreases in positive parenting were associated with increases in parental depressive symptomatology.

In addition, two longitudinal studies on these data are reported in the current volume. DeLucia, Paikoff, and Holmbeck (this volume) use our longitudinal data to discuss methods of studying individual growth curves and trajectories of experience for our youth. Tolou-Shams, Paikoff et al., (this volume) talk about the role of parenting and adolescent mental health problems in contributing to adolescent HIV risk during the transition from early to late adolescence. Each of these studies takes advantage of the wealth of longitudinal data to conduct research which has direct implications for HIV prevention program development.

The basic CHAMP study has thus provided the background data and experiences for the development of the CHAMP family-based interventions. Additional findings from studies using baseline data from the intervention study have further helped to refine the intervention (Miller et al.; Traube et al.; McKay, Bannon et al.; in current volume).

CHAMP II:
FAMILY BASED INTERVENTION
TO PREVENT ADOLESCENT HIV RISK

Funding to study the design, delivery and outcome of the CHAMP Family Program is now in its' ninth year. The initial proposal requested funding to involve African American pre-adolescents (4th and 5th graders) and their families in a test of a three-year preventive intervention. The CHAMP Family Program was delivered at the 4th and 5th grade (at an age where the vast majority of youth were not expected to have engaged in sexual behavior) and then the same cohort of children and families were followed to early adolescence (6th/7th grade) to participate in a second exposure of the program. Program effects are being tested within a longitudinal, experimental design with random assignment to the CHAMP Family Program or a longitudinal interview condition occurring in the fall of 4th/5th grade for youth in 4 elementary schools on the southside of Chicago. The impact of the program in relation to proximal outcomes (e.g., family process, parent and child AIDS knowledge and attitudes, use of social supports for assistance with parenting, child assertiveness and peer social problem solving skills) and distal outcomes (time spent in sexual possibility situations at pre-adolescence and sexual activity and HIV risk exposure behavior at early adolescence) continue to be examined.

To date, the following goals have been met: (1) Two CHAMP curricula (pre and early adolescence) have been developed; (2) A sample of 4th and 5th graders and their families have been recruited to participate in the study, randomly assigned to receive the CHAMP Family Program or a longitudinal interview condition and followed over time; (3) Preliminary analyses of programmatic effects are underway; (4) A CHAMP Collaborative Board, consisting of parents, school staff, community-based agencies and university-based researchers has met at least monthly over the last nine years and overseen the development, delivery and evaluation of the research study; (5) Opportunities to increase the leadership and research capacities of CHAMP Collaborative Board Members have been created; (6) A CHAMP Collaborative Board have been developed in the Bronx, New York; (7) There has been an ongoing translation of research to inform program development; and (8) Investigators and Board members have been involved in dissemination activities.

More specifically, two family-based HIV prevention curricula have been developed, extensively pilot tested and delivered. A 12-week 4th/5th grade family intervention and guiding protocol was created in collaboration with urban parents. The 4th/5th grade curriculum was pilot tested in three separate trials, with the final pilot involving Collaborative Board members and their children as participants. This was done for two reasons. First, the Board was committed to providing the community with an intervention of the highest quality, therefore, they wanted to experience firsthand the content and format of the program to ensure that it would be acceptable. Second, their participation was seen as the first step in training Board members to co-deliver the program with mental health interns when the CHAMP Family Program was brought to the field.

Next, a sample of 4th and 5th graders and their families were recruited to participate in the study, randomly assigned to receive the CHAMP Family Program or a longitudinal interview condition and followed longitudinally. A sample of 500 4th and 5th graders and their families were identified for participation in the study, with 324 children randomly assigned to receive the CHAMP Family Program and the remaining youth and their families assigned to a comparison condition. Of the 324 youth assigned to CHAMP, 274 (85%) could be located and invited to participate in the program. Factors that interfered with location included: (1) demolition of four of sixteen high-rise housing units within the target community; and (2) relocation of hundreds of families out of the community due to massive re-vitalization efforts by the city.

Of the 274 families located, 214 came to at least one meeting of the program (78%); 211 attended more than 3 sessions (77%); and 201 families

(73% of families located) completed the program. In order to achieve these high rates of participation within the target inner-city community, university researchers and community parents developed intensive outreach strategies (McCormick et al., 2000). Involvement strategies included: (1) community parents in leadership roles making initial contacts with participant families (either via home visits or telephone calls), (2) multiple contacts with families prior to the first CHAMP meeting to establish familiarity and trust, (3) extensive discussions of purpose of study, funding sources, privacy issues, informed consent and prior experiences with universities and researchers to address hesitancies to participate, and (4) joint training (both mental health interns and community parents) in the use of systematic engagement strategies developed within other urban focused research projects (McKay et al., 2004).

In addition, a study to examine the impact of specific barriers, both within the family and the community, as well as resources that predicted program attendance in order to fine tune recruitment strategies was conducted. Data collected from CHAMP staff regarding their initial contacts with the first three cohorts of families ($n = 227$) invited to participate in CHAMP were analyzed to identify barriers and facilitators of program attendance and retention (Pinto et al., this volume). Briefly, parental concerns related to discussions about sex or HIV/AIDS was negatively related to total number of CHAMP sessions attended ($r = -.47; p = .00$), as well as presence of family stressors ($r = -.16; p = .04$). Multivariate analyses revealed parental motivation to participate ($b = .97; p = .00$) and parental understanding of the purpose of CHAMP ($b = -1.5; p = .02$) to be significant predictors of ongoing attendance ($R^2 = .24; p = .00$). Based upon these findings, outreach and engagement strategies were developed in order to enhance participation. Preliminary analyses of programmatic effects have begun.

Delivery of the 4th and 5th grade intervention has been completed in Chicago. Preliminary effects are reported in McKay et al. (2004), and in this volume (McBride et al.). At the proximal level, preliminary findings already offer encouragement for the continued development and refinement of the CHAMP Family Program (McKay et al. 2004). More specifically, preliminary analyses reveal significant increases from pre to post assessment in the following domains: family decision making; attitudes regarding HIV/AIDS; family comfort related to discussions of sensitive topics; parental off-site monitoring (e.g., via phone, neighborhood supports; and disruptive behavioral difficulties. Parental anxiety and depression also decreased significantly from pre to post test (Paikoff, 1997). When posttest scores of families in the CHAMP Family Program are compared to those in the no treatment control condition, program effects for family decision making, with parents more likely to make decisions within the family, were significant (CHAMP mean 27.1 vs. control mean 34.0). In addition, families in CHAMP held significantly more positive attitudes about interacting with persons with AIDS (mean = 5.3) in comparison to control families (mean = 5.8). Off-site monitoring scores also significantly favored participation in the CHAMP program (mean = 6.2) in comparison to families in the control condition (mean = 5.0) (McKay et al., 2004).

Community collaboration has been critical to every aspect of CHAMP. This is an area where we have learned an enormous amount and at this point have reached a level of community partnerships where community members participate in the direction and focus of the research. More specifically, the entire program development, delivery and current evaluation phase of our project has been overseen by the CHAMP Collaborative Board. Since its inception, the Board has met at least monthly. Board members and other community parents have been trained along with mental health interns (e.g., undergraduate and graduate level social work and psychology students) to implement the program at schools and community sites. In addition to delivering the program, community members participate on committees that make key personnel and budget decisions, create project policies concerning personnel and data collection, design the intervention curriculum, and review proposals for research using the intervention data (see McKay, Hibbert et al., in this volume). Additionally, community Board members have participated in new "professional" roles as conference presenters, and as part-time and full-time project staff.

In addition, opportunities to increase the leadership and research collaboration capacities of CHAMP Collaborative Board Members have been created over the course of the projects. For example, in the second and third year of the initial funding cycle, the investigative team, including the CHAMP Collaborative Board received a small grant, "Strengthening Inner-city Communities Research Capacity: A Collaborative Partnership Model." The primary purpose was to enhance urban parents, teachers and researchers' capacities to collaborate in the development of community-based programming and research. In order to achieve this goal, a series of seminars and technical assistance workshops (a total of 36 hours) were conducted for all members of the CHAMP Collaborative Board. These seminars provided information and practical experience in identifying pressing community needs, exploring options for programming and understanding the program evaluation processes. In addition, homework writing and discussion exercises were developed. Small working groups of parents, teachers and researchers were formed and bi-monthly contacts were scheduled in order to facilitate development of writing skills and grant proposal development skills. A key outcome of the project was the development of small grant proposals. In addition to knowledge and skill acquisition related to research, the project provided an opportunity for Board members to develop personal leadership skills. A model developed by Carl Bell, M.D., for the development of human capabilities was used to encourage: (1) development of self (motivation, awareness, confidence, positive expectancy); (2) goal directedness; and (3) enhancement of skills (problem solving, decision making and communication).

A series of assessment measures and goal attainment rating scales were developed explicitly to assist Board members in tracking their learning and skill development. In addition, two grant proposals have been funded as a result of these efforts. First, funding was received from the NIMH for a longitudinal study, "Informed consent in urban AIDS and mental health research." This project examines factors that influence the process of informed consent, initial and ongoing involvement in prevention research efforts for inner-city children and their adult caregivers. A particular emphasis of this study is to examine the influence of perceptions of racism and historical events such as the Tuskegee Syphilis Study. The project is co-directed by a university trained staff member and a community parent. All project interviews are conducted by community parents (see Kerkorian et al., in this volume).

CHAMP III:
IMPACT OF COLLABORATIVE PARTNERSHIPS

Next, Dr. McKay's move to New York precipitated an opportunity to test the community collaborative model of HIV prevention along with the program. Thus, new funding from the National Institute of Mental Health was obtained to study the development and impact of CHAMP Collaborative Boards in two urban epicenters of the virus (New York and Chicago). At both sites, 2 major research aims will be addressed: Program design, adaptation to particular community need, delivery, outcome and transfer of ownership of the CHAMP Family Program are being examined.

The project is a multi-site study, jointly conducted by the current investigative team of CHAMP. The P.I. (McKay) coordinates the Bronx, New York site where a new CHAMP Collaborative Board has been formed in consultation with current Chicago Collaborative Board Members. The Co-P.I. (Paikoff) coordinates the expansion of CHAMP to a new urban community on the westside of Chicago with the current CHAMP Board providing primary leadership.

At both sites, the CHAMP Collaborative Boards now meet bi-monthly to review and adapt the CHAMP Family Program content to respond to emerging research data from the CHAMP Family Study and pressing community needs related to HIV risk. In addition, at both sites, the CHAMP Collaborative Board oversees the replication test of the impact of CHAMP with 4th and 5th grade children randomly assigned to the 3 year, developmentally focused intervention or longitudinal follow-up (see McKay, Hibbert et al., in this volume). Finally, the CHAMP Collaborative Boards are in the process of creating and executing a longitudinal plan for sustainability and linkage with existing resources (see Baptiste et al., in this volume).

A two site study was necessary in order to understand the process of replication of the Collaborative Board as a vehicle for urban, HIV prevention programming within diverse (e.g., geographically, racially/culturally) low-income communities. Two sites also provide the opportunity to examine issues related to local primacy (e.g., specific adaptations made to HIV prevention programs to ensure high cultural and contextual sensitivity) vs. the ability to transport a protocol-driven HIV preventive intervention from one community to another. This is particularly important as community level characteristics could impact the development of community-university partnerships (e.g., moving from a Midwestern city with high levels of racial segregation and concentrated high rise public housing to a large, eastern city with similar high concentrations of poverty, yet higher levels of racial/ethnic integration).

As the HIV epidemic began devastating other parts of the world, CHAMP investigators began to consider how adaptation the family-based approaches to HIV prevention could be made via collaborations within international contexts (see Bell et al., and Baptiste et al., in this volume for a description of CHAMP projects in Trinidad and South Africa). In all, the CHAMP projects have proven to be both a serious opportunity to create knowledge regarding youth HIV prevention, but also a journey about learning how to conduct research that has cultural and contextual relevance, recognized the strengths and protective influences of families and communities and provide maximum opportunities for collaboration among investigators and with communities.

REFERENCES

Aponte, H.J., Zarski, J., Bixenstene, C., & Cibik, P. (1991). Home/community based services: A two-tier approach. *American Journal of Orthopsychiatry*, 61, 3, 403-408.

Baptiste, D., Paikoff, R., McKay, M., Madison-Boyd, S., Coleman, D., & Bell, C. (2005). Collaborating w/ an urban community to develop an HIV and AIDS Prevention Program for black youth & families. *Behavior Modification, 29*, pp. 370-416.

Boyd-Franklin, N. (1993). Black Families. In F. Walsh (Ed.). *Normal Family Process*. New York: Guilford Press.

Brooks-Gunn, J., Phelps, E., and Elder, G.H. (1991). Studying lives through time: Secondary data analyses in developmental psychology. *Developmental Psychology, 27*(6), 899-910.

Center for Disease Control (1998). New Study Profiles Hispanic Births in America. National Center for Health Statistics. Released February 13, 1998. Retrieved from the World Wide Web: *http://www.cdc.gov/cchswww/releases/98/facts/98sheets/hisbirth.htm*

Center for Disease Control (2000). Tracking the hidden epidemics: Trends in STDs in the United States, 2000, Atlanta, Georgia: Center for Disease Control.

Center for Disease Control (2001). HIV/AIDS Surveillance Report. Atlanta, GA Center for Disease Control and Prevention.

Chase-Lansdale, P. L., Mott, F.L., Brooks-Gunn, J., and Phillips, D.A. (1991). Children of the National Longitudinal Survey of Youth: A unique research opportunity. *Developmental Psychology, 27*(6), 918-931.

Cicchetti, D. and Garmezy, N. (1993). Prospects and promises in the study of resilience. *Development & Psychopathology, 5* (4), 497-502.

Dalton, H.L. (1989). AIDS in Blackface. *Daedalus*, 118. 3. 205-227

Delucia, C., Paikoff, R. L., & Holmbeck, G. N. (2007). Individual growth curves of frequency of sexual intercourse among urban, adolescent, African American youth: Results from the CHAMP Basic Study. Published simultaneously in *Social Work in Mental Health, 5*(1/2) pp. 59-80 and M. McKay and R. Paikoff (eds.) *Community Collaborative Partnerships and Empirical Findings: The Foundation for HIV Prevention Research Eforts*. The Haworth Press, Inc.

DiLorenzo, T. & Hein, K. (1993). Adolescents: The leading edge of the next wave of the HIV epidemic. In J.L. Wallender, L. J. (Eds.)., *Adolescent Health Problems: Behavioral Perspectives* (pp. 117-140). New York: Guilford Press.

Donahue, B.B., Parfenoff, S. H., and Holmbeck, G. N. (1998). Oppositional-defiant disorder and risk for early sexual experience in preadolescents. Presentation submitted to Biennial Meeting of the Society for Research on Adolescence, San Francisco, CA.

Fullilove, M. T. & Fullilove, R.E. (1993). Understanding sexual behaviors and drug use among African Americans: A case study of issues for survey research. In D.G. Ostrow & R.C. Kessler (Eds.). *Methodological Issues in AIDS Behavioral Research*. (pp. 117-132). New York: Plenum Press.

Galbraith, J., Stanton, B., Feigelman, S., Ricardo, I., Black, M., & Kalijee, K. (1996). Challenges and rewards of involving community in research: An overview of the "Focus on Kids" HIV-Risk Reduction Program. *Health Education Quarterly, 23*(3) pp. 383-94.

Garmezy, N. (1993). Vulnerability and resilience. In D.C. Funder and R.D. Parke (Eds), *Studying lives through time: Personality and development. APA science volumes.* (pp. 377-398). Washington, DC, US: American Psychological Association.

Garmezy, Norman. Developmental psychopathology: Some historical and current perspectives. (1993). In D. Magnusson and P. Casaer (Eds). *Longitudinal research on individual development: Present status and future perspectives. European network on longitudinal studies on individual development* (pp. 95-126). New York, NY, US: Cambridge University Press.

Hill, J.P. (1987). Research on adolescents and their families: Past and prospect. In C.E. Irwin (ed.) *Adolescent social behavior and health. New Directions for Child Development no.37.* San Francisco: Jossey-Bass.

Jemmott, J.B. & Jemmott, L.S. (1992). Increasing condom-use intentions among sexually active Black adolescent women. *Nursing Research,* 41, 273-279.

Jemmott, J.B., Jemmott, L. & Fong, G.T. (1998). Abstinence and safer sex HIV risk reduction interventions for African American Adolescents. *Journal of the American Medical Association,* 270, 1529-1536.

Madison, S., Bell, C., Sewell, S., Nash, G., McKay, M. & Paikoff, R. (in press). "True community/academic partnerships." *Psychiatric Services.*

Madison, S., McKay, M., Paikoff, R.L. & Bell, C. (2000). "Community collaboration and basic research: Necessary ingredients for the development of a family-based HIV prevention program." *AIDS Education and Prevention,* 12, 281-298.

Masten, Ann S; Powell, Jenifer L. A resilience framework for research, policy, and practice. (2003) In S. Luthar (Ed). *Resilience and vulnerability: Adaptation in the context of childhood adversities* (pp. 1-25). New York, NY, US: Cambridge University Press.

Masten, A.S & Curtis, W. J. (2000). Integrating competence and psychopathology: Pathways toward a comprehensive science of adaption in development. *Development & Psychopathology, 12*(3), 529-550.

McBride, C. K., Paikoff, R. L., & Holmbeck, G. N. (2003). Individual and Familial Influences on the Onset of Sexual Intercourse Among Urban African American Adolescents. *Journal of Consulting and Clinical Psychology,* 71(1), 159-167.

McCormick, A., McKay, M., Gilling, G., & Paikoff, R. (2000). "Involving families in an urban HIV preventive intervention: How community collaboration addresses barriers to participation." *AIDS Education and Prevention,* 12, 299-307.

McKay, M. M., Chasse, K. T., Paikoff, R. L., McKinney, L., Baptiste, D., Coleman, D., Madison, S., & Bell, C. C. (under review) Family-level impact of the CHAMP family program: A community collaborative effort to support urban families and reduce youth HIV risk exposure.

McKay, M., Hibbert, R., Hoagwood, K., Rodriguez, J. & Murray, L. (2004). "Integrating evidence-based engagement interventions into 'real world' child mental health settings. *Journal of Brief Treatment and Crisis Intervention,* 4, 177-186.

McKay, M., Paikoff, R., Baptiste, D., Bell, C., Coleman, D., Madison, S., McKinney, L. & CHAMP Collaborative Board. (2004). "Family-level impact of the CHAMP Family Program: A community collaborative effort to support urban families and reduce youth HIV risk exposure." *Family Process,* 77-91.

McKay, M., Paikoff, R., Bell, C., Madison, S., & Baptiste, D. (2000). *Community Partnership to Reduce Urban Youth HIV Risk.* National Institute of Mental Health, Office on AIDS funded grant.

McLoyd, V. C. (1990). The impact of economic hardship on Black families and children: Psychological distress, parenting, and socioemotional development. *Child Development*, 61, 311-345.

Paikoff, R.L. (1997). Applying developmental psychology to an AIDS prevention model for urban African American youth. *Journal of Negro Education*, 65,44-59.

Paikoff R., McKay M., & Bell C., (1994). The Chicago HIV prevention and adolescent mental health project (CHAMP) family-based intervention. National Institute of Mental Health, office on AIDS and William T. Grant Foundation funded grants.

Paikoff, R.L., Parfenoff, S.H., Williams, S.A., McCormick, A., Greenwood, G.L., & Holmbeck, G.N. (1997). Parenting, parent-child relationships, and sexual possibility situations among urban African American Pre-Adolescents: Preliminary Findings and Implications for HIV Prevention. *Journal of Family Psychology*, 11, 11-22.

Parfenoff, S. H. & McCormick, A. (1997). Parenting preadolescents at risk: Knowledge, attitudes, and communication about HIV/AIDS. Presentation at the Biennial meeting of the Society for Research in Child Development, Washington, D.C.

Rotheram-Borus, M. J., Mahler, K. A., & Rosario, M. (1995). AIDS prevention and adolescents families. *AIDS Education and Prevention*, 7 (4), 320-336

Sagrestano, L.M., et al. (1997). The role of depression in family relationships among inner-city African American adolescents. *Journal of Research on Adolescence.*

Sagrestano, L.M., McCormick, S.H., Paikoff, R.L., & Holmbeck, G.N. (1999). Pubertal development and parent-child conflict in low-income, urban, African American Adolescents. *Journal of Research on Adolescence*, 9 (1), 85-107.

Sagrestano, L.M., Paikoff, R. L., Hombeck, G. N., & Fendrich, M. (2003). A longitudinal examination of familial risk factors for depression among inner-city African American adolescents. *Journal of Family Psychology*, 17(1), 108-120.

Spencer, M. B. & Dornbusch, S. M. (1990). Challenges in studying minority youth. In S.S. Feldman and G. R. Elliott (Eds.) *At the Threshold: The Developing Adolescent*, (pp. 123-146). Cambridge, MA: Harvard University Press.

Steinberg, L. (1987). Impact of puberty on family relations: Effects of pubertal status and pubertal timing. *Developmental Psychology*, 23(3), 451-460.

Steinberg, L., Lamborn, S.D., Dornbusch, S.M., Darling, N. (1992) Impact of parenting practices on adolescent achievement: Authoritative parenting, school involvement, and encouragement to succeed. *Child Development, 63*(5), 1266-1281.

Stevenson, H. C. & White, J. J. (1994). AIDS prevention struggles in ethnocultural neighborhoods: Why research partnerships with community based organizations can't wait. *AIDS Education & Prevention*, 6, 126-139.

Thomas, S.B. & Quinn, S.C. (1991). The Tuskegee syphilis study, 1932 to 1972: Implications for HIV education and AIDS use education programs in the black community. *American Journal of Public Health*, 81 (11), 1495-1505.

Tolan, P.H. & Gorman-Smith, D. (2002). What violence prevention research can tell us about developmental psychopathology. *Developmental & Psychopathology*, 14(4), 713-729.

Tolan, P.H. (2001). Emerging themes and challenges in understanding youth violence involvement. *Journal of Clinical and Child Psychology*, 30(2), 233-239.

Tolan, P.H., Gorman-Smith, D., & Loeber, R. (2000). Developmental timing of onsets of disruptive behaviors and later delinquency of inner-city youth. *Journal of Child& Family Studies, 9(2)*, 203-220.

Tolou-Shams, M., Paikoff, R. L., McKirnan, D. J., & Holmbeck, G. N. (2005). Mental health and HIV risk among African American Adolescents: The role of parenting. *Social Work in Mental Health* 5 (1/2), 25-56.

Mental Health and HIV Risk Among African American Adolescents: The Role of Parenting

Marina Tolou-Shams
Roberta Paikoff
David J. McKirnan
Grayson N. Holmbeck

SUMMARY. The family system is integral to adolescent mental health and HIV risk. However, few studies have addressed family variables and adolescent outcomes among African American families. This study tested a longitudinal model of parenting, adolescent mental health, and adoles-

Marina Tolou-Shams, PhD, is affiliated with Brown University Medical School/ Rhode Island Hospital. Roberta Paikoff, PhD, is affiliated with the University of Illinois at Chicago, Department of Psychiatry/Institute For Juvenile Research. David J. McKirnan, PhD, is affiliated with the University of Illinois at Chicago, Department of Psychology. Grayson N. Holmbeck, PhD, is affiliated with Loyola University, Chicago, Department of Psychology.

Address correspondence to: Marina Tolou-Shams, PhD, Brown University Medical School/Rhode Island Hospital, Bradley/Hasbro Research Center, Coro West, One Hoppin Street, Suite 204, Providence, RI 02903 (E-mail: mtoloushams@lifespan.org).

Without the contributions of CHAMP Collaborative Board members and participants, this work would not have been possible.

Funding from the National Institute of Mental Health (R01 MH 63662, R01 MH 50423-08) and the W. T. Grant Foundation is gratefully acknowledged.

[Haworth co-indexing entry note]: "Mental Health and HIV Risk Among African American Adolescents: The Role of Parenting." Tolou-Shams, Marina et al. Co-published simultaneously in *Social Work in Mental Health* (The Haworth Press, Inc.) Vol. 5, No. 1/2, 2007, pp. 27-58; and: *Community Collaborative Partnerships: The Foundation for HIV Prevention Research Efforts* (ed: Mary M. McKay, and Roberta L. Paikoff) The Haworth Press, Inc., 2007, pp. 27-58. Single or multiple copies of this article are available for a fee from The Haworth Document Delivery Service [1-800-HAWORTH, 9:00 a.m. - 5:00 p.m. (EST). E-mail address: docdelivery@haworthpress.com].

cent HIV risk, among a community sample of low-income, urban African American families from the Collaborative HIV prevention and Adolescent Mental Health Project (CHAMP). Consistent with general adolescent population data, we expected less parental monitoring, greater psychological control and less positive parenting to increase risk for adolescent depression and conduct problems. We hypothesized that these variables would in turn increase rates of HIV risk.

We followed one hundred and thirty-four African American youth and their maternal caregivers as part of the CHAMP project. Study variables included: positive parenting, parental monitoring, psychological control, adolescent distress, conduct problems, and recent HIV risk. We examined the relationship among these variables via longitudinal path analysis.

Age was strongly associated with increased adolescent HIV risk. Contrary to hypotheses, more parental psychological control was marginally associated with less HIV risk, while positive parenting was marginally associated with greater HIV risk. Adolescent depression was associated with more conduct problems, but unrelated to HIV risk. Thus, parenting practices generally considered negative might actually be protective among some lower SES African-American families. This underscores the importance of extending studies of family context and adolescent risk behaviors to diverse social and ethnic groups. Designing prevention programs for diverse groups will require articulating culturally specific effects for different parenting practice. doi:10.1300/J200v05n01_02 *[Article copies available for a fee from The Haworth Document Delivery Service: 1-800-HAWORTH. E-mail address: <docdelivery@haworthpress.com> Website: <http://www.HaworthPress.com> © 2007 by The Haworth Press, Inc. All rights reserved.]*

KEYWORDS. Parental monitoring, positive parenting, adolescent distress, conduct problems, recent HIV risk

Low-income, urban African American adolescents are at high risk for contracting HIV (Centers for Disease Control [CDC], 2002). African Americans account for approximately 12% of the total US population, but make up almost 38% of all AIDS cases reported in this country (CDC, 2002). Females comprise 47% of HIV cases in this age group (reports from 2000; CDC, 2002). Thus, African American youth, particularly females, are at great risk for HIV infection.

Many African American youth live in communities with chronic stressors such as discrimination, inadequate health care, and high crime rates that negatively affect both parenting practices and mental health; this places African American families at heightened risk for depression and other psychiatric disorders (Klebanov, Brooks-Gunn & Duncan, 1994; Myers & Sanders Thompson, 2000). Psychological difficulties in adolescents may themselves lead to other health vulnerabilities, such as behavioral risk for HIV infection (Brown, Danovsky, Lourie, Di- Clemente & Ponton, 1997).

Among the many precursors of HIV risk in young men and women, the conditions of inner city, minority areas may make these parenting variables particularly important to the development of risk among young African Americans. This study tested a longitudinal model of late adolescent HIV risk among urban, low-income African Americans. It was hypothesized that early parenting practices–specifically lack of positive parenting, lack of parental monitoring, and high levels of psychological control–underlie mid-adolescent distress and conduct problems, that themselves induce HIV risk behavior (see Figure 1). These variables were chosen because they have been well studied in general samples, although very few studies have attempted to examine the effect of these practices among inner-city African American families.

HIV RISK AMONG AFRICAN AMERICAN ADOLESCENTS

Historical trends have indicated a steady growth in the percentage of youth who initiated sexual intercourse as teenagers, with a possible leveling off in the mid-1990s (Brooks-Gunn & Furstenberg, 1989; Singh & Darroch, 1999). The most recent data suggest that between the ages of 15-19, 51% of females and 56% of males have had sexual intercourse [Alan Guttamacher Institute (AGI), 1999]. African American youth have generally shown earlier sexual activity than have Caucasians, although that gap appears to be narrowing (Brooks-Gunn & Furstenberg, 1989; Singh & Darroch, 1999).

Adolescent contraceptive use has generally increased over time, mainly due to the massive surge in condom use post HIV/AIDS epidemic (AGI, 1999). Despite this, of the 33% of high school students nationwide who describe themselves as currently sexually active, 42% report that they did not use a condom during last intercourse [Youth Risk Behavior Surveillance (YRBS), 2001]. Thus, many adolescents are sexually active, yet condom use is inconsistent over sexual episodes

FIGURE 1. Framework of Initial Model

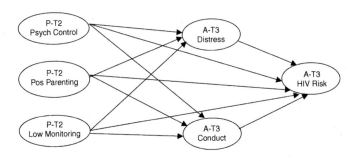

(Piccinino & Mosher, 1998; Wellings & Mitchell, 1998). With respect to trends in age, gender and ethnicity, African American girls have more recently marginally surpassed Caucasian girls with respect to condom use rates (38% versus 36%, respectively; Piccinino & Mosher, 1998). This increase in condom use among some of the more at-risk youth likely reflects the impact of larger HIV prevention campaigns that targeted low-income, communities of color in the late 80s and early 90s. While these trends are encouraging, rates of condom use among these at-risk youth are still less than desirable (Roderigue, Tercyak & Lescano, 1997), especially for African American youth, who comprised 65% of all HIV diagnoses among ages 13-24 (CDC, 2002).

MENTAL HEALTH STATUS AMONG AFRICAN AMERICAN ADOLESCENTS

In community samples psychological distress and "externalizing" behaviors such as conduct disorder are associated with early sexual activity and lower rates of condom use (e.g., Ary et al., 1999a, 1999b; Bachanas et al., 2002; Jessor & Jessor, 1977; Jessor, 1998). The association of distress with HIV risk may be greater for girls, whether Caucasian (Smith, 1997) or African American (DiClemente et al., 2001). Capaldi, Stoolmiller, Clark, and Owen (2002) reported a longitudinal effect of conduct problems on HIV risk among Caucasian males, and Lanctot and Smith (2001) showed cross-sectional associations between conduct disorder, substance use, HIV risk and pregnancy among African American girls.

African American adolescents may be at greater risk for psychological distress than are Caucasian adolescents (Garrison, Schluchter, Schoenbach & Kaplan, 1989; Nettles & Pleck, 1994; Schoenbach, Kaplan, Grimson & Wagner, 1982), although other studies suggest the opposite (e.g., Schraedley, Gotlib & Hayward, 1999), especially when controlling for socioeconomic status (Samaan, 1998). Females of all ethnicities are at heightened risk for psychological distress, especially during mid-adolescence (Cicchetti & Toth, 1998; Cyranowski, Frank, Young & Shear, 2000; Nolen-Hoeksama, 1994; Siegel, Aneshensel, Taub, Cantwell, & Driscoll, 1998).

African American youth are disproportionately represented with respect to rates of conduct disorder and antisocial behavior; yet, they are also more likely to be arrested, convicted and kept in prison than Caucasian youth that commit the same acts (Gibbs, 1998). African American males and females are also more likely to report having engaged in physical fights than Caucasian youth, potentially due to psychological effects of their greater exposure to violence and other chronic stressors throughout childhood (Gibbs, 1998; Myers & Sanders Thompson, 2000).

PARENTING STRATEGIES
OF URBAN AFRICAN AMERICAN PARENTS

Consistent with Patterson and colleagues (1989; 1992), it was hypothesized that distress, conduct problems and HIV risk in adolescence stem from ineffective parenting practices within a context of chronic neighborhood violence and socioeconomic disadvantage. Studying African American families, Pittman and Chase-Lansdale (2001) found low parental warmth and monitoring to induce severe internalizing and externalizing problems among adolescent girls, and Weis (2002) showed dismissive and distressed parents to have the worst psychosocial outcomes among their children at two-year follow-up. Thus, a lack of positive parenting combined with distress and anger creates significant risk for mental health problems African American youth (Weis, 2002).

Parental support has both indirect and direct effects on risky sexual behavior (Miller, Benson, & Galbraith, 2001). Whitbeck et al. (1992, 1993) found less parental support and warmth to underlie depressed affect among girls, which itself related to more adolescent sexual activity. Lower parental support has been directly related to more sexual risk, including less condom use, among Caucasian male and female samples (Jaccard, Dittus & Gordon,1996; Luster and Small, 1994). The effects of parental support have been less clear among African American youth. Crosby et al. (2001) found direct effects of maternal support on adolescent HIV risk among African American adolescent females, including an increased likelihood of communicating with sexual partners and of using a condom (Crosby et al., 2001). In contrast, Lauritsen (1994) and Perkins, Luster, Villarruel, and Small (1998) found no effect of parental support on HIV risk among African American youth.

Findings from multiple longitudinal studies in both African American (Kilgore et al., 2000) and multiethnic (Herman et al. 1997) samples support the hypothesis that decreased parental monitoring predicts the later development of antisocial behavior, as well as greater HIV risk (Metzler, Noell, Biglan, Ary & Smolkowski, 1994; Miller, Forehand & Kotchick, 1999; Rodgers, 1999). However, several studies (e.g., Fox & Inazu, 1980; East, 1996; Resnick & Burt, 1996), found no association between parental monitoring and sexual risk when simultaneously considering race (East, 1996) or parent knowledge and attitudes about teen sex (Resnick & Burt, 1996).

"Psychologically controlling" parenting (defined as demanding, hostile, or overprotective; Barber & Harmon, 2002) has consistently been related to distress and anxiety in mainly Caucasian, but also some African American families (Barber and Harmon, 2002; Baron & MacGillivray, 1989; Bean, 1998; Barber, Olsen & Shagle, 1994; Barber, 1996; Eccles, Early, Frasier, Belansky, & McCarthy, 1997; Petit et al., 2001). Few studies have linked parental psychological control to teenage HIV risk (Miller et al., 2001), although psychological control has been related to earlier age of sexual intercourse (see Barber, 1996), and to lessened condom use among daughters of highly controlling fathers (Rodgers, 1999). Since psychological control has clear effects on adolescent distress symptoms (Barber & Harmon, 2002), at least among Caucasian families, and there is evidence for an association between psychological distress and adolescent sexual behavior (Whitbeck et al., 1992; 1993), it is plausible that psychological control might indirectly increase adolescent HIV risk vis-à-vis an increase in depressive symptoms.

In sum, three general hypotheses were tested in a community sample of African American families: (1) ineffective parenting practices, traditionally defined as less positive parenting, less parental monitoring and greater psychological control, would increase the risk for the development of late adolescent distress and conduct problems; (2) late adolescent distress and conduct problems would themselves increase HIV risk; and, (3) parenting during mid-adolescence would have both direct effects on later adolescent HIV risk as well as indirect effects via late adolescent distress and conduct problems.

METHOD

Participants

Participants were 311 African American youth and their caregivers recruited into the Chicago HIV Prevention and Adolescent Mental Health Project (CHAMP) during the 4th and 5th grades, from elementary schools in urban, low-income neighborhoods (see Procedures). Schools were selected near public housing projects in neighborhoods with high rates of HIV infection.

Participants were interviewed at three separate time points over the course of 7-8 years total, with an average of 2-3 years between Time 1 and Time 2 and an average of 5 years between Time 2 and Time 3. At Time 1, 304 of the 311 parent-adolescent dyads initially recruited had complete study data on variables of interest. By Time 3, 209 adolescents and 215 parents (69% and 71% of original samples) returned for study follow-up, representing 188 complete dyads. The primary reason for loss to follow-up was the scattering of participants after demolition of many of the target housing projects. Of the 188 parent-adolescent dyads[1] retained for Time 3, seven were dropped because they involved only a paternal caregiver. Of the 181 remaining mother-adolescent dyads, 134 dyads had complete data on variables of interest across all study time points. Current analyses focused on parenting at Time 2 (early adolescence) and adolescent mental health and HIV risk at Time 3, approximately five years later (late adolescence). T-tests showed no systematic differences in mental health measures between dyads with complete study data ($n = 134$) and those who were lost to follow-up or had missing data ($n = 169$); all analyses $t (301) <$ .5, $p >$ .05. Final analyses used the 134 mother-adolescent dyads that had complete study data across Time 2 and Time 3.

Measures

Core variables consisted of maternal psychological control, parental monitoring, positive parenting, adolescent distress, adolescent conduct problems, and adolescent HIV risk. Maternal psychological control was assessed via an observational scale of parent-child interactions. Adolescent distress and HIV risk were assessed via adolescent report only. Both parental and adolescent self-reports of maternal monitoring, positive parenting, and adolescent conduct problems were collected. For each of these variables the parent and adolescent measures if significantly correlated were, at best, modestly associated (eg., $r = .23, p < .01$ for positive parenting). We therefore decided to not combine the adolescent and parental versions of these measures. Where available, general findings from the literature guided our decision about who would be the best single reporter (Angold et al., 1987). Thus, for positive parenting and adolescent conduct problems we used maternal self-report measures. Although some data (Stattin & Kerr, 2000) suggest that the child's disclosure of parental knowledge of their whereabouts and rules is a better predictor than parent report, to maintain consistent reporters across parenting measures, we chose to rely on parental report of monitoring.

Time 2 Measures

Maternal Psychological Control: Observational. Parents were not asked to complete a self-report measure of psychological control at this study time point and therefore only an observational measure of maternal psychological control was available for analysis. Mothers and children participated in a 10 minute videotaped conflict interaction task wherein they were asked to try resolving a mutually conflictual topic. Details about these interactions and the coding methodology are reported elsewhere (see McBride, Paikoff & Holmbeck, 2003). The psychological control scale was derived from 6-point likert scale [0 (not at all) to 5 (very much)] ratings of the extent to which each (1) pressured the other(s) to agree; (2) frequently blamed other family members for problems, and (3) requested change in the other family member (codes were chosen to represent the definition of psychological control, see Barber, 1996, Barber & Harmon, 2002; Holmbeck, Shapera & Hommeyer, 2002; Steinberg, 1990). The average rating across two raters for each scale item was used to comprise the final scale score for parent psychological control. Higher scores indicated more maternal psychological control. Average inter-rater reliability for the full scale was .43 (ranging from .28 to .56 depending on scale item) and psychological control scale reliability was good (scale $\alpha = .83$).

Maternal Monitoring: Parent Report. Behavioral control was assessed by a 17-item parental report measure adapted from the Pittsburgh Youth Study interview (Gorman-Smith et al., 1996; Lamborn et al., 1991; Stouthamer-Loeber & Loeber, 1986). Items addressed parents' enforcement of house rules (e.g., " . . . on school nights, I expect my child to be in bed by a certain time . . . "), and awareness of their child's behaviors, and whereabouts. Responses were made on a Likert scale ranging from always true (1) to always false (4), with a "does not apply" option. Higher average scores represent less parental monitoring and behavioral control. The inter-item reliability for the parent scale was alpha = .66.

Positive Parenting: Parent Report. This 6-item scale measured the amount of parents' positively reinforcing activities with their children, e.g., warmth, support and praise. It was adopted from a 12-item scale (Gorman-Smith et al., 1996), e.g., "In the past 12 months, when your child did something that you liked or approved of, how often did you: give a wink or a smile, say something nice about it, and give a reward for it." Responses were made on a 3-point scale, ranging from 1 (almost never) to 3 (almost always). Higher scores indicate more positive parenting. Inter-item reliability for the parent scale was .78.

Time 3 Measures

Psychological Distress: Adolescent Report: An abbreviated version (29 items) of the Levonn (40 items; Martinez & Richters, 1993), a scale based on the work of Valla et al. (1994) was used to measure internalizing symptoms in adolescents. This scale has been previously used to measure symptoms of distress in younger children living in an urban environment (Martinez & Richters, 1993) and was adapted to ask adolescents about how often they find themselves in various distressing situations, e.g., witnessing violence, feeling sad about people you know who have died. Responses are made on a 3-point likert scale, ranging from 0 (never) to 2 (a lot of times). Higher average scores indicate greater adolescent distress. This scale demonstrated good scale reliability across study time points (α = .89 for Time 2, α = .93 for Time 3).

Conduct Problems: Parent Report. Mothers in the study filled out an abbreviated (53-item) version of the Child Behavior Checklist (CBCL; Achenbach, 1991). Data from the delinquency and aggression subscales (33-items) were used as indicators of conduct problems. Higher scores indicate worse conduct problems. This conduct problem subscale demonstrated good scale reliability across study time points (α = .92 for Time 2, α = .91 for Time 3).

HIV risk: Adolescent report. Scales adapted from the NIMH multi-site prevention trials and Rotheram-Borus and colleagues (e.g., Rotheram-Borus, Murphy, Reid, & Coleman, 1996; Rotheram-Borus et al., 1997) were used to assess HIV risk behavior. Adolescents were asked generally about lifetime risk (e.g., have you ever had sex?) as well as more detailed partner-by-partner questions regarding recent (past 90 days) sexual risk and condom use. Based on response patterns, a four-level HIV risk variable was created. A score of 0 indicated 'no sex ever (no risk)'; 1 indicated 'no sex in the past 90 days (no recent risk)'; 2 indicated 'protected sex in past 90 days (some recent risk)'; and 3 indicated 'unprotected penile-vaginal intercourse past 90 days (recent high risk).' Higher scores indicated increased HIV risk.

Procedure

Families were originally recruited for the CHAMP study when the child was in fourth and fifth grade through six public schools on the South and West sides of Chicago located in African American communities with particularly high rates of poverty and above average rates of HIV infection. Trained graduate research assistants and project staff spent time developing rapport with students and school staff. Flyers about the study were then sent home to 740 parents. Of these parents, 311 families completed initial interviews on-site at the University of Illinois at Chicago.

Upon signing an IRB-approved informed consent, mother and child were each interviewed separately and privately by extensively trained project staff. Every effort was made to match the ethnicity and gender of interviewer to family member. Interview questions were read aloud and participants were given a copy of the interview booklet and responses so that they could follow along and select their responses more easily. After the interview, parents were asked to complete videotaped observational tasks. Project staff then had an additional private, individual interview with the young adolescent, which was conducted at their school. The school was not involved with the interviews at all and had no access to the information given to CHAMP by the young adolescent. Young adolescents were reminded that everything remained confidential and that they could refuse to answer anything that made them feel uncomfortable (particularly since these interviews included potentially very sensitive information about sexual behavior). At Time 3 (approximately five years later), the aforementioned procedures and compensation were repeated. However, at Time 3, all procedures were conducted at the university site, the sexual behavior interview was more detailed (given that adolescents were now in the late adolescent stage of development) and was conducted face-to-face with a same-sex interviewer. At each study time point, all mother and adolescent procedures took approximately 4-6 hours to complete. Mothers and adolescents were compensated for their time and transportation expenses at each time point.

Data Analysis

LISREL 8.52 (Joreskog & Sorbom, 1996a, 1996b) was used to test the goodness-of-fit and structural coefficients of recursive path models of maternal parenting, adolescent mental health and HIV risk. The models were "recursive" in that all causal effects were considered to be unidirectional (Kline, 1998). Prior to analysis, all data were screened and adjusted for normality (skew, kurtosis, outliers), missing observations, linearity, homoscedasticity, and multicollinearity.

A nested model trimming approach (Kline, 1998) that employed both a priori theoretical and empirical considerations was used to determine the best-fitting, most parsimonious model. Nested models refer to successive tests of the same observed variables that estimate differed numbers of paths. Three measures were used to assess absolute model fit, the χ^2 statistic, the root mean square of approximation (RMSEA; Steiger, 1991) and the goodness-of-fit index (GFI; Joreskog & Sorborn, 1996a). The χ^2 statistic is used as a test of significance of the difference in fit between the observed and predicted covariance structure, derived from a maximum likelihood (ML) estimation. Thus, a low and nonsignificant χ^2 indicates good model fit. The RMSEA and GFI indices are more standardized and less sensitive to sample size than the χ^2 statistic. An RMSEA of .05 or lower represents close fit; RMSEA between .05 and .08 represents reasonably close fit; and RMSEA above .10 represents an unacceptable model (Browne & Cudeck, 1989). The GFI indicates the proportion of observed covariances explained by the model, ranging from 0 to 1, where 1 indicates an optimal model fit. It is recommended that the GFI value be greater than .90 for acceptable model fit (Kline, 1998).

Two measures of relative model fit, the Bentler-Bonett Non-Normed Fit Index (NNFI; Bentler, 1990; Bentler & Bonett, 1980), and the Standardized Root Mean Squared Residual (SRMR; Joreskog & Sorbom, 1996a) were also used. The NNFI is a version of the Normed Fit Index (NFI; Bentler & Bonett, 1980) that corrects for the number of parameters in the model and NNFI values of .90 or greater are desired. The SRMR represents a summary of the standardized covariance residuals, which are the differences between the observed and model-estimated covariances (Kline, 1998). As the average discrepancy between observed and expected covariances increases, so does the SRMR value. Therefore, SRMR values closer to 0 are desired and indicate a better model fit. There is no significance test for the NNFI or SRMR indices.

To test alternative models (i.e., models that were not originally hypothesized but may be of equal or superior statistical fit) of parenting, mental health and HIV risk, "nonnested" comparisons were conducted, wherein entire variables were removed from the model. For this, the Akaike Information Criterion (AIC) fit index was used (Akaike, 1987). The AIC is similar to the χ^2 statistic, but adjusts for differences in the number of model parameters (Kline, 1998). There is no significance test for the AIC comparison, but the model with the lowest AIC is preferred (Akaike, 1987; Kline, 1998). Finally, path coefficients in the various models were examined using a critical ratio statistic. A significant critical ratio indicated that a particular pathway among variables was statistically significant. Standardized path coefficients with absolute values less than .10 indicate a "small" effect; coefficients around .30 indicate a "medium" effect; and those greater than .50 indicate a "large" effect (Cohen, 1988; Kline, 1998).

Gender, Age and Baseline Adolescent Mental Health

The statistical relationship between age, adolescent mental health and HIV risk was first examined in simple correlational analyses. Age was then included as a model covariate if significantly associated with an outcome. Sample size was not adequate to test gender as a moderator of the proposed overall model. Therefore, gender differences in outcome variables were first examined using MANOVA. Based on MANOVA results, gender was then included as a covariate of adolescent outcomes in the final best-fitting models to determine if there were shifts in path coefficients and/or explained variance in outcomes above and beyond gender. Models were also tested controlling for baseline adolescent mental health.

RESULTS

Demographics

The average age of the 134 maternal caregivers at Time 2 and 3 was 37 years ($SD = 6.98$) and 42 years ($SD = 6.61$), respectively. Ninety percent ($n = 121$) were birth mothers, 5% ($n = 7$) were grandmothers, 4% ($n = 5$) were aunts, and .7% ($n = 1$) were female guardians. Fifty-two percent had graduated from high school or received a GED and 40% reported having been employed sometime during the past year. Thirty-four percent ($n = 45$) of maternal caregivers endorsed receiving public assistance and 52% endorsed living in government-subsidized housing. Including public aid assistance, 89% reported receiving a yearly total income of less than $15,000.

The average age of 83 female and 51 male adolescents at Time 2 and 3 was 13 years ($SD = .71$) and 18 years ($SD = 1.02$), respectively. By Time 3, 17% ($n = 23$) had completed high school or received their GED and 78% ($n = 103$) were still living in their parent/guardian's home. By Time 3, 24% ($n = 31$) had a child (26 females and 5 males; two adolescents were missing data on this item). Those who had a child were significantly older ($M = 18.55$, $SD = 1.05$) than those who did not have a child ($M = 17.76$, $SD = .95$), $t_{(130)} = 3.95$, $p < .001$.

Descriptive Statistics

Descriptive statistics of late adolescent outcomes across each study time point are presented in Table 1. Parenting descriptive statistics are presented in Table 2. An examination of missing data patterns showed no systematic differences between those who had missing observations across time points and those who did not. Given that missing observations were primarily due to subject attrition, imputation with estimated scores was not appropriate (Kline, 1998; Raymond & Roberts, 1987; Ward & Clark, 1991). Thus, only participants with valid values on all variables for analysis were considered.

Nineteen percent of participants had a change in maternal caregiver across time-points. To rule out the possibility that this change affected the adolescent outcomes, participants who had a consistent maternal caregiver ($n = 109$) were compared to those who did not ($n = 25$). There were no differences in parenting practices between these groups (all p's > .05). These groups were combined for all analyses. In most cases "maternal caregiver" represented the biological mother, but could also refer to a foster mother, grandmother, aunt or other legal guardian.

TABLE 1. Longitudinal Descriptives of Adolescent Distress, Conduct Problems and HIV Risk ($N = 134$)

Variable	Time 2	Time 3
Age M(SD)	13.00 (.71)	17.94 (1.02)
Adolescent Mental Health M(SD)		
Distress score	.59 (.29)	.43 (.32)
# symptoms	14.26 (6.23)	10.82 (7.29)
Conduct problems score	.43 (.31)	.35 (.29)
# symptoms	11.03 (6.70)	8.92 (6.77)
Lifetime HIV risk (n,%)		
Ever had vaginal sex	26 (24%)	107 (80%)
Ever had oral sex	---	48/107 (36%)
Ever had anal sex	---	13/107 (10%)
Used condom (last intercourse)	23/26 (88%)	77/107 (72%)
Only 1 partner	10/26 (38%)	25/107 (23%)
> 1 partner[a]	16/26 (62%)	82/107 (77%)
Past 90 days HIV risk (n,%)		
Vaginal sex		85/107 (79%)
unprotected		32/85 (38%)
Oral sex		34/85 (40%)
unprotected		21/34 (62%)
Anal sex		10/85 (12%)
unprotected		2/10 (20%)
Only 1 risky partner >1 risky		29/32 (91%)
partner (range= 2-3)		3/32 (9%)

[a] range of partners for time 1 = 1-10 (2 adolescents had 2-3; 1 had between 4-10); for time 2 = 1-5 (2 had 8 partners, 3 had 7 partners, 1 had 5 partners; for time 3 = 2-8 (23 adolescents had 4-10 partners; 11 had more than 10 partners

Model of Parenting, Adolescent Mental Health and HIV Risk

Descriptive Findings

During early adolescence, maternal caregivers generally self-reported high rates of parental monitoring and positive parenting (see Table 2).

Yet, per observer ratings, they also engaged in moderate rates of psychologically controlling behavior during that same time period. Overall, late adolescent distress symptoms and conduct problems declined from early to late adolescence (Table 1). Sixty-five percent ($n = 87$) of late adolescents were reported by their parents to have engaged in at least one form of aggressive or delinquent behavior "most often or all of the time" during the past 6 months. These were generally not severe

TABLE 2. Means, Standard Deviations and Cronbach Alphas for Model Variables (N = 134)

Reporter-Variable[1]	M	SD	Skewness	Kurtosis	# items	Alpha[2]
Time 2						
P- Monitoring	1.37	.25	.62	−.07	17	.66
P-Psych Control	2.47	.57	−.01	.08	3	.83
P- Positive Parenting	2.50	.35	−.50	.16	6	.78
Time 3						
A-Distress	.43	.32	1.20	1.72	29	.93
P-Adolescent Conduct Problems	.35	.29	1.22	1.43	33	.91
A-HIV risk [0 (no risk)-3 (high risk)]	1.60	1.04	−.37	−1.05		
A- Age (years)	17.94	1.02	.07	−.46		

[1] P represents parent report; A represents adolescent report.
[2] *n*'s for alphas vary slightly due to certain scale items randomly missing across participant

conduct problems (e.g., substance use, truancy) and were instead more related to arguing, demanding attention, preferring to be with older kids and talking too much. On the Levonn measure, 55% (*n* = 74) of late adolescents endorsed at least one distress symptom as occurring "all of the time" and 22% (*n* = 29) reported 3 or more chronic distress symptoms. Commonly endorsed symptoms included: "you get really mad or upset easily, even about things that do not bother other people or make them angry (11%)," "you feel sad about people you know have died (32%)," and "when the teacher is trying to teach something in class, you think about something else (11%)."

Lifetime HIV Risk at Time 3

Eighty percent of participants (*n* = 107) reported having had vaginal intercourse by Time 3. Sixty percent (*n* = 64/107) reported using condoms "every time" and 72% (*n* = 77) reported using condoms at last intercourse. Twenty-three percent (*n* = 25) reported having had one lifetime sexual partner, 45% (*n* = 48) reported having had "two or three," 22% (*n* = 23) reported having had between 4-10, and 10% (*n* = 11) reported having had more than 10 lifetime partners.

Recent HIV Risk at Time 3

Of the 107 sexually active adolescents, 79% (*n* = 85) had been sexually active during the past 90 days. Fifty percent (*n* = 53) of sexually active participants reported protected vaginal intercourse, and 30% ($n = 32$) reported at least one episode of unprotected vaginal intercourse (range = 1-40 unprotected vaginal sex episodes). Ninety-one percent of those reporting unprotected vaginal sex had only one partner ($n = 29/32$); two adolescents had risky sex with two partners in the past 90 days, and one adolescent had recent risky sex with three different partners. For analyses, HIV risk was operationalized within four categories: 0 = 'no sex ever' ($n = 27$); 1 = 'no sex in the past 90 days' ($n = 22$); 2 = 'protected sex in past 90 days' ($n = 53$), and; 3 = 'unprotected vaginal sex past 90 days' ($n = 32$). Table 1 shows specific sexual activity data across all study time points, including more specific sexual risk activity during the past 90 days.

All variables tested in this model fit assumptions of normality (Table 2). Intercorrelations are presented in Table 3.

None of the Time 2 parental variables–psychological control, monitoring, and positive parenting–were significantly associated with Time 3 HIV risk. In addition, neither Time 3 adolescent distress nor conduct problems was significantly correlated with Time 3 HIV risk (all $ps > .05$). Age was significantly associated with HIV risk ($r = .39, p < .001$); older adolescents reported more HIV risk. Since older age was also associated with increased odds of having had a child, recent HIV risk among sexually active adolescents *with* children was compared to that among sexually active adolescents *without* children. Adolescents with children ($n = 31$) were at slightly greater risk for HIV and other STDs during the past 90 days ($M = 2.32, SD = .79$) than adolescents without children ($n = 74; M = 2.00, SD = .66$), $p = .05$.

Model Testing: Adolescent Mental Health and HIV Risk

Table 4 presents goodness-of-fit indices for a series of models examining the effects of parenting variables and adolescent mental health on HIV risk.

The initial hypothesis was that Parental Psychological Control, Parental Monitoring, and Positive Parenting at Time 2 would directly lead to HIV risk at Time 3, and would indirectly lead to HIV risk by influencing Time 3 adolescent distress and conduct problems, which themselves would predict HIV risk. Given the strong association between parental monitoring and positive parenting demonstrated via simple correlational analyses, the path between these Time 2 parenting variables was also estimated and all other paths between Time 2 parenting variables were constrained to zero. This framework is given in Figure 2.

TABLE 3. Intercorrrelations for Model Variables

Subscales	1	2	3	4	5	6	7
Adolescents (N = 134)							
Parent report Time 2							
1. Parental Monitoring (House Rules)	1.00	2.31**	.12	.19*	.12	.10	--- [a]
2. Positive Parenting		1.00	−.07	−.27**	−.24**	.08	---
Observational Data Time 2							
3. Parental Psychological Control			1.00	.04	.02	−.15	---
Parent report Time 3							
4. Adolescent Conduct Problems (Youth Behavior Profile)				1.00	.28**	.10	.08
Adolescent report Time 3							
5. Adolescent Distress (Levonn scale)					1.00	−.03	−.07
6. Adolescent HIV Risk						1.00	.39***
7. Age at Time 3							1.00

[a]The relationship between Age at Time 3 and other model variables was only tested with Time 3 adolescent outcomes.
** p < .01; *** p < .001

TABLE 4. Goodness-of-Fit Statistics for Path Models 1-8 Predicting Late Adolescent Mental Health and HIV Risk (N = 134)

Model Type	Outcome Measures	Number of Variables	Measures of Absolute Fit					Measures of Relative Fit	
			χ^2	df	RMSEA	GFI	SRMR	NNFI	R^2
Model 1	Distress	6	6.80*	3	.10	.98	.05	.54	.06
	Conduct	6							.09
	HIV risk	6							.07
Model 2	Distress	6	6.81*	5	.05	.98	.05	.87	.06
	Conduct	6							.09
	HIV risk	6							.07
Model 3	Distress	6	7.20*	6	.04	.98	.05	.93	.06
	Conduct	6							.09
	HIV risk	6							.07
Model 4	Distress	6	7.53*	7	.02	.98	.05	.97	.06
	Conduct	6							.09
	HIV risk	6							.06
Model 5	Distress	6	9.17*	8	.03	.98	.05	.95	.06
	Conduct	6							.09
	HIV risk	6							.05
Model 6	Distress	6	10.05*	8	.04	.98	.06	.91	.06
	Conduct	6							.09
	HIV risk	6							.04
Model 7	Distress	6	9.47*	8	.04	.98	.05	.93	.06
	Conduct	6							.07
	HIV risk	6							.06
Model 8[1]	**Distress**	**6**	**.72***	**6**	**.00**	**.998**	**.01**	**1.00**	**.06**
	Conduct	**6**							**.13**
	HIV risk	**6**							**.06**

*p > .05
[1]bold type represents "best-fitting" model

FIGURE 2. Model 4

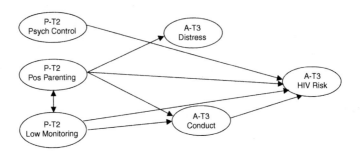

Per the χ^2 difference test, nested *Models 1 through 7* (see Table 4) did not significantly differ in terms of overall model fit. However, of Models 1 through 7, Model 4 (see Figure 2) was retained as the best-fitting model because it was the most parsimonious model with strong goodness-of-fit indices ($\chi^2 = 7.53$, $df = 7$, $p > .05$; RMSEA = .02; GFI = .98; NNFI = .97).

Given that Time 3 distress was not significantly associated with Time 3 HIV risk, but Time 3 conduct problems were marginally associated with Time 3 HIV risk ($\beta = .11$, $p < .10$), the hypothesis that Time 3 adolescent distress was associated with HIV risk via Time 3 conduct problems was tested. Time 3 adolescent distress symptoms and conduct problems were significantly associated in preliminary correlational analyses ($r = .28$, $p < .001$); therefore, the test of this hypothesis was both empirically and theoretically justified. Of all nested model comparisons, Model 8 (see Figure 3) was the best-fitting model ($\chi^2 = .72$, $df = 6$, $p > .05$; RMSEA = .00; GFI = .998; NNFI = 1.00), and was a statistically significant improved fit over Model 4 (χ^2 difference = 6.81, df difference = 1, $p < .01$).[2]

The final model explained 6% of the variance in late adolescent distress, 13% of the variance in late adolescent conduct problems, and 6% of the variance in adolescent HIV risk. The links between Time 2 parental monitoring and Time 3 conduct problems (standardized $\beta = .11$, $p < .10$), Time 2 parental monitoring and Time 3 HIV risk ($\beta = .14$, $p < .10$), and Time 2 positive parenting and Time 3 HIV risk ($\beta = .15$, $p < .10$) represented only trends toward being significantly different from zero. Paths between Time 2 positive parenting and Time 3 distress ($\beta = -.24$, $p < .01$) and conduct problems ($\beta = -.18$, $p < .05$) were significantly

FIGURE 3. Best-Fitting Model (Model 8)

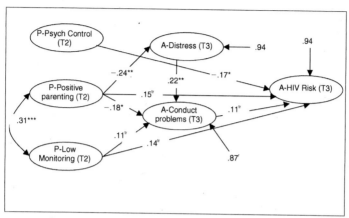

***p < .0001; ** p < .01 *p < .05 all one-tailed p's; tr = trend toward significance, i.e., p < .10

different from zero, as was the relationship between Time 2 parental psychological control and Time 3 HIV risk ($\beta = -.17, p < .05$).

The direction of the relationships between Time 2 positive parenting and psychological control to Time 3 HIV risk was in the opposite of the hypothesized direction, such that more positive parenting during early adolescence was marginally associated with more late adolescent HIV risk, and more parental psychological control during early adolescence was significantly associated with decreased late adolescent HIV risk. Relationships between Time 3 outcomes in the final model were consistent with hypotheses; more late adolescent distress was associated with increased conduct problems ($\beta = .22, p < .05$) and more conduct problems were marginally associated with increased HIV risk ($\beta = .11, p < .10$). Additionally, there was a significant indirect effect of Time 2 positive parenting on Time 3 conduct problems via Time 3 adolescent distress ($\beta = -.05, p < .05$), such that more positive parenting predicted less adolescent distress, which was associated with less adolescent conduct problems.[3]

Gender and Age

Based on an initial MANOVA, girls were more likely to be distressed ($M = .48, SD = .34$) than boys ($M = .34\ SD = .27$), F $(1,134) = 6.23, p <$

.05) and older adolescents were more likely to have recent HIV risk ($r =$ .39, $p < .001$). Therefore, a form of Model 8 was tested that included the effect of gender on distress as well as the effect of age on HIV risk. This model fit the data well ($\chi^2 = 5.06$, $df = 17$, $p > .05$; RMSEA $= .00$; GFI $= .99$; NNFI $= 1.00$), but had a larger AIC value than Model B8 ($AIC_{gender/age}$ 59.02 versus $AIC_{Model\ 8} = 42.72$). There was a strong positive association between Time 3 age and Time 3 HIV risk ($\beta = .36$, $p < .0001$). Gender also had a significant indirect effect on Time 3 adolescent conduct problems via Time 3 adolescent distress ($\beta = .04$, $p < .05$); adolescent girls were more likely to have conduct problems because they were also more likely to report depressive symptoms. Overall, the AIC results suggested that this more complex model was a slightly less accurate fit to the data than was Model 8, despite strong age effects.

Including age, however, in Model 8 shifted the magnitude of direct relationships between Time 2 parenting and Time 3 HIV risk. When age was included in the model the association between Time 2 parental psychological control and Time 3 HIV risk diminished (excluding age, $\beta = -.17$, $p < .05$; including age, $\beta = -.11$, $p < .10$), as did the previously marginal association between Time 2 parental monitoring and Time 3 HIV risk (excluding age, $\beta = .14$, $p < .10$; including age, $\beta = .10$, ns.). These results suggest that parenting variables did not directly or indirectly predict HIV risk above and beyond the effects of age. Further, the percentage of variance the model accounted for in HIV risk went from 6% to 18% in the model that included age as a predictor. In sum, although including age and gender led to a slightly more complex model without improved overall fit indices, this model was still an adequate to good fit of the data and explained up to three times more variance in late adolescent HIV risk.

DISCUSSION

This study found that, among low-income, urban African American families, maternal monitoring, psychological control and positive parenting in mid-adolescence directly affected late adolescent rates of distress, conduct problems and HIV risk. However, contrary to prior findings, adolescent distress and conduct problems did not significantly heighten HIV risk. In addition, there were no differences between adolescent males and females with respect to HIV risk, but older adolescents were more sexually risky.

African American adolescents in this study had a greater frequency of sexual intercourse, but were more likely to protect themselves from HIV and other STDs than the general adolescent population. Specifically, between the ages of 15-20, 80% of adolescents in this study had sexual intercourse, versus some 51% of females and 56% of males surveyed by the Alan Guttmacher Institute (1999). These results support the perspective that early sexual activity may be more normative among African American adolescents (Black, Ricardo & Stanton, 1997; Dittus, Miller, Kotchick & Forehand., 2004; Ensminger, 1990). But, compared to a Youth Risk Behavior Survey (YRBS, 2001) sample, a greater proportion of the youth in this study used condoms at last intercourse (72% versus 58%). In addition, self-reported rates of condom use during the past 90 days was 62%, which was substantially higher than the 38% condom use rate reported by Piccinno and Mosher (1998) for their sample of African American females. These trends may reflect an increased focus the development and implementation of more culturally congruent adolescent HIV primary prevention interventions for African American youth and families (e.g., Parents Matter Program, Dittus et al., 2004).

With regard to adolescent mental health, symptom counts of distress supported the emerging consensus that inner-city African American adolescents are at risk for internalizing disorders (e.g., Samaan, 2000). Consistent with the larger depression literature, African American late adolescent girls reported greater distress than did late adolescent boys. Yet, contrary to studies (with predominantly Caucasian youth) that indicate rates of psychological distress or depression increasing over age (Harrington et al., 1996; Schraedley et al., 1999), average rates of distress declined by late adolescence. Another recent longitudinal study of distress symptoms among inner-city African American children and adolescents similarly found a decrease in symptoms over time (Shaffer, Forehand, Kotchick, & Family Health Project Research Group, 2002), suggesting that developmental trajectories of psychological distress may differ between ethnic minorities in disadvantaged environments and more general Caucasian samples. One possible explanation is that the chronic stressors affecting African American youth in impoverished communities lead to relatively high rates of distress during early adolescence, that decline over time as adolescents develop more mature coping strategies to counteract environmental stressors (Jones & Forehand, 2003).

Similar to adolescent distress, adolescent conduct problems declined over time. Overall, however, this sample showed a relatively low rate of conduct problems, with no gender difference. In addition, parents rarely, if ever, endorsed more severe conduct problems, such as theft, setting fires or physical aggression towards others. There are three reasons why the unexpectedly low rate of conduct problems in this sample must be interpreted with caution. First, adolescent conduct problems were assessed by their mother's behavioral reports taken when the adolescents were approximately 18 years old. The mothers' lessening awareness of their children's' actions at 18 versus 13 years of age (i.e., age at Time 2) might account for the observed average decline in conduct problems at Time 3. Second, the Child Behavior Checklist (CBCL; Achenbach, 1991) may not be as relevant for measuring externalizing behaviors among African American adolescents as for Caucasians. For example, Lambert et al. (2002) found a range of externalizing symptoms shown by African American youth that did not match any CBCL items (e.g., uncooperative, mischievous, easily frustrated, bad attitude, refuses to do school work). Thus, the CBCL may miss externalizing symptoms relevant to this youth population, which might help to explain the relatively low rate of conduct problems reported in this sample. Third, the current data may provide a more accurate representation of symptom rates in a non-clinical, community sample. Previous research that has found higher rates of conduct problems in African American adolescents generally focused on clinical samples of youth who had some form of legal involvement (e.g., juvenile detainees; Teplin, Abram, McClelland, Dulcan, & Mericle, 2002). In this light, previous findings of high rates of conduct disorder among African American youth may reflect a "problem-oriented" sample bias.

Although adolescent distress and conduct problems were positively associated, neither was strongly linked to HIV risk. This finding suggests that unprotected sexual intercourse is not part of a larger, unitary construct of risk behavior for a community sample of urban, low-income African American adolescents and runs counter to the co-occurrence of problem behaviors observed in other studies (e.g., Jessor & Jessor, 1977). From a public health standpoint, given the density of HIV infection in these adolescents' community and rates of unprotected sex (despite mainly being with only one partner), these youth are still at high-risk for HIV infection. Yet, these data suggest that other factors besides mental health, e.g., parenting and peer influence, might be more relevant determinants of their recent HIV risk.

In fact, consistent with most prior literature across various racial or ethnic samples (Borawski, Levers-Landers, Lovegreen, & Trapl, 2003; Huebner & Howell, 2003), less parental monitoring marginally predicted greater future HIV risk. However, contrary to prior findings (e.g., Dittus et al., 2004) positive parenting was related to increased HIV risk.

It is possible that mothers who are positive parents are just generally more positive and accepting, even of behaviors that may lead to eventual HIV risk (e.g., sexual exploration). This might especially be true if their adolescents are reporting unprotected sex with only one main partner (e.g., a steady boy or girlfriend), which is seemingly "safer" behavior. A more positive, reinforcing parent may also provide license for the adolescent to take risks via being generally more permissive, perhaps to the extent of acting more like a peer than a parent.

Another unexpected finding was that maternal psychological control was related to less HIV risk. Only five prior studies have examined psychological control within samples including some proportion of African American families (Barber & Harmon, 2002). While such studies have suggested effects of psychological control are similar to Caucasian families, it is possible that psychological control could have different effects on adolescent risk among low-income, urban African American families versus middle-income Caucasian families. Previous data suggest that parental "over"-involvement or authoritarianism might be more beneficial than authoritative parenting for low income ethnic minority youth (Baumrind, 1972; Deater-Deckard, Dodge, Bates & Petit, 1998) and that parenting needs to be examined in the context of these family's lives (Steinberg, Dornbusch, & Brown, 1992). This contrasts with the more typical perception that high control represents a negative "over"-involvement with the child (Baumrind, 1968). It is plausible that having a more psychologically controlling maternal caregiver helps rebut some of the environmental press toward problem behaviors in neighborhoods where problem behavior is more common or even quasi-normative. The parenting behavior that a child in a more organized, less stressful environment would view as intrusive may be experienced as protective in a more disorganized setting. Less psychological autonomy between mother and adolescent could also create a stronger parental psychological presence, reminding the adolescent more readily of how their mother might "blame" them if they were to get pregnant or get an STD. These interpretations are tentative, however, and warrant more in-depth study.

Parenting also had direct effects on adolescent mental health; positive parenting and parental monitoring during early adolescence led to less distress and conduct problems during late adolescence. This finding is consistent with data that suggest, among African American and other ethnic minority families, parental warmth, support and monitoring buffer against the development of child mental health difficulties (e.g., Pittman & Chase-Lansdale, 2001). Parental monitoring and positive parenting were also strongly associated, suggesting a protective effect on adolescent mental health for mothers who were more knowledgeable about their adolescents' whereabouts, peer group, and had stricter "house rules" (Ary et al., 1999a; Ary et al., 1999b; Herman et al., 1997). Maternal psychological control, however, was unrelated to late adolescent distress, conduct problems or any other parenting practice. These findings were inconsistent with previous findings that parental psychological control exacerbates the development of adolescent mental health problems (Barber & Harmon, 2002).

Study Limitations

The ability to test relatively complex models of adolescent mental health and HIV risk, incorporating measures from two time points, was severely limited by a small sample size. It is possible that a number of conceptually important associations could not be detected in these models, particularly once variables such as age or baseline mental health status were considered. When conducting longitudinal analyses, both subject attrition and varying incomplete measures across time points can account for large amounts of missing data. Fortunately, patterns of missing data in this study were not associated with baseline values of the key outcome measures.

While parent and adolescent reports of many study measures were available for analysis, the small sample dictated a path analysis approach, using only parent or adolescent measures. With a larger sample a more powerful latent variable modeling approach could be used to combine variance from both parent and adolescent reports. However, the correlations between the parent and adolescent measures were weak enough that it is not clear that an adequate measurement model could have been derived with these variables, even with a larger sample. Clearly more research is warranted to develop more valid ways of measuring parenting and mental health African American youth and families.

There is some question as to whether standard mental health measures in the field hold the same content and construct validity across different racial or ethnic groups (e.g., Lambert et al., 2002). Some adolescent mental health rates were comparable to previously published sample data on predominantly Caucasian families. However, other findings in this study question whether measures such as the CBCL are as valid for African American community samples. One strength of this study was it used an adolescent distress measure developed specifically to address mental health among low-income, ethnic minority youth living in communities with chronic environmental stressors. This study also used a more unique observational measure of parental psychological control. While it is beneficial to utilize multi-method measurement, the unexpected direction of the relationship between psychological control and HIV risk and the lack of findings between psychological control and adolescent mental health may have been due to measure limitations (i.e., the observational measure used in this study was more limited in scope than self-report measures used in prior studies, such as the CPRBI; Schaefer, 1965).

Future Directions

The findings of this study underscore the importance of focusing on improving maternal mental health and parenting early in the child's development, to protect youth from developing mental health difficulties and HIV infection. This study, one of the first to examine the longitudinal effects of early maternal parenting factors on adolescent mental health and HIV risk within an entirely low-income, urban African American sample, suggests more promising areas of future research. These findings call for further investigation on how to define "effective" parenting practices across diverse social and ethnic groups since what constitutes "best" parenting practices appears to be different for low-income, urban African American families than the more traditionally studied Caucasian families. The continued development and refinement of adolescent mental health assessment measures for African American youth is also a critical area for future research. Consistent with recent recommendations by Tinsley, Lees and Sumartojo (2004), designing successful family-based mental health and HIV prevention interventions requires a greater understanding of what constitutes protective parenting practices across various ethnic and social subgroups.

Some parents returned for Time 3 assessment without their adolescent and vice versa. These data were therefore not included because they did not represent a complete dyad, i.e., 188 dyads represent complete family assessments.

Controlling for baseline mental health in this model led to similar fit indices ($\chi^2 = 1.22$, $df = 6$, $p > .05$; RMSEA = .00; GFI = .997; NNFI = 1.00) and only a marginally higher AIC value (43.22 vs. 42.72). However, prior marginal associations between Time 2 parental monitoring and Time 3 conduct problems (Model $_{ignore}$ α = .11, p < .10 vs. Model $_{controlled}$ α = .02, ns.) and Time 3 conduct problems and Time 3 HIV risk (Model $_{ignore}$ α = .11, p < .10 vs. Model $_{controlled}$ α = .07, ns.) diminished. Thus, while not necessarily accounting for better overall model fit, controlling for baseline adolescent mental health demonstrates how relationships between certain earlier parenting practices, such as parental monitoring, and subsequent late adolescent HIV risk might shift as a function of controlling for prior adolescent mental health difficulties.

Given that directions between Time 3 cross-sectional outcomes could differ (e.g., HIV risk could lead to distress instead of distress leading to HIV risk) equivalent models were tested that altered the direction of the associations between Time 3 outcomes. Goodness-of-fit indices and AIC value of these models were the same as those of Model 8. Since Model 8 was originally hypothesized, we retained it as the best-fitting model of late adolescent HIV risk. However, these results suggest that statistically it is still equally plausible that HIV risk in adolescents induces, rather then results from, conduct problems or distress.

REFERENCES

Achenbach, T. M. (1991). *Manual for the Child Behavior Checklist and 1991 Profile.* Burlington, VT: University of Vermont, Department of Psychiatry.

Akaike, H. (1987). Factor analysis and AIC. *Psychometrika, 52,* 317-322.

Alan Guttmacher Institute. *Teen sex and pregnancy.* (1999). Retrieved 8/15/02, 2002, from *http://www.agi-usa.org/index.html*

Angold, A. (1988). Childhood and adolescent depression: II. Research in clinical populations. *British Journal of Psychiatry, 153,* 476-492.

Angold, A., Weissman, M.M., John, K. Merikangas, K.R. et al. (1987). Parent and child reports of depressive symptoms in children at low and high risk of depression. *Journal of Child Psychology & Psychiatry & Allied Disciplines, 28*(6), 901-915.

Ary, D. V., Duncan, T. E., Biglan, A., Metzler, C. W., Noell, J. W., & Smolkowski, K. (1999a). Development of adolescent problem behavior. *Journal of Abnormal Child Psychology, 27*(2), 141-150.

Ary, D. V., Duncan, T. E., Duncan, S. C., & Hops, H. (1999b). Adolescent problem behavior: The influence of parents and peers. *Behaviour Research & Therapy, 37*(3), 217-230.

Bachanas, P. J., Morris, M. K., Lewis-Gess, J. K., Sarett-Cuasay, E. J., Flores, A. L., Sirl, K. S. et al. (2002). Psychological adjustment, substance use, HIV knowledge, and risky sexual Behavior in at-risk minority females: Developmental differences during adolescence. *Journal of Pediatric Psychology, 27*(4), 373-384.

Barber, B. K. (1996). Parental psychological control: Revisiting a neglected construct. *Child Development, 67*(6), 3296-3319.

Barber, B. K., & Harmon, E. L. (2002). Violating the self: Parental psychological control, and youth problem behavior. In B. K. Barber (Ed.), *Intrusive parenting: How psychological control affects children and adolescents* (pp. 15-52). Washington DC: American Psychological Association.

Barber, B. K., Olsen, J. E., & Shagle, S. C. (1994). Associations between parental psychological and behavioral control and youth internalized and externalized behaviors. *Child Development, 65*(4), 1120-1136.

Baron, P., & MacGillivray, R. G. (1989). Depressive symptoms in adolescents as a function of perceived parental behavior. *Journal of Adolescent Research, 4*(1), 50-62.

Baumrind, D. (1968). Authoritarian vs. authoritative parental control. *Adolescence, 3*, 255-272.

Baumrind, D. (1972). An exploratory study of socialization effects on Black children: Some Black-White comparisons. *Child Development, 43*, 261-267.

Bean, R. A. (1998). *Academic grades, delinquency, and depression among ethnically diverse youth: The influences of parental connection, regulation, and psychological control.* Brigham Young U, US.

Bentler, P.M. (1990). Comparative fit indexes in structural models. *Psychological Bulletin, 107*, 238-246.

Bentler, P.M. & Bonett, D.G. (1980). Significant tests and goodness of fit in the analysis of covariance structures. *Psychological Bulletin, 88*, 588-606.

Black, M. M., Ricardo, I. B., & Stanton, B. (1997). Social and psychological factors associated with AIDS risk behaviors among low-income, urban, African American adolescents. *Journal of Research on Adolescence, 7*(2), 173-195.

Borawski, E. A., Levers-Landis, C. E., Lovegreen, L. D., & Trapl, E. S. (2003). Parental monitoring, negotiated unsupervised time, and parental trust: The role of perceived parenting practices in adolescent health risk behaviors. *Journal of Adolescent Health, 33*, 60-70.

Brooks, T. L., Harris, S. K., Thrall, J. S., & Woods, E. R. (2002). Association of adolescent risk behaviors with mental health symptoms in high school students. *Journal of Adolescent Health, 31*, 240-246.

Brooks-Gunn, J., & Furstenberg, F. F. (1989). Adolescent sexual behavior. *American Psychologist, 44*(2), 249-257.

Browne, M. W. & Cudeck, R. (1989). Single sample cross-validation indices for covariance structures. *Multivariate Behavioral Research, 24*(4), 445-455.

Brown, L.K, Danovsky, M.B., Lourie,K. J., DiClemente, R. J. & Ponton, L. (1997). Adolescents with psychiatric disorders and the risk of HIV. *Journal of the American Academy of Child & Adolescent Psychiatry, 36*(11), 1609-1617.

Capaldi, D. M., Stoolmiller, M., Clark, S., & Owen, L. D. (2002). Heterosexual risk behaviors in at-risk young men from early adolescence to young adulthood: Prevalence, prediction, and association with STD contraction. *Developmental Psychology, 38*(3), 394-406.

Centers for Disease Control. *Sexual Behavior and HIV risk among African American Adolescents.* (2002). Retrieved August 29, 2002, from *www.cdc.gov*

Cicchetti, D., & Toth, S. L. (1998). The development of depression in children and adolescents. *American Psychologist, 53*(2), 221-241.

Cohen, J. (1988). *Statistical power analysis for the behavioral sciences* (2nd ed.). New York: Academic Press.

Crosby, R. A., DiClemente, R. J., Wingood, G. M., Cobb, B. K., Harrington, K., Davies, S. L. et al. (2001). HIV/STD-protective benefits of living with mothers in perceived supportive families: A study of high-risk African American female teens. *Preventive Medicine, 33*(3), 175-178.

Cyranowski, J. M., Frank, E., Young, E., & Shear, K. (2000). Adolescent onset of the gender difference in lifetime rates of major depression: A theoretical model. *Archives of General Psychiatry, 57*(1), 21-27.

Deater-Deckard, K., Dodge, K. A., Bates, J. E., & Petit, G. S. (1998). Multiple risk factors in the development of externalizing behavior problems: Group and individual differences. *Development & Psychopathology, 10*(3), 469-493.

DiClemente, R.J., Wingood, G.M., Crosby, R.A., Sionean, C., Brown, L.K., Rothbaum, B. et al. (2001). A prospective study of psychological distress and sexual risk behavior among black adolescent females. *Pediatrics, 108*(5), e85.

Dittus, P., Miller, K. S., Kotchick, B. A., & Forehand, R. (2004). Why parents matter!: The conceptual basis for a community-based HIV prevention program for the parents of African American youth. *Journal of Child and Family Studies, 13*(1), 5-20.

East, P. L. (1996). The younger sisters of childbearing adolescents: Their attitudes, expectations, and behaviors. *Child Development, 67*(2), 267-282.

Eccles, J. S., Early, D., Frasier, K., Belansky, E., & McCarthy, K. (1997). The relation of connection, regulation, and support for autonomy to adolescents' functioning. *Journal of Adolescent Research, 12*(263-286).

Ensminger, M. E., (1990). Sexual activity and problem behaviors among black, urban adolescents. *Child Development, 61*, 2032-2046.

Fox, G. L., & Inazu, J. K. (1980). Patterns and outcomes of mother-daughter communication about sexuality. *Journal of Social Issues, 36*(1), 7-29.

Garrison, C. Z., Schluchter, M. D., Schoenbach, V. J., & Kaplan, B. K. (1989). Epidemiology of depressive symptoms in young adolescents. *Journal of the American Academy of Child and Adolescent Psychiatry, 28*, 343-351.

Gibbs, J. T. (1998). High-risk behaviors in African American youth: Conceptual and methodological issues in research. In *McLoyd, Vonnie C; Steinberg, Laurence. (1998). Studying minority adolescents: Conceptual, methodological, and theoretical issues* (pp. 55-86). Mahwah, NJ, US; Mahwah, NJ, US: Lawrence Erlbaum Associates, Inc., Publishers; Lawrence Erlbaum Associates, Inc., Publishers.

Gorman-Smith, D., Tolan, P. H., Zelli, A., & Huesmann, L. R. (1996). The relation of family functioning to violence among inner-city minority youths. *Journal of Family Psychology, 10*, 115-129.

Harrington, R., Rutter, M., & Fombonne, E. (1996). Developmental pathways in depression: Multiple meanings, antecedents, and endpoints. *Development & Psychopathology, 8*(4), 601-616.

Herman, M. R., Dornbusch, S. M., Herron, M. C., & Herting, J. R. (1997). The influence of family regulation, connection, and psychological autonomy on six measures of adolescent functioning. *Journal of Adolescent Research, 12*(1), 34-67.

Holmbeck, G. N., Shapera, W.E., & Hommeyer, J.S. (2002). Observed and perceived parenting behaviors and psychosocial adjustment in preadolescents with spina bifida. In B. K. Barber (Ed.), *Intrusive parenting: How psychological control affects children and adolescents* (pp. 191-234). Washington DC: American Psychological Association.

Huebner, A. J. & Howell, L. W. (2003). Examining the relationship between adolescent sexual risk-taking and perceptions of monitoring, communication, and parenting styles. *Journal of Adolescent Health, 33,* 71-78.

Jaccard, J., Dittus, P. J., & Gordon, V. V. (1996). Maternal correlates of adolescent sexual and contraceptive behavior. *Family Planning Perspectives, 28,* 159-165.

Jessor, R. (Ed.). (1998). *New perspectives on adolescent risk behavior.* New York, NY, US: Cambridge University Press. (1998). xii, 564 pp.

Jessor, R., & Jessor, S. (1977). *Problem behavior and psychosocial development: A longitudinal study of youth.* New York: Academic Press.

Jones, D.J., & Forehand, G. (2003). The stability of child problem behaviors: A longitudinal analysis of inner-city African American children. *Journal of Child and Family Studies, 12*(2), 215-227.

Jöreskog, K. G., & Sörbom, D. (1996a). *LISREL8: User's reference guide.* Chicago: Scientific Software International.

Jöreskog, K. G., & Sörbom, D. (1996b). *PRELIS2: User's reference guide.* Chicago: Scientific Software International.

Kilgore, K., Snyder, J., & Lentz, C. (2000). The contribution of parental discipline, parental monitoring, and school risk to early-onset conduct problems in African American boys and girls. *Developmental Psychology, 36*(6), 835-845.

Klebanov, P. K., Brooks-Gunn, J., & Duncan, G. J. (1994). Does neighborhood and family poverty affect mothers' parenting, mental health, and social support? *Journal of Marriage & the Family, 56*(2), 441-455.

Kline, R. B. (1998). *Principles and Practice of Structural Equation Modeling.* New York: Guilford Press.

Lambert, M. C., Rowan, G. T., Lyubansky, M., & Russ, C. M. (2002). Do problem of clinic-referred African American children overlap with the Child Behavior Checklist? *Journal of Child and Family Studies, 11*(3), 271-285.

Lamborn, S., Mounts, N., Steinberg, L., & Dornbusch, S. (1991). Patterns of competence and adjustment among adolescent from authoritative, authoritarian, indulgent, and neglectful homes. *Child Development, 62,* 1049-1065.

Lanctot, N., & Smith, C. A. (2001). Sexual activity, pregnancy, and deviance in a representative urban sample of African American girls. *Journal of Youth and Adolescence, 30*(3), 349-372.

Lauritsen, J. L. (1994). Explaining race and gender differences in adolescent sexual behavior. *Social Forces, 72*(3), 859-883.

Luster, T., & Small, S. A. (1994). Factors associated with sexual risk-taking behaviors among adolescents. *Journal of Marriage & the Family, 56*(3), 622-632.

Maggs, J.L. (1997). Alcohol use and binge drinking as goal-directed action during the transition to postsecondary education. In J. Schulenberg, J.L. Maggs, & K. Hurrelmann (Eds.), *Health risks and developmental transitions during adolescence* (pp. 345-371). New York, NY: Cambridge University Press.

Martinez, R., & Richters, J. (1993). The NIMH community violence project: II. Children's distress symptoms associated with violent exposure. *Psychiatry, 56,* 22-35.

McBride, C.K., Paikoff, R.L., & Holmbeck, G. N. (2003). Individual and familial influences on the onset of sexual intercourse among urban African American adolescents. *Journal of Consulting & Clinical Psychology, 71*(1), 159-167.

Metzler, C. W., Noell, J., Biglan, A., Ary, D., & Smolkowski, K. (1994). The social context for risky sexual behavior among adolescents. *Journal of Behavioral Medicine, 17*(4), 419-438.

Miller, Benson, & Galbraith. (2001). Family relationships and adolescent pregnancy. *Developmental Review, 21*, 1-38.

Miller, K. S., Forehand, R., & Kotchick, B. A. (1999). Adolescent sexual behavior in two ethnic minority samples: The role of family variables. *Journal of Marriage & the Family, 61*, 85-98.

Myers, M. A., & Sanders Thompson, V. L. (2000). The impact of violence exposure on African American youth in context. *Youth & Society, 32*(2), 253-267.

Nettles, S. M., & Pleck, J. H. (1994). Risk, resilience, and development: The multiple ecologies of black adolescents in the United States. In R. J. Haggerty, L. R. Sherrod, N. Garmezy & M. Rutter (Eds.), *Stress, risk, and resilience in children and adolescents: Processes, mechanisms, and interventions* (pp. 147-181). New York, NY: Cambridge Press.

Nolen-Hoeksema, S. (1994). An interactive model for the emergence of gender differences in depression in adolescence. *Journal of Research on Adolescence, 4*(4), 519-534.

Paikoff, R.L. (1990). Attitudes toward consequences of pregnancy in young women attending a family planning clinic. *Journal of Adolescent Research, 5*(4), 467-484.

Patterson, G. R., DeBaryshe, B. D., & Ramsey, E. (1989). A developmental perspective on antisocial behavior. *American Psychologist, 44*, 329-335.

Patterson, G. R., Reid, J. B., & Dishion, T. J. (1992). *Antisocial boys: A social interactional approach*. Eugene, OR: Castalia Publishing Company.

Perkins, D. F., Luster, T., Villaruel, F. A., & Small, S. (1998). An ecological risk-factor examination of adolescents' sexual activity in three ethnic groups. *Journal of Marriage and the Family, 60*, 660-673.

Petit, G. S., Laird, R. D., Dodge, K. A., Bates, J. E., & Criss, M. M. (2001). Antecedents and behavior-problem outcomes of parental monitoring and psychological control in early adolescence. *Child Development, 72*(2), 583-598.

Piccinino, L. J., & Mosher, W. D. (1998). Trends in contraceptive use in the United States:1982-1995. *Family Planning Perspectives, 30*(1), 4-10.

Pittman, L. D., & Chase-Lansdale, P. L. (2001). African American adolescent girls in impoverished communities: Parenting style and adolescent outcomes. *Journal of Research on Adolescence, 11*(2).

Raymond, M. R., & Roberts, D. M. (1987). A comparison of methods for treating incomplete data in selection research. *Educational and Psychological Measurement, 47*, 13-26.

Resnick, G., & Burt, M. R. (1996). Youth at risk: Definitions and implications for service delivery. *American Journal of Orthopsychiatry, 66*(2), 172-188.

Richters, J. E. & Martinez, P. (1993). The NIMH community violence project: I. Children as victims of and witnesses to violence. *Psychiatry, 56*(1), 7-21.

Rodgers, K. B. (1999). Parenting processes related to sexual risk-taking behaviors of adolescent males and females. *Journal of Marriage & the Family, 61*(1), 99-109.

Rotheram-Borus, M. J., Murphy, Reid, & Coleman. (1996). Sexual abuse history and associated multiple risk behavior in adolescent runaways. *American Journal of Orthopsychiatry, 66*(3), 390-400.

Rotheram-Borus, M. J., Murphy, D. A., Coleman, C. L., Kennedy, M., Reid, H. M., Cline, T. R. et al. (1997). Risk acts, health care, and medical adherence among HIV+ youths in care over time. *AIDS & Behavior, 1*(1), 43-52.

Sagrestano, L., Paikoff, R. L., Holmbeck, G. N., & Fendrich, M. (2003). A longitudinal examination of familial risk factors for depression among inner-city African American adolescents. *Journal of Family Psychology, 17*(1), 108-120.

Samaan, R. A. (1998). The influences of race, ethnicity, and poverty on the mental health of children. *Journal of Health Care for the Poor & Underserved, 11*(1), 100-110.

Schaefer, E. S. (1965). Children's reports of parental behavior: An inventory. *Child Development, 36*, 413-424.

Schoenbach, V. J., Kaplan, B. H., Grimson, R. C., & Wagner, E. H. (1982). Use of a symptom scale to study the prevalence of a depressive syndrome in young adolescents. *American Journal of Epidemiology, 116*, 791-800.

Schraedley, P. K., Gotlib, I. H., & Hayward, C. (1999). Gender differences in correlates of depressive symptoms in adolescents. *Journal of Adolescent Health, 25*(2), 98-108.

Shaffer, A., Forehand, R., Kotchick, B. A., & the Family Health Project Research Group (2002). A longitudinal examination of correlates of depressive symptoms among inner-city African American children and adolescents. *Journal of Child and Family Studies, 11*(2), 151-164.

Siegel, J. M., Aneshensel, C. S., Taub, B., Cantwell, D. P., & Driscoll, A. K. (1998). Adolescent depressed mood in a multiethnic sample. *Journal of Youth & Adolescence, 27*(4), 413-427.

Singh, S., & Darroch, J. E. (1999). Trends in Sexual Activity Among Adolescent American Women:1982-1995. *Family Planning Perspectives, 31*(5), 212-219.

Smith, C. A. (1997). Factors associated with early sexual activity among urban adolescents. *Social Work, 42*(4), 334-346.

Stattin, H. & Kerr, M. (2000). Parental monitoring: A reinterpretation. *Child Development, 71*(4), 1072-1085.

Steiger, J. H. (1991). Structural model evaluation and modification: An interval estimation approach. *Multivariate Behavioral Research, 25*(2), 173-180.

Steinberg, L. (1990). Autonomy, conflict, and harmony in the family relationship. In S. S. Feldman & G. R. Elliott (Eds.), *At the threshold: The developing adolescent* (pp. 255-276). Cambridge, MA: Harvard University Press.

Steinberg, L., Dornbusch, S. M., & Brown, B. (1992). Ethnic differences in adolescent achievement: An ecological perspective. *American Psychologist, 47*(6), 723-729.

Stouthamer-Loeber, M., & Loeber, R. (1986). Boys who lie. *Journal of Abnormal Child Psychology, 14*(4), 551-564.

Teplin, L.A., Abram, K. M., McClelland, G. M., Dulcan, M. K., & Mericle, A. A. (2002). Psychiatric disorders in youth in juvenile detention. *Archives of General Psychiatry, 59*(12), 1133-1143.

Tinsley, B. J., Lees, N. B., & Sumartojo, E. (2004). Child and adolescent HIV risk: Familial and cultural perspectives. *Journal of Family Psychology, 18*(1), 208-224.
Valla, J.P., Bergeron, L., Berube, H., Gaudet, N. et al. (1994). A structured pictorial questionnaire to assess DSM-III–R-based diagnoses in children (6-11 years): Development, validity, and reliability. *Journal of Abnormal Child Psychology, 22*(4), 403-423.
Ward, T. J., & Clark, H. T. (1991). A reexamination of public-versus private school achievement: The case for missing data. *Journal for Educational Research, 84,* 153-163.
Weis, R. (2002). Parenting dimensionality and typology in a disadvantaged, African American sample: A cultural variance perspective. *Journal of Black Psychology, 28*(2).
Wellings, K., & Mitchell, K. (1998). Risks associated with early sexual activity and fertility. In J.Coleman & D. Roker (Eds.), *Teenage sexuality: health, risk and education.* Amsterdam, The Netherlands: Harwood Academic.
Whitbeck, L. B., Conger, R. D., & Kao, M. (1993). The influence of parental support, depressed affect, and peers on the sexual behaviors of adolescent girls. *Journal of Family Issues, 14*(2), 261-278.
Whitbeck, L. B., Hoyt, D. R., Miller, M., & Kao, M. (1992). Parental support, depressed affect, and sexual experience among adolescents. *Youth & Society, 24*(2), 166-177.
Youth Risk Behavior Surveillance Report. (2001). Retrieved August 29, 2002, from www.cdc.gov

doi:10.1300/J200v05n01_02

Individual Growth Curves of Frequency of Sexual Intercourse Among Urban, Adolescent, African American Youth: Results from the CHAMP Basic Study

Christian DeLucia
Roberta L. Paikoff
Grayson N. Holmbeck

SUMMARY. In the current study we examined individual growth curves of frequency of sexual intercourse among a sample of urban, low-income, African American youth at increased risk for subsequent HIV/AIDS exposure. Three waves of longitudinal data from the Collaborative HIV-Prevention Adolescent Mental Health (CHAMP) project were utilized. Participant ages ranged from 9 to 12 years ($M = 11$ years) at the first interview wave and from 15 to 19 years ($M = 18$ years) at the final interview wave. As such, we were able to map out true develop-

---

Christian DeLucia, PhD, and Roberta L. Paikoff, PhD, are affiliated with the University of Illinois at Chicago. Grayson N. Holmbeck, PhD, is affiliated with Loyola University of Chicago.

Without the contributions of CHAMP Collaborative Board members and participants, this work would not have been possible.

Funding from the National Institute of Mental Health (R01 MH 50423-08) is gratefully acknowledged.

[Haworth co-indexing entry note]: "Individual Growth Curves of Frequency of Sexual Intercourse Among Urban, Adolescent, African American Youth: Results from the CHAMP Basic Study." DeLucia, Christian, Roberta L. Paikoff, and Grayson N. Holmbeck. Co-published simultaneously in *Social Work in Mental Health* (The Haworth Press, Inc.) Vol. 5, No. 1/2, 2007, pp. 59-80; and: *Community Collaborative Partnerships: The Foundation for HIV Prevention Research Efforts* (ed: Mary M. McKay, and Roberta L. Paikoff) The Haworth Press, Inc., 2007, pp. 59-80. Single or multiple copies of this article are available for a fee from The Haworth Document Delivery Service [1-800-HAWORTH, 9:00 a.m. - 5:00 p.m. (EST). E-mail address: docdelivery@haworthpress.com].

mental trajectories of sexual intercourse over a 10-year period of adolescence (spanning ages 9 to 19 years). Results indicate that the average study participant was sexually abstinent (in terms of intercourse) during the pre-teen years, reported a single episode of sexual intercourse between ages 14 and 15, and by age 19, reported between 3 and 10 episodes of sexual intercourse. Significant variability in the acceleration of growth rates (as captured by a quadratic random effect) was observed, suggesting that some youth accelerated more rapidly (in their sexual intercourse histories) than did others. Participant gender predicted trajectory starting points; boys reported higher rates of sexual intercourse at age 12. Frequency of baseline exposure to sexual possibility situations (i.e., being in mixed-sex company in a private place in the absence of adult supervision) predicted growth curve acceleration, suggesting pre-teens with more exposure to sexual possibility situations accelerated more rapidly in their rates of sexual intercourse over time. Developmental implications of these data are discussed. doi:10.1300/J200v05n01_03

[Article copies available for a fee from The Haworth Document Delivery Service: 1-800-HAWORTH. E-mail address: <docdelivery@haworthpress.com> Website: <http:// www.HaworthPress.com> © *2007 by The Haworth Press, Inc. All rights reserved.]*

KEYWORDS. Developmental trajectories of sexual intercourse, exposure to sexual possibility situations, HIV/AIDS exposure, growth curves of sexual intercourse

Strands of etiological theory on adolescent sexual behavior can be woven into a biopsychosocial fabric of risk factors. In their review of the literature on adolescent sexuality, Brooks-Gunn and Furstenberg (1989) describe a number of putative causal pathways to early sexual debut that involve the interplay of biological, psychological, and social processes. For example, hormonal changes brought about by pubertal development can lead to striking physical changes in young adolescent girls, which in turn elicit attention from older adolescent boys, providing access to an older peer group with norms supportive of sexual intercourse. In the hypothesized causal chan, distal biological variables (e.g., hormonal changes) activate a chain of events that eventually give rise to more proximal contextual factors (e.g., a sexually experienced peer group) conducive to early sexual debut.

Although the social science literature is replete with studies of adolescent sexual behavior, our current knowledge is still limited in important ways (Brooks-Gunn & Furstenberg, 1989; Brooks-Gunn & Paikoff, 1997). This limited knowledge base results partly from the young stage of scientific inquiry in this area and partly from the paucity of investigations with a true developmental focus (Brooks-Gunn & Furstenberg, 1989; CDC, 2000). From a public health perspective, the need to better understand the development of emerging sexual behavior during adolescence has never been more pressing than it is today. Recent estimates suggest that at least half of all new HIV cases in the United States are reported among individuals 25 years of age or younger, the majority of whom were infected sexually during adolescence (Rosenberg, Biggar, & Goederth, 1994) (as cited at http://www.cdc.gov/hiv/pubs/facts/youth.htm).

The current study hopes to fill an important gap in the extant literature by mapping out true developmental trajectories of frequency of sexual intercourse during the preteen and teenage years–i.e., the period of development during which the majority of America's youth initiate sexual intercourse (CDC, 2004). We use individual growth curve methodology to describe change over time in frequency of sexual intercourse among a sample of African American youth at high risk for subsequent HIV/AIDS exposure. This is the first in a series of studies that will allow us to better understand: (a) the developmental course of sexual behavior during adolescence among urban, low income, African American youth, (b) the role of various individual- and family-level processes in shaping this course, and (c) the possible effects of sexual development on subsequent life events.

SEXUAL BEHAVIOR AND RATES OF HIV/AIDS AMONG AFRICAN AMERICANS

Rates of sexual behavior during adolescence and HIV/AIDS during adolescence and young adulthood are disproportionately high among individuals of African American ethnicity. Although it is not well understood why African American children tend to initiate sexual intercourse earlier than do their Caucasian contemporaries, theorizing about possible mechanisms has often centered on biological factors (e.g., on average, African American children experience puberty at earlier ages), familial/social factors (e.g., a disproportionate share of African American children are raised in single-parent, female-headed households, placing greater demands on parental supervision), and broader contextual factors (e.g., a disproportionate share of African American children live in densely populated housing units, which might raise risk for observing sexual acts at younger ages). Moreover, the poor, urban neighborhoods in which African American children disproportionately reside are characterized by high concentrations of individuals living with HIV/AIDS (Stanton et al., 1996), increasing the cumulative probability of exposure to an infected sex partner (Brunswick & Flory, 1998).

When compared with youth of other ethnicities, African American adolescents tend to report higher rates of sexual behaviors. For example, recent national data presented in the Youth Risk Behavior Surveillance report (CDC, 2004) suggest that among ninth through twelfth grade American youth, African American adolescents report the highest rates of sexual intercourse (67% versus 51% among Hispanic and 42% among White youth), the highest rates of having had experienced sex prior to age 13 (19% versus 8% among Hispanic and 4% among White youth), and the highest rates of exposure to four or more sexual partners (29% versus 16% among Hispanic and 11% among White youth).

African American adolescents and adults living in the United States also report the highest rates of HIV/AIDS (see, http://www.cdc. gov/hiv/pubs/Facts/afam.htm). For example, for the period between 1999 and 2002, among women diagnosed with HIV/ AIDS, 72% were Black, 18% were White, 9% were Hispanic, and 1% were classified as Other. Among men diagnosed with HIV/AIDS, 49% were Black, 37% were white, 13% were Hispanic, and 1% were classified as Other. It is worth noting that these rates of HIV/AIDS among African American individuals are alarmingly high, given that African American persons account for 12.3% of the United States population (based on the 2000 Census, as cited at the above Web link).

STUDIES OF SEXUAL BEHAVIOR
AMONG AFRICAN AMERICAN YOUTH

Studies of sexual behavior among African American adolescents can inform preventive interventions designed to reduce risk of eventual exposure to HIV/AIDS among African American youth (Paikoff, Parfenoff, Williams, & McCormick, 1997). This approach is consistent with the more general "Science of Prevention" framework that has been espoused at the National level (Coie et al., 1993). At present, studies that contribute to our understanding of sexual behaviors among African American youth can be generally classified into two broad categories. The first class of studies examines predictors of actual sexual debut or some possible developmental precursor (for example, see Costa, Jessor, Donovan, & Fortenberry, 1995; Lammers, Ireland, Resnick, & Blum, 2000; McBride, Paikoff, & Holmbeck, 2003; Paikoff, 1995; Paikoff et al., 1997; Rostosky, Regnerus, & Wright, 2003). The second class of studies examines the co-occurrence of sexual behavior and other possible youth "problem" behaviors (e.g., substance use and externalizing problems, see Ensminger, 1990; Li et al., 2001; Stanton et al., 1993; Wills, Gibbons, Gerrard, Murry, & Brody, 2003). Some studies have examined these issues simultaneously within a single study (for examples, see Costa et al., 1995; Wills et al., 2003). Although these studies add to our knowledge of sexual development among African American youth, many share a common limitation in that they provide snapshots of a developmental phenomenon that would be much better captured by a moving picture.

Prior research. For example, using two waves of national data (from the ADD Health survey) collected from nearly 3700 adolescents from ethnically diverse backgrounds, Rostosky et al. (2003) found that for both male and female adolescents, age and number of romantic partners were associated with an increased probability of debut, while negative sex beliefs were associated with a decreased probability of debut. For female adolescents, being African American (as opposed to Caucasian), having lower levels of religiosity, and having positive sex beliefs were associated with an increased risk of debut while having more educated mothers was associated with a decreased risk of debut. For males, higher levels of religiosity and taking a virginity pledge interacted with race such that these factors were associated with an increased risk of debut among African American (as opposed to Caucasian) adolescents. Costa, Jessor, and Fortenberry (1995) found that unconventionality (indicated by lower academic expectations, greater reliance on peers, and involvement in other problem behaviors) was a prospective predictor of earlier sexual debut among Hispanic and Caucasian adolescents, but not among African American adolescents. Our own data, drawn from a sample of low-income, African American youth growing up on Chicago's South Side, suggest that familial and individual factors interact in predicting sexual debut among adolescents who were on average 13 years of age (McBride et al., 2003). For example, among those families experiencing increases in observed family conflict during the transition to adolescence, pubertal development was associated with increased rates of sexual debut; whereas for families experiencing decreases in observed family conflict, pubertal development was unrelated to sexual debut.

Other authors have examined patterns of co-occurrences among sexual behavior and other possible youth problem behaviors (e.g., substance use, externalizing problems). For example, in a model examining predictors of risky sexual behavior (ranging from low-risk abstinent youth to high risk youth who reported engaging in sex without condom use and also reported having multiple sexual partners), Li et al. (2001) observed that youth who engaged in both sex and substance use behaviors reported higher rates of risky sex than did youth who engaged in sex-only behavior (although differences between groups might have resulted from factors responsible for selection into the combined sex and substance use group–e.g., sensation seeking). Ensminger (1990) found that the co-occurrence of sex and other problem behaviors might have different meanings for male and female adolescents. Among African American males, "sex-only" and "no-problem" youth were nearly indistinguishable on a number of risk indicators (some of which were measured years earlier), while both groups were reliably differentiated from a "multiple problem" group. For females, however, both the sex-only and the multi-problem youth were reliably differentiated from the no-problem youth (suggesting perhaps that sex is more of a "problem" behavior for females than for males).

Main objective of current study. Although these studies have contributed to our knowledge in meaningful ways, they generally lack the requisite developmental focus needed to better capture growth over time in sexual intercourse during adolescence. As such, basic developmental questions remain unanswered. For example, once sexual intercourse is initiated among African American youth, what do their intercourse histories look like over the next several years? Do they increase in a relatively stable manner over adolescence? Do some adolescents increase more rapidly in their frequency of sexual intercourse than do other adolescents? Are increases in frequency of sexual intercourse accompanied by concomitant increases in number of sexual partners (suggesting a higher-risk trajectory)?

The main objective of the current study is to provide a basic description of change over time in the frequency of sexual intercourse among an urban, low-income, African American sample of children growing up on Chicago's South Side in the 1990s. We will also discuss some real-world implications of these basic trajectories of sexual intercourse, and show how subsequent (more complicated) analyses could be undertaken as a means of providing answers to some of the interesting developmental questions posed above.

METHOD

This research is based on data from the Collaborative HIV-Prevention Adolescent Mental Health Project (CHAMP), a longitudinal study designed to examine family and mental health factors for adolescent HIV risk among urban, low-income, African American families with adolescent children (for a more elaborate discussion of the CHAMP project, see Madison, McKay, Paikoff, & Bell, 2000; Paikoff et al., 1997).

Sample

The CHAMP study involved 313 African American families who were living on Chicago's South Side in 1994, at the study's inception (i.e., baseline). The majority of the children in the study were in the fourth and fifth grades at baseline, although ages ranged from 9 to 12 years ($M = 11, SD = .70$). The overwhelming majority of these children (between 95% and 98%) contributed data to the current study. As such, comparisons between those individuals included and excluded in the current study were not warranted. The majority of the sample was low-income (e.g., 64% had total incomes under $10,000) and unemployed (63% of primary caregivers had not worked in the previous year). Approximately half of the primary caregivers had not completed high school (53%).

Recruitment

Families were recruited from six elementary schools situated in disadvantaged, inner-city neighborhoods. After agreement was received from local school councils and officials to recruit participants for CHAMP in the schools, parents of all 4th and 5th graders were sent flyers ($N = 740$). The flyers described CHAMP and included a form for parents to return, indicating if they wished to be contacted regarding participation in the project. All children, including those whose parents did not want to be contacted about CHAMP, were provided a small prize for returning the forms (a total of 527 flyers were returned). Parents who expressed interest in being contacted ($N = 455$) were either called or visited so that more information about CHAMP could be provided to them. If they wanted to participate after learning more about the project, appointments were made for them to be interviewed. In addition to those families who responded favorably to the flyer, a number of families that did not initially express interest in participating were included either because they later volunteered to participate or were recruited by community consultants to the project. In the final analysis, 238 of the 455 families who said "yes" to the flyer participated (comprising 76% of the final sample), 11 of the 72 families who initially said "no" to the flyer participated (4% of the final sample), and 64 of the 213 families (20% of the final sample) who did not respond to the flyer or did not receive a flyer participated.

Procedure

Four, one hour interviews were conducted for the project: a primary caregiver interview, a child interview, a videotaped family interaction session with both caregiver and child, and a separate school interview for the child. All interviews, other than the school interview, were conducted in a university setting, while the school interview was conducted in a private room in the child's school. Primary caregivers and children were interviewed privately in separate rooms in the initial interviews. These initial (i.e., university-based) interviews usually lasted three to four hours and parents were paid $95 for time and transportation expenses. School interviews, which assessed for the child's exposure to sexual possibility situations and the child's actual sexual behaviors (if appropriate), took place after the university interviews and were conducted by interviewers who were almost always of the same sex (95%) and usually (87%) of the same ethnicity as the child being interviewed. Throughout the interview, children were reminded that the interview was confidential and that they could choose not to respond to any question if it made them uncomfortable. This interview lasted between one and two hours and children were paid $25 for their participation.

Measures

Child self-report data were used in the current investigation. Child gender (0 = female, 1 = male) and child age (at each of the interview waves) were the sole demographic measures. Frequency of sexual intercourse (at each of the interview waves) was measured with the following item: "How many times have you had sexual intercourse?" Response options included the following: 0 (never), 1 (once), 2 (twice), 3 (between 3 and 10 times), and 4 (more than 10 times). Frequency of exposure to sexual possibility situations (i.e., being in mixed-sex company in a private place with no adult supervision) was measured with the following item: "How many time in the past year were you with members of the opposite sex in a private place with no adults around?"

Response options included the following: 0 (never), 1 (once), 2 (only 2 or 3 times), 3 (4 to 8 times), 4 (9 to 15 times), 5 (closer to every other week), 6 (closer to every week), 7 (more like 2 or 3 times a week), and 8 (almost every day). (Although this item was measured at all three waves, only the baseline item was used in the current set of analyses.)

RESULTS

Our primary objective was to describe change over time in the frequency of sexual intercourse over the pre-teen and teenage years. Although the current study involved three repeated assessments of study participants over a seven year period, age heterogeneity present in the sample at study inception (and study completion) allowed us to study change over time in frequency of sexual intercourse over a ten year developmental period spanning ages 9 to 19. At the first interview wave, participants ranged in age from 9 to 12 ($M = 11$). At the second interview wave, participants were on average two years older and their ages ranged from a 11 to 15. At the final interview wave, participant ages ranged from 15 to 19 ($M = 18$).

To assess change over time in frequency of sexual intercourse, we estimated individual growth curve models (Willet, 1997) using the Mixed Procedure in SAS statistical software (for a basic primer on SAS's Mixed Procedure, see Singer, 1998). These statistical models are also known as random effects regression models (Hedeker, Gibbons, & Flay, 1994) and as hierarchical linear models (Bryk & Raudenbush, 1987). Terminology varies by discipline (e.g., psychology versus education) and by software preferences. Statistically, the models are equivalent (given the utilization of the same estimation procedure) and quite flexible allowing the user to estimate change over time in a developmental phenomenon in the presence of missing data and unequal spacing between measurement occasions (Gibbons et al., 1993).

When examining change over time in a phenomenon, the researcher is faced with many preliminary decisions that should be made prior to model fitting (although in reality, model fitting is typically an iterative process). In the present case, our two main preliminary decisions were: (a) how should be we "scale" the time variable (i.e., participant age) and (b) what shape do the trajectories of frequency of sexual intercourse take on in the present study?

The scaling of the time variable has implications for the interpretation of various model parameters. In the present study, for example, the value of the intercept is interpreted as the average frequency of sexual intercourse when participant age equals zero. Because the average frequency of sexual intercourse at an individual's birth (i.e., when his or her age equals zero) is not substantively meaningful (and extends well beyond the range of data collected in the current study), we chose to rescale (i.e., center) participant age such that its zero point corresponded to an age of 12 (mathematically, this is accomplished by subtracting 12 from each individual's age variable). We chose age 12 for two reasons. First, during the study, we were able to observe 140 different individuals when they were 12-years-old, suggesting more than adequate data coverage at this age. Second, by centering age at 12, we were able to be consistent with the CDC's definition of early onset of sexual intercourse (i.e., sex before age 13). As such, higher intercept values in the present study are substantively meaningful and indicate high risk trajectory starting points.

As for the shape of the trajectories in the present study, a visual inspection of plots of change over time in frequency of sexual behavior suggested that trajectory shapes were quadratic (i.e., trends were generally characterized by one bend). In Figure 1, we present raw data trajectories of frequency of sexual intercourse for five individuals (with complete data) chosen at random from the data set. All five individuals reported no intercourse at waves one and two of data collection (i.e., had a value of zero on the response scale). At wave three, two individuals reported having sex 11 or more times (i.e., had a value of 4 on the response scale). (Trajectories are redundant and denoted by a thicker line.) Of the remaining three individuals, one remained abstinent at wave three (dotted line on the horizontal axis), one reported having had sex twice, and one reported having had sex between three and ten times. Although these plots provide useful information about the data, it is worth noting that they lack a true developmental focus because the trends are plotted as a function of assessment wave rather than by participant age. As such, two seemingly identical trajectories might have disparate developmental meanings (e.g., because one individual is much younger than the other when reporting a similar high level of sexual intercourse). Nonetheless, these trajectories were presented to show: (a) several patterns of change over time in frequency of intercourse; and (b) that different individuals tend to have different trajectory curves (e.g., some individuals accelerate more rapidly while others tend to accelerate more gradually).

Although we suspected that trajectories would be characterized by a quadratic component (in addition to a linear component), we began our

FIGURE 1. Raw Data Trajectories of Frequency of Sexual Intercourse

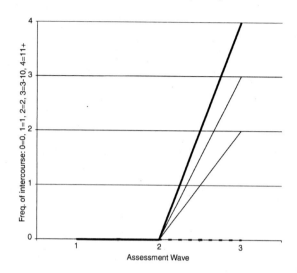

model estimation work with the simplest possible model (i.e., an unconditional means model) and sequentially estimated more complex models. This practice is often recommended by statisticians (e.g., Singer & Willet, 2003) and provides useful information for comparisons between competing models. Consistent with our suspicions, the final model retained for analyses in the present study included a fixed intercept, a fixed linear trend, and a quadratic trend, which included both fixed and random components. (More detailed information about model fitting–including deviance tests between nested models–is available from the authors.) The intercept was specified as a fixed effect because its variance was estimated at near zero in all models (i.e., the vast majority of children reported no sexual intercourse at 12-years-old). We chose to specify the linear component as a fixed effect while specifying the quadratic component as both a fixed and random effect to keep the number of random effects to a minimum (thus avoiding estimation problems), while allowing for individual variability in the rate of trajectory acceleration (which is captured by the quadratic random effect).

Given this specification of the unconditional growth model, the intercept fixed effect of .2271 corresponds to the average frequency of sexual intercourse at age 12–suggesting the average 12-year-old has had sex fewer than one time. The linear fixed effect of .1919 corresponds to the slope of the instantaneous growth rate at age 12. Because this coefficient is positive (i.e., greater than zero), it denotes an increasing linear trend of sexual intercourse among 12-year-olds. Because the intercept and linear trends are specified as fixed effects only, all individuals have the same values for these parameters. Because the quadratic component was specified as both a fixed and random effect, the quadratic fixed effect of .03698 corresponds to the average curvature (in this case, acceleration) of trajectories across study participants. This average acceleration suggests that trajectories are bending upward (i.e., toward higher rates of sexual intercourse). By specifying the quadratic effect as a random effect also, we allowed different individuals to exhibit different rates of trajectory curvature.

Several model-implied developmental trajectories of frequency of sexual intercourse are displayed in Figure 2. The thick line in the middle of the figure represents the average trajectory of frequency of sexual intercourse plotted as a function of the average ages of study participants at the three interview waves (i.e., ages 11, 13, and 18). (The thicker dashes that extend this trajectory represent an extrapolation of this average trajectory across the full range of ages observed in the current study.) This trajectory indicates that at age 11, the predicted value of frequency of intercourse for the average study participant was .07–suggesting that nearly all individuals are abstinent at age 11. By age 13, this value had increased to .46–suggesting that the average 13-year-old has had sex less than one time. By age 18, the value had increased still further to 2.71–suggesting that the average 18-year-old has had between 3 and 10 experiences with sexual intercourse (if 2.71 is rounded up to 3).

The five remaining trajectories depicted in Figure 2 are the model-implied trajectories for the individuals whose raw data were plotted in Figure 1. Four of the trajectories are easily seen, while the fifth is partly obscured by the average trajectory. Although these five trajectories have the same intercept and slope values (because these values are fixed for all individuals in the sample), they vary in their quadratic trends. For example, the thin line characterized by smaller dashes (displayed in the lower part of the figure) is the model-implied trajectory for study participant # 23. The empirical Bayes estimate for this individual's quadratic component is −.01917, suggesting a downward curvature in this individual's trajectory (as seen in Figure 2). The thin line characterized by larger dashes (displayed in the upper part of the figure) is the model-implied trajectory for study participant # 137. The empirical Bayes estimate for this individual's quadratic component is .08251, which is the largest quadratic coefficient depicted in the figure, suggesting the most dramatic upward curvature (or acceleration). All of

FIGURE 2. Model-Implied Trajectories of Frequency of Intercourse

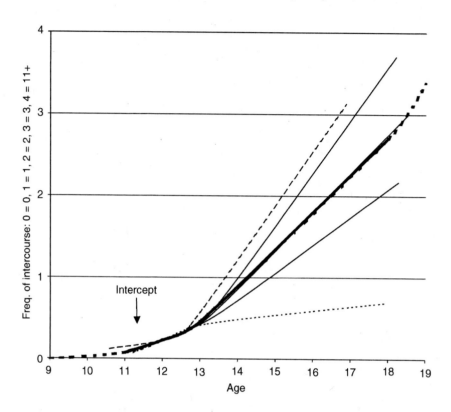

these model-implied trajectories pass through the same intercept (i.e., .2271 at age 12) and then begin to diverge, based on that individual's rate of acceleration or deceleration. For example, by approximately age 16, participant # 137 is reporting between 3 and 10 experiences with sexual intercourse while participant # 23 is reporting less than 1 sexual intercourse experience.

A final characteristic of these model-implied trajectories is worthy of mention. The correlation between the model-implied predicted scores and the observed (i.e., raw) data is .89, suggesting that over 75% of the variance in frequency of sexual intercourse was captured by the specified model (for a description of this and other means of assessing model fit, see chapter 4 in Singer & Willet, 2003). Practically speaking, this suggests that a large portion of the variance in frequency of sexual intercourse during adolescence is captured by the linear and quadratic effects of age (or the passage of time).

Although the model we have presented provides a basic descriptive account of growth in frequency of sexual intercourse among the participants in our study, it is possible to expand this model in many ways to capture more specific information about this developmental phenomenon, thus further augmenting our current understanding. For example, we could introduce a number of predictor variables in this model to see if they have an impact on the trajectory starting points (i.e., the trajectory intercept), or to see if they have an impact on the rate of change (e.g., the quadratic component). In this instance, some of the parameters from this initial model would become the outcomes of interest in other models (at least conceptually, although all effects could be derived from one large simultaneous model). It is also possible to take the random quadratic effect from this model and use it as a predictor of some other outcome of interest. For example, we could treat the empirical Bayes estimates of each individual's quadratic component as a new (predictor) variable in a subsequent model predicting high risk sexual behaviors (e.g., unprotected sex). Such an analysis would test whether individuals with higher rates of trajectory acceleration were more likely to report higher levels of unprotected sexual intercourse as well.

As an illustration of one of these more comprehensive models, we examined whether participant gender and frequency of exposure to sexual possible situations at study inception impacted trajectory starting points (i.e., intercepts) and/or trajectory rates of change (i.e., quadratic components). In this model we found that being male was associated with a .15 increase in trajectory starting points, $t(297) = 2.31$, $p < .05$. In other words, among 12 year-olds, boys, on average, reported higher rates of frequency of sexual intercourse than did girls. Although exposure to sexual possible situations was unrelated to trajectory starting points, it was a marginally significant predictor of trajectory rates of change, $t(419) = 1.77$, $p = .08$, suggesting that for every one unit increment in exposure to sexual possibility situations, quadratic components (i.e., rates of trajectory acceleration) increased by .00282. Although this predictor was only marginally significant, its inclusion in the model explained 5.7% of the variance in the quadratic random effect.

To place the results of this final model in context, three model-implied trajectories are presented in Figure 3. These are average trajectories in that frequency of sexual intercourse is plotted according to average age at the three study waves (i.e., 11, 13, and 18) and also according to overall model parameters (rather than by empirical Bayes estimates). The top (i.e., solid) line denotes the highest risk trajectory (based on the current model) and includes boys who reported the maximum value on frequency of exposure to sexual possibility situations at study inception. The bottom line (comprised of larger dashes) denotes the lowest risk trajectory and includes girls who reported no exposure to sexual possibility situations at study inception. The middle line (comprised of smaller dashes) denotes an intermediary risk trajectory and includes boys who reported no exposure to sexual possibility situations at study inception. A few observations are worthy of mention. At age 12 (the intercept in the current model), trajectories are differentiated as a function of participant gender and exposure to sexual possibility situations. The intercept difference between the bottom two lines is solely a function of gender (because all of these girls and boys reported no exposure to sexual possibility situations). The intercept difference between the top two lines is solely a function of exposure to sexual possibility situations (because both lines are plotted for boys) and is rather small (and nonsignificant). The bottom two trajectories are parallel. Practically speaking, these trajectories are quite similar and indicate that on average both boys and girls who were not exposed to sexual possibility situations at baseline were abstinent at age 11. By age 18, these boys and girls reported approximately two experiences with sexual intercourse. The top line is not parallel with the other two, because its rate of acceleration (i.e., quadratic component) is more dramatic. By age 15, these participants are reporting approximately two experiences with sexual intercourse while by age 18, these participants are reporting between 3 and 10 experiences with sexual intercourse.

DISCUSSION

The primary objective of the current study was to examine the emergence of sexual intercourse behaviors among an urban, low-income sample of African American youth at increased risk for subsequent HIV/AIDS exposure. Through the use of longitudinal data and individual growth curve methodology, we were able to estimate and describe

FIGURE 3. Gender as Predictor of Intercept and SPS as Predictor of Quadratic

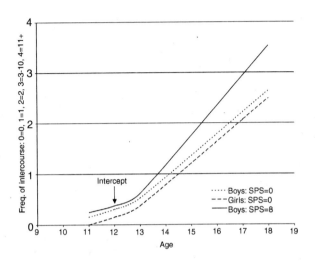

true developmental trajectories of frequency of sexual intercourse during the pre-teen and teenage years.

One of the strengths of individual growth curve methodology is that it allows the user to simultaneously estimate an average growth rate or trajectory for all study participants, while also examining whether variability in the growth rate exists (e.g., whether individuals are growing at different rates). Data from the current study suggest that the average study participant was sexually abstinent during the pre-teen years (at least in terms of intercourse), reported a single episode of sexual intercourse between ages 14 and 15, and by age 19, reported between 3 and 10 episodes of sexual intercourse. These data suggest that the *average* rate of growth in frequency of sexual intercourse during adolescence is relatively gradual. Data from the current study also suggest that meaningful variability exists in growth in sexual intercourse during adolescence. Some adolescents appear to remain abstinent throughout the teenage years, while others show a much more gradual increase in number of sexual episodes, and still others show a more dramatic increase, reporting greater than 10 episodes of sexual intercourse by the latter teenage years.

As a means of trying to explain some of this variability in the trajectories of sexual intercourse during adolescence, we introduced two covariates (i.e., participant gender and frequency of exposure to sexual possibility situations at baseline) as predictors of trajectory starting points and rates of change. Participant gender was a significant predictor of trajectory starting points, suggesting that boys reported higher initial levels of frequency of sexual intercourse at age 12. Frequency of exposure to sexual possibility situations at baseline was a significant predictor of rates of trajectory change, suggesting that more exposure to sexual possibility situations at baseline was associated with faster acceleration in sexual intercourse trajectories.

Practically speaking, the gender effect on trajectory starting points was relatively minor in that average boys and girls reported a similar level of sexual intercourse over the age range studied. The effect of baseline exposure to sexual possibility situations on rates of trajectory acceleration had the potential to have a more dramatic impact on trajectories of sexual intercourse. In other words, differences in rates of trajectory acceleration among those youth who reported no exposure to sexual possibility situations at baseline (i.e., reported a 0 on the scale) relative to youth who reported daily exposure to sexual possibility situations (i.e., reported an 8 on the scale) could be quite dramatic–suggesting differences between 2 and greater than 10 episodes of sexual intercourse by the latter teenage years.

To the extent that growth in frequency of sexual intercourse during adolescence is indicative of a high risk process (e.g., is associated with concomitant growth in number of sexual partners and/or unprotected sex), the combination of pre-teen peer group composition and decreased parental monitoring (as captured by the exposure to sexual possibility situations item) could place youngsters on risky sexual trajectories that eventually raise risk for subsequent HIV infection. In these instances, increments in exposure to sexual possibility situations (as pre-teens) would actually be associated with increments in exposure to subsequent HIV/AIDS. There is reason to suspect that exposure to multiple sexual partners is associated with increased risk of HIV infection among adult African Americans. For example, in a study assessing changing HIV infection rates (as measured by saliva antigen assay) among an adult sample of African Americans residing in metropolitan New York, exposure to multiple partners (over the past several years) was associated with a five-fold increase in the odds of HIV infection among both men and women (even after the effects of other powerful risk factors–e.g., intravenous drug use–were statistically controlled) (Brunswick & Flory, 1998). At present, however, the association between the individual growth curves of sexual intercourse discussed in the present investigation and more explicit high risk sexual behaviors await future investigation.

In subsequent studies we hope to build more comprehensive predictive models to explain additional variability in growth in sexual intercourse during adolescence. Hopefully, further understanding of the variability in the developmental course of sexual behaviors will allow us to create better (i.e., more ecologically valid) preventive interventions designed to reduce high risk sexual behaviors among urban, low-income, African American youth. A number of interesting possibilities remain, some of which are simple extensions of our present work (e.g., simply adding more theoretically meaningful predictors to our current model), while some of which would involve slightly different conceptualizations. For example, we might attempt to form several groups of relatively homogenous trajectories of sexual intercourse and then test the potency of several predictors in distinguishing among these trajectory classes. In other words, we might empirically identify three classes of trajectories: (a) the abstainers, (b) adolescents showing more gradual growth in sexual intercourse, and (c) adolescents showing more accelerated growth in sexual intercourse. Although trajectory identification is interesting and informative in its own right because it suggests several possible "patterns" of a developmental phenomenon, it is perhaps more interesting to examine the antecedents and possible developmental consequences of membership in the different trajectory classes.

Although the present study fills a gap in the extant literature by placing the study of sexual behavior during adolescence in an explicit developmental context (through the use of individual growth curve methodology), it is worth recognizing some of its limitations. First, although we examined multiple competing growth models before choosing our final model, all models were based on a normal-distribution theory of growth. Given that our outcome measure can also be conceptualized as an ordered categorical variable, it might have been useful to analyze these developmental trajectories under different distributional assumptions (Hedeker & Gibbons, 1996). Second, our statistical methods assume that missing data were missing at random, an assumption that is often violated in the behavioral sciences. Although we were able to retain the overwhelming majority of our original sample for the present analyses, some of these individuals had more missing data than did others (e.g., some were observed at one data point only). Given that the most problematic youth tend to have more missing data, it is possible that our methods actually underestimated the rate of growth in frequency of sexual intercourse in the current sample of youth. Third, although we examined growth in sexual intercourse over the develop- mental period spanning ages 9 to 19, our data coverage was sparse at certain ages (e.g., 15), suggesting that estimation of the rates of sexual intercourse might be less reliable at these ages. Finally, it is worth noting that our individual growth curves are based on a single interview item assessed at three different interview waves. Although some individual items capture a construct as well as a multiple-item scale, scales with fewer items tend to be less reliable, increasing the possible impact of measurement error on study results.

In summary then, in the current study we examined individual growth curves of frequency of sexual intercourse during adolescence among a sample of urban, low-income, African American youth at increased risk for subsequent HIV/AIDS exposure. Results indicated that the average study participant was sexually abstinent (in terms of intercourse) during the pre-teen years, reported a single episode of sexual intercourse between ages 14 and 15, and by age 19, reported between 3 and 10 episodes of sexual intercourse. Significant variability in the acceleration of growth rates (as captured by a quadratic random effect) was observed, suggesting that some youth accelerated more rapidly (in their sexual intercourse histories) than did others. Participant gender predicted trajectory starting points; boys reported higher rates of sexual intercourse at age 12. Frequency of baseline exposure to sexual possibility situations predicted growth curve acceleration, suggesting pre-teens with more exposure to sexual possibility situations accelerated more rapidly in their rates of sexual intercourse over time.

Implications for HIV Prevention Programming

To the extent that growth in frequency of sexual intercourse during adolescence is indicative of a high risk process (e.g., is associated with experience with multiple sexual partners and/or unprotected sexual experiences), the combination of pre-teen peer group composition and decreased parental monitoring could place youngsters on risky sexual trajectories that eventually raise risk for subsequent HIV/AIDS exposure. Numerous studies have shown that children's peer groups offer a significant source of support, comparison and pressure to engage in sexual risk taking and other types of behavior that can increase the risk of contracting HIV (Lewis & Lewis, 1984; Fuemmeler, Taylor, Metz, & Brown, 2002). Conversely, there is also evidence that family influences, particularly those related to parental supervision and monitoring of youth activities (Romer et al., 1994; Pick & Palos, 1995; Hutchinson &

Cooney, 1998) and family communication (Muller & Powers, 1990; Kafka & London, 1991; Pick & Palos, 1995; Jackson, Bijstra, & Oostra, 1998) play a critical role in delaying youth sexual involvement, reducing early adolescent sexual risk taking behaviors, and potentially reducing the risk of HIV transmission.

Therefore, HIV prevention programs may benefit from developing programs to increase parental monitoring and family communication as well as skills training for children around peer pressure situations. Given that the frequency of sexual intercourse and, in turn, HIV risk increases developmentally, prevention programs should develop interventions that are also developmentally driven. Parents should be instructed on strategies for monitoring their children as their children age and begin to demand greater independence. Likewise, as children gain greater independence from their parents they will need to develop strategies to handle their peers in the absence of adult supervision. These protective factors may aid in decreasing the alarming rate of HIV transmission among African American youth.

REFERENCES

Brooks-Gunn, J., & Furstenberg, F. F., Jr. (1989). Adolescent sexual behavior. *American Psychologist, 44*(2), 249-257.

Brooks-Gunn, J., & Paikoff, R. (1997). Sexuality and developmental transitions during adolescence. In J. Schulenberg & J. L. Maggs & K. Hurrelmann (Eds.), *Health risks and developmental transitions during adolescence* (pp. 190-219). New York: Cambridge University Press.

Brunswick, A. F., & Flory, M. J. (1998). Changing HIV infection rates and risk in an African American community cohort. *AIDS Care, 10*(3), 267-281.

Bryk, A. S., & Raudenbush, S. W. (1987). Application of hierarchical linear models to assessing change. *Psychological Bulletin, 101*(1), 147-158.

Centers for Disease Control and Prevention. Surveillance Summaries, May 21, 2004. MMWR 2004:53(No. SS-2)

Centers for Disease Control (2000). *Tracking the hidden epidemics: Trends in STD's in the United States, 2000.* Atlanta, Georgia: Center for Disease Control.

Coie, J. D., Watt, N. F., West, S. G., Hawkins, J. D., Asarnow, J. R., Markman, H. J., Ramey, S. L., Shure, M. B., & Long, B. (1993). The science of prevention: A conceptual framework and some directions for a national research program. *American Psychologist, 48*, 1013-1022.

Costa, F. M., Jessor, R., Donovan, J. E., & Fortenberry, J. D. (1995). Early initiation of sexual intercourse: The influence of psychosocial unconventionality. *Journal of Research on Adolescence, 5*, 93-121.

Ensminger, M. E. (1990). Sexual activity and problem behaviors among Black, urban adolescents. *Child Development, 61*(6), 2032-2046.

Fuemmeler, B.F., Taylor, L.A., Metz, A.E.J., & Brown, R.T. (2002). Risk-taking and smoking tendency among primarily African American school children: Moderating influences of peer susceptibility. *Journal of Clinical Psychology and Medical Settings, 9* (4), 323-330.

Gibbons, R. D., Hedeker, D., Elkin, I., Watermaux, C., Kraemer, H. C., Greenhouse, J. B., Shea, T., Imber, S. D., Sotsky, S. M., & Watkins, J. T. (1993). Some conceptual and statistical issues in analysis of longitudinal psychiatric data. *Archives of General Psychiatry, 50,* 739-750.

Hedeker, D., & Gibbons, R. D. (1996). MIXOR: A computer program for mixed-effects ordinal probit and logistic regression analysis. *Computer Methods and Program in Biomedicine, 49,* 157-176.

Hedeker, D., Gibbons, R. D., & Flay, B. R. (1994). Random effects regression models for clustered data with an example from smoking prevention research. *Journal of Consulting & Clinical Psychology, 62*(4), 757-765.

Hutchinson, M.K., & Cooney, T.M. (1998). Patterns of parent-teen sexual risk communication: Implications for intervention. *Family Relations, 47* (2), 185-194.

Jackson, S., Bijstra, J., & Oostra, L (1998). Adolescents' perceptions of communication with parents relative to specific aspects of relationships with parents and personal development. *Journal of Adolescence, 21,* 305-322.

Kafka, R.R., & London, P. (1991). Communication in relationships and adolescent substance use: the influence of parents and friends. *Adolescence, 26* (103), 587-598.

Lammers, C., Ireland, M., Resnick, M., & Blum, R. (2000). Influences on adolescents' decision to postpone onset of sexual intercourse: A survival analysis of virginity among youths aged 13 to 18 years. *Journal of Adolescent Health, 26*(1), 42-48.

Lewis, C.E., & Lewis, M.A. (1984). Peer pressure and risk-taking behaviors in children. *American Journal of Public Health, 74* (6), 172-194.

Li, X., Stanton, B., Cottrell, L., Burns, J., Pack, R., & Kaljee, L. (2001). Patterns of initiation of sex and drug-related activities among urban low-income African American adolescents. *Journal of Adolescent Health, 28*(1), 46-54.

Madison, S. M., McKay, M. M., Paikoff, R., & Bell, C. C. (2000). Basic research and community collaboration: Necessary ingredients for the development of a family-based HIV prevention program. *AIDS Education and Prevention, 12*(4), 281-298.

McBride, C. K., Paikoff, R. L., & Holmbeck, G. N. (2003). Individual and familial influences on the onset of sexual intercourse among urban African American adolescents. *Journal of Consulting & Clinical Psychology, 71*(1), 159-167.

Mueller, K.E., & Powers, W.G. (1990). Parent-child sexual discussion: perceived communication style and subsequent behavior. *Adolescence, XXV* (98), 469-482.

Paikoff, R. L. (1995). Early heterosexual debut: Situations of sexual possibility during the transition to adolescence. *American Journal of Orthopsychiatry, 65*(3), 389-401.

Paikoff, R. L., Parfenoff, S. H., Williams, S. A., & McCormick, A. (1997). Parenting, parent-child relationships, and sexual possibility situations among urban African American preadolescents: Preliminary findings and implications for HIV prevention. *Journal of Family Psychology, 11*(1), 11-22.

Pick, S., & Palos, P.A. (1995). Impact of the family on the sex lives of adolescents. *Adolescence, 30* (119), 667-675.

Romer, D., Black, M., Ricardo, I., Feigelman, S., Kalijee, L., Galbraith, J. et al. (1994). Social influences on the sexual behavior of youth at risk for HIV exposure. *American Journal of Public Health, 84* (6), 977-985.

Rosenberg, P. S., Biggar, R. J., & Goederth, J. J. (1994). Declining age at HIV infection in the United States. *New England Journal of Medicine, 330,* 789-790.

Rostosky, S. S., Regnerus, M. D., & Wright, M. L. C. (2003). Coital Debut: The Role of Religiosity and Sex Attitudes in the Add Health Survey. *Journal of Sex Research, 40*(4), 358-367.

Singer, J. D. (1998). Using SAS PROC MIXED to fit multilevel models, hierarchical models, and individual growth models. *Journal of Educational and Behavioral Statistics, 24*(4), 323-355.

Singer, J. D., & Willet, J. B. (2003). *Applied Longitudinal Data Analysis: Modeling Change and Event Occurrence.* NY, New York: Oxford University Press.

Stanton, B., Romer, D., Ricardo, I., Black, M., Feigelman, S., & Galbraith, J. (1993). Early initiation of sex and its lack of association with risk behaviors among adolescent African Americans. *Pediatrics, 92*(1), 13-19.

Stanton, B. F., Li, X., Black, M. M., Ricardo, I., Galbraith, J., Feigelman, S., & Kaljee, L. (1996). Longitudinal stability and predictability of sexual perceptions, intentions, and behaviors, among early adolescent African Americans. *Journal of Adolescent Health, 18,* 10-19.

Willet, J. B. (1997). Measuring change: What individual growth modeling buys you. In E. Arnsel & K. A. Reninger (Eds.), *Change and Development* (pp. 213-243). Mahwah, NJ: Erlbaum.

Wills, T. A., Gibbons, F. X., Gerrard, M., Murry, V. M., & Brody, G. H. (2003). Family communication and religiosity related to substance use and sexual behavior in early adolescence: A test for pathways through self-control and prototype perceptions. *Psychology of Addictive Behaviors, 17*(4), 312-323.

doi:10.1300/J200v05n01_03

Understanding African American Youth HIV Knowledge:
Exploring the Role of Racial Socialization and Family Communication About "Hard to Talk About Topics"

Mary M. McKay
William M. Bannon, Jr.
James Rodriguez
Kelly Taber Chasse

Mary M. McKay, PhD, is Professor of Social Work in Psychiatry & Community Medicine, Mount Sinai School of Medicine. William M. Bannon, Jr., MSW, and Kelly Taber Chasse, PhD, are affiliated with the Columbia University School of Social Work. James Rodriguez, PhD, is affiliated with the New York State Psychiatric Institute.

Address correspondence to: Mary M. McKay, PhD, Professor of Social Work in Psychiatry & Community Medicine, Mount Sinai School of Medicine, One Gustave L. Levy Lane, New York, NY 10029 (E-mail: mary.mckay@mssm.edu).

The contributions of the following people are especially recognized: co-investigators Carl C. Bell, MD, and Roberta Paikoff, PhD; staff members Sybil Madison-Boyd, PhD, Anthony McCormick, PhD, Sheila Parfenoff, PhD, Gloria Coleman, MA, and Ida Coleman; the CHAMP Collaborative Board members and participants.

Funding from the National Institutes of Mental Health (R01 MH 63662) is gratefully acknowledged. William Bannon is currently a pre-doctoral fellow at the Columbia University School of Social Work supported by a training grant from the National Institutes of Mental Health (5T32MH014623-24).

[Haworth co-indexing entry note]: "Understanding African American Youth HIV Knowledge: Exploring the Role of Racial Socialization and Family Communication About "Hard to Talk About Topics"." McKay et al. Co-published simultaneously in *Social Work in Mental Health* (The Haworth Press, Inc.) Vol. 5, No. 1/2, 2007, pp. 81-100; and: *Community Collaborative Partnerships: The Foundation for HIV Prevention Research Efforts* (ed: Mary M. McKay, and Roberta L. Paikoff) The Haworth Press, Inc., 2007, pp. 81-100. Single or multiple copies of this article are available for a fee from The Haworth Document Delivery Service [1-800-HAWORTH, 9:00 a.m. - 5:00 p.m. (EST). E-mail address: docdelivery@haworthpress.com].

SUMMARY. This article presents the results of a study examining correlates of urban African American youth HIV knowledge. The influence of family level factors (e.g., family communication, parental AIDS knowledge and myths regarding HIV transmission, along with family composition and family income) are examined. In addition, the current study explores the influence of racial socialization processes, specifically the influence of religious/spiritual coping, extended family caring, cultural pride reinforcement and racial awareness teaching (Stevenson, 1994; 1995; 1997) on youth HIV knowledge. Multivariate analyses revealed a significant association between youth HIV knowledge and being reared in a single parent home. Further, in every model, controlling for all types of racial socialization processes, family communication was significantly associated with youth HIV knowledge. Implications are drawn regarding the development of culturally and contextually specific HIV prevention programming for African American youth and their families. doi:10.1300/J200v05n01_04 *[Article copies available for a fee from The Haworth Document Delivery Service: 1-800-HAWORTH. E-mail address: <docdelivery@haworthpress.com> Website: <http://www.HaworthPress.com> © 2007 by The Haworth Press, Inc. All rights reserved.]*

KEYWORDS. Urban African American youth HIV knowledge, parental myths regarding HIV transmission, influence of racial socialization processes, influence of family level factors, culturally and contextually specific HIV prevention programs

As the AIDS epidemic enters its third decade, the demographic characteristics of those most at risk for infection has shifted considerably. In fact, our nation's youth have become significantly more vulnerable to HIV exposure. More specifically, African American adolescents are fast approaching one of the most at risk populations for HIV infection (Centers for Disease Control, 2001; 2000; 1998). African American youth residing in inner-city neighborhoods appear to be significantly impacted by accumulated contextual risk factors, including higher overall rates of neighborhood prevalence, along with poorer access to preventive health care, early detection and treatment services (Centers for Disease Control, 2001; Miller, Clark, & Moore, 1997; Rotheram-Borus, Wilson, 1987). Thus, HIV preventative interventions developed over the last decade have targeted urban, African American adolescents and their families (see Jemmott, Jemmott & Fong, 1997 for an exemplar; Centers for Disease Control, 2001).

In addition to HIV prevention programs targeting youth directly (Jemmott, Jemmott & Fong, 1997), a number of interventions have adopted family-based approaches (Boyd-Franklin, 1995; McKay, Baptiste et al., 2000; Madison, McKay et al., 2000; Pequegnat & Szapocznik, 2000). The premise behind these programs is that adult caregivers play important roles in providing health, sexuality and HIV prevention information to their children (McKay et al., 2000). In addition, specific parent level practices, such as supervision and monitoring of the child (Anderson, 1989; Clarke, 1983; Furstenburg, 1993; Garbarino, 1993; Jarret, 1995) and family level processes, such as family communication may have a protective influence on urban African American adolescents and, thereby, reduce sexual risk taking behavior (Baumesiter, Flores, & Marin, 1995; Fox & Inazu, 1980; Kotchick et al., 199; McNeeley et al., 2002; O'Sullivan et al., 1999; Pick & Palos, 1997).

As the number of family-based HIV prevention programs targeting minority youth and their families grow, findings from basic research studies involving participants representing these groups is needed to inform program development (Paikoff, 1997). More specifically, population specific information is needed in order to understand the influence of more traditionally studied families processes, such as family communication on African American youth HIV prevention outcomes. This is critical in light of the serious questions raised about applying findings from the existing family process literature to populations of color, including African American families. For example, there is significant evidence that parental communication about health behaviors and risk prevention can vary by race, ethnicity and community setting, particularly within inner-city contexts (Jaccard et al., 1998).

Therefore, knowledge is needed regarding processes that may be unique to African American families as adult caregivers attempt to protect children from contextual risks, including HIV exposure (Jarrett, 1990; 1995). Racial socialization, both the overt and subtle messages that African Americans parents convey to their children that reinforces cultural pride and attempts to prepare youth for navigating a world characterized by racism, is hypothesized to be critical in understanding the outcomes of African American youth. However, this construct has not yet been explored extensively within the HIV prevention literature.

Thus, the primary purpose of this article is to present the results of a study that examines correlates of urban African American youth HIV knowledge. The influence of typically studied family level factors (e.g., family communication, parental AIDS knowledge and myths regarding HIV transmission, along with family composition and family income) are examined. In addition, the current study focuses on the influence of racial socialization processes, specifically the influence of religious/spiritual coping, extended family caring, cultural pride reinforcement and racial awareness teaching (Stevenson, 1994; 1995; 1997) on youth HIV knowledge. Implications are drawn regarding the development of culturally and contextually specific HIV prevention programming for African American youth and their families.

URBAN YOUTH HIV RISK

Young urban African American adolescents living in poverty are at an increased risk for HIV infection (Centers for Disease Control, 1992; 2001). Inner-city African Americans represent 50% of all new AIDS cases diagnosed (Centers for Disease Control, 1992; 2001). African American females are disproportionately affected by the AIDS epidemic (Centers for Disease Control, 1992; 2001). This may be due to the unfortunate combination of an increased likelihood of residing in poor neighborhoods with higher rates of infection, elevated psychosocial stressors associated with poverty and urban living and limited access to health-oriented prevention and treatment resources (Paikoff, 1995; Rotheram- Borus et al., 1995; Wilson, 1987). Further, urban African American adolescents may be at heightened risk due in part to earlier onset of sexual intercourse (Brooks-Gunn & Paikoff, 1993; Santelli, Lindberg, Abma et al., 2000; Sonenstein, Pleck, & Klu, 1991; Sonenstein, Pleck, & Klu, 1989) and increased number of sexual partners (Ford, Sohn, & Lepkowski, 2002; Sonenstein, Pleck, & Klu, 1989). Given that early involvement takes place within urban communities evidencing rising HIV infection rates, the consequences for engaging in sexual risk taking are quite serious.

YOUTH HIV KNOWLEDGE AND MYTHS

Many HIV prevention efforts targeting youth at risk are based upon the premise that increases in knowledge about HIV infection, patterns of transmission and behaviors that increase risk of HIV exposure are necessary to protect youth (Lefkowitz et al., 1998; Segelman et al.,

1993). Further, there is evidence that youth do endorse a number of serious myths and negative attitudes related to HIV (Cole et al., 1996; DeLoye, Henggeler, & Daniels, 1993). For example, prior studies have suggested that children's attitudes toward people with HIV/AIDS, even those who are knowledgeable about the disease, are more negative than toward people with other serious illnesses (DeLoye, Henggeler, & Daniels, 1993). There is also evidence to suggest that children rate other children with AIDS as more responsible for the disease than children with diabetes, asthma or cystic fibrosis (Cole, Roberts, & McNeal, 1996). For African American youth, there has only been one study conducted with findings suggesting that African American youth were less willing to interact with a child infected with AIDS in comparison to white youth (Kistner et al., 1997).

TRANSMITTING ADULT HIV KNOWLEDGE TO YOUTH

Previous studies have argued for the importance of parent-child communication in relation to preventing youth HIV risk. For example, Sigelman, Derenowski, Mullaney and Siders (1993) found a strong positive relationships between parents' myths regarding the transmission of AIDS and their children's endorsement of those same myths in high communication families. However, in low communication families, a significant correspondence between the myths of parents and children was not found. In another study that examined the content, as well as the frequency of mother-child communication regarding AIDS, Lefkowitz and colleagues (1998) found that more frequent conversations about AIDS were related to less discrepancy in AIDS knowledge between mothers and their adolescents children. However, this study also revealed that about a third of the mothers never discussed either transmission or prevention of AIDS with their adolescents.

FAMILY COMMUNICATION
AND HIV RISK EXPOSURE PREVENTION

Adolescents who communicate with their parents about high-risk behavior have been found to more successfully negotiate peer pressure social situations and resist engaging in high-risk behavior than adolescents who do not communicate with their parents (Romer et al., 1994; Pick & Palos, 1995; Somers & Paulson, 2000). In addition, in families where adolescents report open and attentive communication with their parents, the adolescents reported more satisfaction with their families and less risk taking behavior than those teens who do not communicate with their parents (Kafka & London, 1991; Pick & Palos, 1995).

Prior research indicates that caregiver-child communication has also been found to be a protective factor against high-risk behavior (Kafka & London, 1991). For example, a study involving African American late adolescents conducted by Pretorius, Ferreira, and Edwards (1999) found that inadequate parent-child communication contributed to substance use and sexual risk taking, particularly teenage pregnancy and sexually transmitted disease.

FAMILY PROCESSES SPECIFIC TO AFRICAN AMERICANS: RACIAL SOCIALIZATION

Emerging research suggests that African American parents adjust their parenting practices to buffer youth from the impact of racism (Stevenson, 1994; 1995; 1997). This process of racial socialization is considered to be both reactive, in response to racism, and proactive, as an effort to promote positive identify development (Stevenson, 1995). Racial socialization as it relates to African Americans has been conceptualized by Stevenson (1994) to include values of African American cultural pride and religiosity. Religiosity encompasses religious beliefs and practices employed in coping approaches.

Findings from prior studies suggest that racially socializing youth is a routine part of the way African American parents choose to rear their children (Thorton, 1997; Thornton, Chatters, Taylor, & Allen, 1990). Yet, only a limited number of studies have examined parent reports of racial socialization practices in relation to youth outcomes. The majority of these have focused on the link between parental racial socialization practices and youth racial or ethnic attitudes, beliefs and awareness (Barnes, 1980; Branch & Newcombe, 1986; Johnson, 2001; Knight, Cota, Bernal, Garza, & Ocampo, 1993; Kofkin, Katz & Downey, 1995; Qunitana & Vera, 1999; Spencer, 1983). Only three prior studies have examined parental racial socialization practices relative to youth adjustment or mental health outcomes (Bowman & Howard, 1985; Marshall, 1995). However, findings are mixed regarding whether these practices are related to successful outcomes for youth, suggesting the need for additional study. No studies have examined racial socialization practices in relation to health-related and risk preventative knowledge of African American youth.

In sum, the current study examines the relative influence of traditionally studied family process characteristics, family communication, parental AIDS knowledge and myths regarding HIV transmission, along with family composition and family income, on understanding African American youth HIV knowledge. Further, the impact of racial socialization processes, specifically the influence of religious/spiritual coping, extended family caring, cultural pride reinforcement and racial awareness teaching (Stevenson, 1994; 1995; 1997) on youth HIV knowledge is also explored here. Thus, the current study will answer the following research question: Will the presence of racial socialization variables make a unique contribution to parent-child communication in explaining degrees of child HIV/AIDS knowledge?

METHODS

The current study is a secondary data analysis from baseline data collected as part of the KAARE (Knowledge about the African American Research Experience) and CHAMP (Chicago HIV prevention and Adolescent Mental Health Project) Family Program Study. The CHAMP Family Program is a family-based HIV prevention project targeting 4th and 5th grade African American, low-income youth and their families in a high HIV infection rate community. The sample drawn for the current study represents a random sample of youth and their families involved in the CHAMP Family Program that also were selected to participate in KAARE, (Knowledge about the African American Research Experience) described next ($n = 140$). All CHAMP Family program participants were chosen randomly from a roster of 550 youth and their families attending four inner-city public elementary schools. A 92% consent rate for inclusion in the random assignment process of the CHAMP Family Program study was obtained (see McKay, Baptiste, Coleman, Madison, Paikoff, & Scott, 2000, for details regarding the CHAMP Family Program study). Approximately 60% of the sample was girls, ages 9 to 11 years, and 40% were boys in the same age range. Almost 82% of parents reported a family income of less than $14,000. Three quarters of adult caregivers completed high school and 8% of parents had attended some college. Approximately 17% of the adult caregivers are between 25 and 29 years, indicating that they were teenagers at the time of the target child's birth.

KAARE supported additional data collection from a random sample of CHAMP participants. Thus, in the current study 140 African American families participated in this cross-sectional study. One hundred percent of caregivers and youth were African American. Ninety-two percent of adult caregivers were female. The typical caregiver was single (77%; $n = 77$), unemployed (58%; $n = 80$), and received public assistance (71%; $n = 99$) with the average annual family income reported between $5,000-$9,000. Eighty percent of caregivers ($n = 110$) had a high school/GED level of education, with 20% ($n = 28$) of caregivers having an education level beyond high school (i.e., trade school, community college, graduate school). Children ranged from 9-15 years ($M = 11.8$; $SD = 1.22$) of age. Sixty percent ($n = 70$) of youth were female.

Data Collection Procedures

Data for the current study was derived from baseline assessment information prior to the start of the family-based intervention and a second interview completed as part of the KAARE project. All information was obtained from parents and youth separately. Each child or adult participant completed paper-pencil instruments in small groups, 6 to 8 participants, with research staff reading each item aloud. Informed consent materials were distributed and completed prior to data collection. Institutional Review Board approval was obtained.

Measures

Independent Variables

Basic information was collected from adult caregivers concerning *child and family demographics characteristics* (e.g., age, gender, marital status, education and income levels).

Family communication was be measured using an adaptation of the FES/FAM designed for urban African American and Latino families (Tolan, Gorman-Smith, Huesmann, & Zelli, 1997). This is a 34-item measure normed on over 600 urban minority families. Statistically derived subscales to be used assess: family cohesion, beliefs about family, and family communication. Inter-item reliability on these subscales ranges from .74 (family communication) to .87 (beliefs about the family).

Parent knowledge of HIV/AIDS prevention was measured via the Beliefs About Preventing AIDS instrument (Koopman et al., 1990). This instrument contains 38-items that assess overall individual beliefs concerning activities that lead to HIV/AIDS infection that are measured along a 4-point Likert scale (*strongly agree* to *strongly disagree*). Items represent five domains: (1) self-efficacy (e.g., It would not be embarrassing to carry a condom with me); (2) peer support for safe sex acts (e.g., Most people probably practice unsafe sex); (3) self-control (e.g., I have no control over my sexual urges); (4) expectation to act to prevent pregnancy (e.g., In the future I plan to make sure we are using condoms); and (5) perceived threat (e.g., AIDS is the scariest disease I know). The child report has good internal consistency (alpha = .81) with higher scores representing a better knowledge of HIV/AIDS issues (possible range = 38-152).

Parent Cultural Beliefs About HIV/AIDS Myths were measured on the Cultural Beliefs About HIV/AIDS Test (Stevenson, 1995). This 8-item scale measures the level of belief in myths about the origin, spread, and contraction of HIV/AIDS. Two sample items from this scale are: (1) AIDS was started as a CIA government plot to kill Black and Hispanic people; and (2) There is a cure for AIDS, but it is only available to the rich. Items are measured along a 4-point Likert scale (*strongly disagree* to *strongly agree*) with higher scores representing a greater belief in HIV/AIDS related myths (possible range = 8-32; alpha = .64).

Parent reports of *racial socialization* were measured on The Scale of Racial Socialization for African American Adolescents (Stevenson, 1994). This instrument contains 45 items scored along a 4-point Likert scale (*strongly disagree* to *strongly agree*). This measure assesses the degree of adult caregiver acceptance of multiple racial socialization attitudes or race-related messages central to child rearing within the African American culture, subscales include: spirituality and religious coping (e.g., A belief in God can help a person deal with tough life struggles; possible range = 7-28, alpha = .71), extended family caring (e.g., Relatives can help Black parents raise their children; possible range = 9-36, alpha = .69), cultural pride reinforcement (e.g., Schools should be required to teach all children about Black history; possible range = 7-28, alpha = .71), and racism awareness teaching (e.g., A Black child or teenager will be harassed simply because she or he is Black; possible range = 6-24, alpha = .59). Higher scores represent a greater degree of racial socialization.

Outcome Variable

Child's knowledge of HIV/AIDS was measured via an adapted version of the Beliefs About Preventing AIDS instrument (Koopman et al., 1990). The original 38-item instrument, which was completed by adult caregivers, was reduced to a 14-item scale to facilitate completion by youth. Items were also answered on a 4-point Likert scale (*strongly agree* to *strongly disagree*) that represent identical domains of beliefs concerning HIV/AIDS prevention (i.e., self-efficacy, peer support for safe sex acts, self-control, expectation to act to prevent pregnancy, perceived threat). The child report has reliable internal consistency (alpha = .71) with higher scores representing a better knowledge of HIV/AIDS issues (possible range = 14-56).

Statistical Analysis

There were three steps involved in analysis of these data. First, we conducted a series of bivariate analyses to examine the association between youth HIV/AIDS knowledge and child, parent, and family demographic characteristics. Second, we examined the relationship between independent variables (demographic characteristics parental AIDS myths and family communication) and child knowledge about AIDS. Third, each racial socialization variable was separately entered into a multivariate model to examine how the relationships between the independent variables and the dependent variable changed in the presence of racial socialization. Finally, we conducted a series of post hoc analyses to examine possible interactions between independent variables.

Bivariate analysis revealed that the two variables, parent beliefs in cultural myths about AIDS and parent beliefs about preventing AIDS, were significantly correlated at a level that violated assumptions of multicollinearity, $r = (90) = -.64 \, p < .01$. As a result, the variable parent beliefs about preventing AIDS was excluded from further analysis. Checks for multicollinearity among remaining independent variables revealed no significant problems (Menard, 1995).

RESULTS

Description of Study Variables

Level of knowledge about preventing AIDS were fairly high for both children ($M = 26.5$; $SD = 4.74$; range = 11-32) and parents ($M = 134.5$; $SD = 10.0$; range = 38-152). On average, parent reported low levels of beliefs concerning cultural myths about AIDS ($M = 11.7$; $SD = 3.51$; range = 8-22) and a high degree of family communication about sensitive topics ($M = 21.7$; $SD = 4.38$; range = 12-28). In terms of racial socialization, parents endorsed using significant amounts of spiritual/religious coping ($M = 22.7$; $SD = 3.17$; range = 15-28), extended family caring ($M = 29.9$; $SD = 3.34$; range = 22-36), cultural pride reinforcement ($M = 23.0$; $SD = 2.70$; range = 17-28) and racial awareness teaching ($M = 22.7$; $SD = 4.13$; range = 12-30) within their families.

The results of bivariate analyses revealed that child knowledge about HIV did not differ by child gender, t (106) = $-.78$, p = .44, parent education level (greater than high school–yes/no), t (124) = -1.47, p = .14, if parents were employed (yes/no), t (122) = -1.23, p = .22, or if families received public assistance (yes/no), t (123) = -1.71, p = .09. However, bivariate analyses revealed that older children tended to have more accurate beliefs concerning knowledge about HIV, r (110) = .27, $p <$ .01. Furthermore, child knowledge about HIV was associated with single parent status with the mean score of two parent families (M = 28.4) being significantly higher than one parent families (M = 25.3), t (90) = -2.63, p < .01. Table 1 provides a summary of bivariate findings.

Multivariate Results

Table 2 summarizes the results of the OLS hierarchical linear regression with more traditionally examined independent variables, family income, family composition, parental AIDS cultural beliefs and family communication about sensitive topics entered into regression equations as independent variables first. Results from these analyses indicate that single parent status significantly contributed to explaining youth HIV knowledge with 14% of the variance in youth HIV knowledge explained, $R^2 = .14$, $F = 2.57$, $p < .05$.

In the second regression model (summarized in Table 3), when religious/spiritual coping was entered into the model, an additional 9% of the variance in youth HIV knowledge was explained, $R^2 = .23$, $F = 2.78$, $p < .05$. Statistical analysis indicated that the increment in R^2 was statistically significant ($p < .05$).

In the next regression model (Table 4), when extended family care was entered into the model, an additional 5% of the variance in youth HIV knowledge was explained, $R^2 = .19$, $F = 2.41$, $p < .05$. Statistical analysis indicated that the increment in R^2 was statistically significant ($p < .05$).

Table 5 summarizes the results when cultural pride reinforcement was added to the multiple regression model. An additional 5% of the variance in youth HIV knowledge was explained, $R^2 = .19$, $F = 2.45$, $p <$

TABLE 1. Interrcorrelations Between Subscales

	1	2	3	4	5	6	7	8	9
1. Child AIDS knowledge	--	-.14	.12	-.27*	.16	.13	-.08	-.12.	10
2. Parent AIDS knowledge		--	-.64**	-.06	-.14	.26*	.06	.09	.27*
3. Parent AIDS myth beliefs			--	.04	.18	.04	.12	.05	-.47**
4. Single parent status				--	-.02	-.20	-.11	.06	.09
5. Family communication					--	.28*	.05	.06	-.13
6. Spiritual/religious coping						--	.49**	.42**	-.23
7. Extended family caring							--	.62**	-.31**
8. Cultural pride reinforcement								--	-.19
9. Racial awareness teaching									--

*$p < .05$, **$p < .01$.

TABLE 2. OLS Linear Regression of Child HIV/AIDS Knowledge

Variable	B	SE B	β
Income	-.37	.44	-.11
Single parent status	-4.16	1.69	-.32*
Parent cultural beliefs about AIDS myths	.11	.18	.08
Family communication	.23	.14	.20

Note. For overall model, $R^2 = .14$, Adjusted $R^2 = .09$, df = 65, F = 2.57, $p < .05$. *$p < .05$

.05. Statistical analysis indicated that the increment in R^2 was statistically significant ($p < .05$).

Finally, in the last regression model (Table 6), when racial awareness teaching was added, an additional 14% of the variance in youth HIV knowledge was explained, $R^2 = .28$, $F = 2.61$, $p < .05$. Statistical analysis indicated that the increment in R^2 was statistically significant ($p < .05$).

Post hoc analysis did not reveal significant interactions between any of the racial socialization variables and family communication.

DISCUSSION

Findings from the current study revealed high HIV knowledge and relatively low levels of endorsement of HIV oriented myths for a sample of inner-city African American youth and their adult caregivers. Further, findings revealed that adult caregivers endorsed engaging in high levels of racial socialization of their children. Multivariate findings revealed that being reared in a single parent household was significantly

TABLE 3. OLS Linear Regression of Child HIV/AIDS Knowledge

Variable change	**B**	**SE B**	**β**	**R²**
Income	−.62	.50	−.18	.09*
Single parent status	−4.74	1.77	−.38**	
Parent cultural beliefs about AIDS myths	.06	.19	.05	
Family communication	.32	.16	.28*	
Religious/Spiritual Coping	.03	.21	.02	

Note. For overall model, R^2 = .23, Adjusted R^2 = .14, df = 53, F = 2.78, $p < .05$. *$p < .05$, ** $p < .01$.

TABLE 4. OLS Linear Regression of Child HIV/AIDS Knowledge

Variable change	**B**	**SE B**	**β**	**R²**
Income	−.15	.48	−.05	.05*
Single parent status	−4.02	1.73	−.34*	
Parent cultural beliefs about AIDS myths	.06	.18	.05	
Family communication	.30	.15	.27*	
Extended family caring	−.18	.17	−.14	

Note. For overall model, R^2 = .19, Adjusted R^2 = .11, df = 55, F = 2.41, $p < .05$. *$p < .05$.

TABLE 5. OLS Linear Regression of Child HIV/AIDS Knowledge

Variable change	**B**	**SE B**	**β**	**R²**
Income	−.37	.51	−.10	.05*
Single parent status	−4.67	1.92	−.34*	
Parent cultural beliefs about AIDS myths	.05	.19	.04	
Family communication	.32	.16	.27*	
Cultural Pride Reinforcement	−.18	.26	−.09	

Note. For overall model, R^2 = .19, Adjusted R^2 = .11, df = 57, F = 2.45, $p < .05$. *$p < .05$.

associated with youth HIV knowledge. Family communication about sensitive topics was only found to be significantly associated with youth HIV knowledge after controlling for multiple types of racial socialization processes. In fact, as much as 28% of the variance in youth HIV knowledge was explained when parental reports of racism awareness teaching were added to the regression model.

TABLE 6. OLS Linear Regression of Child HIV/AIDS Knowledge

Variable change	B	SE B	β	R^2
Income	.09	.76	.02	.14*
Single parent status	−4.28	2.45	−.33	
Parent cultural beliefs about AIDS myths	.39	.27	.25	
Family communication	.45	.21	.36*	
Racial awareness teaching	.07	.21	.06	

Note. For overall model, $R^2 = .28$, Adjusted $R^2 = .18$, df = 38, $F = 2.61$, $p < .05$, *$p < .05$.

Thus, it appears important that family communication around sensitive topics such as HIV and AIDS be reinforced in order to ensure adequate youth context. However, it also appears that the racially socializing context within which a child is reared plays an important role in understanding youth HIV knowledge. Further research efforts need to focus on the role, particularly the unique influences, that family processes unique to African American youth and their families play in explaining youth outcomes. This is a critical area of future investigation so that findings may be used to inform youth-oriented prevention and intervention programs.

To date, HIV prevention programs are increasingly recognizing the importance of involving adult caregivers in the process of increasing youths' awareness of HIV exposure risks and their knowledge regarding models of transmission and means of protection (Pequegnat & Szapocznik, 2000). Although efforts have been made to design this set of family-based HIV prevention programs to be maximally culturally and contextually sensitive, additional empirical findings to inform these family-focused efforts is needed. In particular, findings focused on both process, content, and context for family communication within specific racial, ethnic, and geographic groups appears to be needed to inform the next generation of family-focused youth HIV prevention activities.

Limitations

The limitations of this study reflect the same methodological limitations found in many of other studies that examine the effects of family level factors on youth outcomes. For example, the current study employed single informant reports (i.e., parent reports) of racial socialization processes. Therefore, the data did not allow for the examination of interaction effects between youth and parent reports or youth reports of racial socialization associated with youth outcomes. Additionally, data were not available concerning child reports of how well messages of racial socialization were internalized. Therefore, it was not entirely clear if parental reports of racial socialization accurately reflected the degree of racial socialization internalized by their respective children and its association with adolescent mental health.

Additionally, the study utilized a small sample. A larger sample would both enhance statistical power and our confidence in the generalizability of findings. Lastly, the study was based on cross-sectional data only. These types of data, pose issues of unclear relationship between cause and effect that make it impossible to discern the temporal ordering between family processes and the acquisition of youth HIV knowledge. In order to accurately assess the association between family processes and associated youth outcomes, prospective longitudinal cohort studies need to be conducted that document the levels of racial socialization, exposures to risk factors and subsequent youth outcomes of African American youth. To date, only the National Survey of Black Americans has gathered similar data using a nationally representative probability sample. However, this data was gathered during the 1960s and 1970s, which may limit application currently.

Conclusion and Practice Recommendations

Despite these limitations, the present study expands knowledge about urban African American youth HIV knowledge in a significant way. The present research study goes beyond an emphasis on the consideration of conventional family-based influences and to identify the correlates to African American youth HIV knowledge. This knowledge can be useful in expanding the development models of urban HIV knowledge and risk and informing interventions designed to prevent HIV risk behavior. Additional research in this area should be pursued that examines how culturally relevant practices, such as racial socialization, can be integrated at various stages of the prevention research to strengthen family processes and enhance outcomes.

Policy Implications

Perhaps the strongest policy implication of the current study is that the data support the creation and implementation of curricula designed to increase the cultural competence of health care workers, including medical students, social workers, and nurses. These curricula are emerging in an attempt to ameliorate the vast racial health disparities that exist in the United States. A well-established body of research that indicates that ethnic minority populations in the United States lag behind European Americans (whites) on almost every health indicator, including health care coverage, access to care, and life expectancy, while surpassing whites in rates of almost all mental health and physical health problems (IOM, 2002; William, 2001) and being disproportionately impacted by the HIV/AIDS epidemic (CDC, 2001). While it is clear that these disparities are not completely understood or well explained, they have all been attributed at least in some way to low levels of cultural competence and even racist notions, among the health care professionals in providing care (Bhopal, 1998; Smith, 1999).

Subsequently, many mental health policy experts, and most recently the Institute of Medicine, suggest that a well-conceptualized focus on culture in the education of all health care professionals could serve as one of several important national strategies to eliminate racial and ethnic mental health disparities through increasing cultural competence within health care systems (AMA, 1999; Brach & Fraser, 2000; Horowitz, Davis, Palermo, & Vladeck, 2001; Morrison, Wallenstein, Natale, Sensei, & Huang, 2000; Rathmore, Lenert, & Weinfurt et al., 2000; Williams, 1999). The current study supports this notion by indicating that measurable cultural variables exist (e.g., racial socialization) that do relate to health outcomes (i.e., child HIV/AIDS knowledge). Therefore, the creation of such educational tools may help health care professionals understand how various mechanisms within urban families of color function and contribute to health related outcomes, which may help them bolster preferred outcomes, such as child HIV/AIDS knowledge.

Practice Implications

A major practice implication of the current study is that racial socialization variables should be considered when structuring and delivering HIV/AIDS preventative services. Since the creation of culturally competent (and culturally relevant) services became a goal within the past few decades, a primary objective of care has been to design services that value differences and integration of cultural attitudes, beliefs, and practices into diagnostic and treatment (intervention) methods. A major obstacle to this goal is that relatively little research exists that documents the relation of cultural variables and health outcomes. Therefore, without the empirical knowledge of how cultural variables impact care, the creation of services that consider cultural variables is somewhat precarious. In other words, researchers, practitioners, and policy makers were not sure how to treat cultural variables because they did not know how they affected care (or erroneously believed that they were not relevant). The data in the current study provide empirical evidence indicating that racial socialization variables play a unique and measurable role in family communication and child HIV/AIDS knowledge. Therefore, when structuring services, these variables should be considered, especially when considering how to increase child HIV/AIDS knowledge in certain communities.

REFERENCES

American Medical Association (1999). *Introduction. In: Cultural Competence Compendium.* New York: American Medical Association.

Barnes, E.J. (1980). The Black community as a source of positive self concept for Black children: A theoretical perspective. In R. Jones (Ed.). *Black Psychology.* New York: Harper & Row.

Baumeister, L.M., Flores, E., & Martin, B.V. (1995). Sex Information given to Latina adolescents by parents. *Health Education Research,* 10: 233-239.

Bhopal, R. (1998). Spectre of racism in health and health care: lessons from history and the United States. *British Medical Journal, 316*(7149), 1970-3.

Bowman, P.J. & Howard, C. (1985). Race-related socialization, motivation, and academic achievement: A study of Black youth in three-generation families. *Journal of the American Academy of Child Psychiatry, 24,* 134-141.

Boyd-Franklin, N., Aleman, J., Jean-Gilles, M.M., & Lewis, S.Y. (1995). Cultural sensitivity and competence: African American, Latino and Haitian families with HIV/AIDS. In N. Boyd-Franklin, G.L., Steiner, & M.G. Boland (Eds.), *Children, families, and HIV/AIDS: Psychosocial and therapeutic issues* (pp. 53-77). New York: Guilford.

Brach, C. & Fraser, I. (2000). Can cultural competency reduce racial and ethnic health disparities? A review and conceptual model. *Medical Resident Review, 57,* 181-217.

Branch, C.W. & Newcombe, N. (1986). Racial attitude development among youth children as a function of parental attitudes: A longitudinal and cross-sectional study. *Child Development, 57,* 712-721.

Brooks-Gunn, J. & Paikoff, R. L. (1993). Sex is a gamble, kissing is a game: Adolescent sexuality, contraception, and pregnancy. In S. Millstein, A. C. Petersen and E. Nightingale (Eds.), *Promotion of healthy behavior during adolescence* (pp. 180-208). New York, Oxford Press.

Centers for Disease Control. (1992). HIV/AIDS Surveillance Report. Atlanta, GA: Center for Disease Control and Prevention.

Centers for Disease Control. (1998). New Study Profiles Hispanic births in America. National Center for Health Statistics. Released February 13, 1998. Retrieved from the World Wide Web: http://www.cdc.gov/nchswww/relases/98facts/98sheets/hisbirth.htm

Center for Disease Control (2000). Tracking the hidden epidemics: Trends in STD's in the United States, 2000. Atlanta, Georgia: Center for Disease Control.

Centers for Disease Control and Prevention. (2000). Tobacco use among middle and high school students-United States, 1999. MMWR 2000; 49: 49-53.

Centers for Disease control (2001). HIV/AIDS Surveillance Report. Atlanta, GA: Center for Disease Control and Prevention.

Cole, K.L., Roberts, M.C., & McNeal, R.E. (1996). Children's perceptions of ill peers: Effects of disease, grade, and impact variables. *Children's Health Care, 25,* 107-115.

DeLoye, G.J., Henggeler, S.W., & Daniels, C.M. (1993). Developmental and family correlates of children's knowledge and attitudes regarding AIDS. *Journal of Pediatric Psychology, 18,* 209-219.

Ford, K., Sohn, W., & Lepkowski, J. (2002). American adolescents: sexual mixing patterns, bridge partners, and concurrency. *Sexually Transmitted Diseases, 29,* pp. 13-19.

Fox, G.L., Inazu, J.K. (1980). Patterns and outcomes of mother-daughter communication about sexuality. *Journal of Social Issues, 36(1),* 7-29.

Horowitz, C. R., Davis, M. R., Palermo, A. Y., & Vladeck, B. C. (2001). Approaches to eliminating sociocultural disparities in health. *Minority Health Today, 2*(2), 33-43.

Institute of Medicine (IOM). (2002). *Examining Unequal Treatment in American Health Care.* Washington, DC: National Academy of Sciences.

Jaccard, J., Dittus, P., & Gordon, V. (1998). Parent-adolescent congruency in reports of adolescent sexual behavior and in communications about sexual behavior. *Child Development, 69,* 247-261.

Jemmott, J.B., Jemmott, L. & Fong, G.T. (1998). Abstinence and safer sex HIV risk reduction interventions for African American *Adolescents. Journal of the American Medical Association, 270,* 1529-1536.

Johnson, D.J. (2001). Parental characteristics, racial stress and racial socialization processes as predictors of racial coping in middle childhood. In Neal-Barnett (Ed.). Forging Links: clinical/Developmental Perspective of African American Children, pp. 57-74. Westport, CT: Greenwood Press.

Kistner, J., Eberstein, I.W. Quadagno, D., Sly, D., Sitting, L., Foster, K., Balthazor, M., Castro, R., & Osborne, M. (1997). Children's AIDS-related knowledge and attitudes: Variations by grade, race, gender, socioeconomic status, and size of community. *AIDS Education and Prevention, 9,* 285-298.

Knight, G.P., Bernal, M.E., Garza, C.A., Cota, M.K., & Ocampo, K.A. (1993). Family socialization and the ethnic identify of Mexican-American children. *Journal of Cross Cultural Psychology, 24,* 99-114.

Kofkin, J.A., Katz, P.A. & Downey, E.P. (1995). Family discourse about race and the development of children's racial attitudes. Paper presented at the meeting of the Society for Research on Child Development, Indianapolis, IN.

Kotchick, B.A., Dorsey, S., Miller, K.S., Forehand, R. (1999) Adolescent sexual-risk taking behavior in single-parent ethnic minority families. *Journal of Family Psychology, 31*(1), 93-102.

Lefkowitz, E.S., Kahlbaugh, P., Kit-fong Au. T., & Sigman, M. (1998). A longitudinal study of AIDS conversations between mothers and adolescents. *AIDS Education and Prevention, 10*, 351-365.

Madison, S.M., McKay, M., Paikoff, R., & Bell, C. (2000). Community collaboration and basic research: Necessary ingredients for the development of a family-based HIV prevention program. AIDS *Education and Prevention, 12*, 281-298.

Marshall, S. (1995). Ethnic socialization of African American Children: Implications for parenting, identity development, and academic achievement. *Journal of Youth and Adolescence, 24*, 377-396.

McKay, M., Baptiste, D., Coleman, D., Madison, S., McKinney, L., Paikoff, R., & CHAMP Collaborative Board. (2000). Preventing HIV risk exposure in urban communities: The CHAMP family program. in W. Pequegnat & Jose Szapocznik (Eds). *Working with families in the era of HIV/AIDS*. California: Sage Publications.

McNeely, C.A., Shew M.L., Beuhring, T., et al. (2002). Mother's influence on adolescents sexual debut. *Journal of Adolescent Health, 31*, 2002.

Miller, K., Forehand, R., Kotchick, B.A. (1997). Adolescent sexual behavior in two ethnic minority samples the role of family variables. *Journal of Marriage and the Family, 61*: 85-98, 1998.

Morrison, R.S., Wallenstein, S., Natale, D., Sensei, R., & Huang, L.L. (2000). "We don't carry that"–failure of pharmacies in predominately nonwhite neighborhoods to stock opioid analgesics. *New England Journal of Medicine, 342*, 1023-6. Rathmore, Lenert, & Weinfurt et al., 2000.

O'Sullivan, L., Jaramillo, B.M.S., Moreau, D., Meyer-Bahlburg, H.L. (1999). Mother-daughter communication about sexuality in clinical sample of Hispanic adolescent girls. *Hispanic Journal of Behavioral Sciences, 21*: 447-469, 1999.

Paikoff, R.L., Parfenoff, S.H., Williams, S.A., McCornick, A., Greenwood, G.L., & Holmbeck, G.L. (1997). Parenting, parent-child relationships, and sexual possibility situations among urban African American preadolescents: Preliminary findings and implications for HIV prevention. *Journal of Family Psychology, 11*, 1-12.

Paikoff, R. L. (1995). Early heterosexual debut: Situations of sexual possibility during the transition to adolescence. *American Journal of Orthopsychiatry, 65(3)*, 389-401.

Paikoff, R.L. (1997). Applying developmental psychology to an AIDS prevention model for urban African American youth. *Journal of Negro Education, 65*, 44-59.

Pick, S., Palos, P.A. (1995). Impact of the families on the sex lives of adolescents. *Adolescence, 30*, 667-675.

Qunitana, S.M. & Vera, E. M. (1999). Mexican American children's ethnic identity, understanding of ethnic prejudice, and parental ethnic socialization. *Hispanic Journal of Behavioral Sciences, 21*, 387-404.

Romer, D., Black, M., Ricardo, I., Feigelman, S., Kaljee, L., Galbraith, J., Nesbit, R., Homik, R., & Stanton, B. (1994). Social Influences on the Sexual Behavior of Youth at Risk of HIV Exposure. *American Journal of Public Health, 84*(6), 977-985.

Santelli, J.S., Lindberg, L.D., Abma J. et al. (2000). Adolescent sexual behavior: Estimates and trends from four nationally representative surveys. *Family Planning Perspectives, 32*, 156-165.

Sigelman, C.K., Derenowski, E.B., Mullaney, H.A., & Siders, A.T. (1993). Mothers' contributions to knowledge and attitudes regarding AIDS. *Journal of Pediatric Psychology, 18,* 221-235.

Spence, M.B. (1983). Children's cultural values and parental child rearing strategies. *Developmental Review, 3,* 351-370.

Stevenson, H.C. (1994). Validation of the scale of racial socialization of African American adolescents: Steps toward multidimensionality. *Journal of Black Psychology, 20,* 445-468.

Stevenson, H.C. (1995). Relationships of adolescent perceptions of racial socialization to racial identity. *Journal of Black Psychology, 21,* 49-70.

Stevenson, H.C., Reed, J., Bodison, P. & Bishop, A. (1997). Racism stress management: Racial socialization beliefs and the experience of depression and anger in African American youth. *Youth and Society, 29,* 172-222.

Stevenson, H.C., Cameron, R., Herrero-Taylor, T., Davis, G.Y. (2002). Development of the teenage experience of racial socialization scale: Correlates of race-related socialization from the perspective of Black youth. *Journal of Black Psychology, 28,* 84-106.

Thornton, M.C. (1997). Strategies of racial socialization among Black parents: Mainstream, minority, and cultural messages. In R.J. Taylor, J.S. Jackson, & L.M. Chatters (eds.). *Family life in Black America,* Thousand Oaks: Sage.

Thornton, M.C., Chatters, L.M., Taylor, R.J. & Allen, W.R. (1990). Sociodemographic and environmental correlates of racial socialization by Black parents. *Child Development, 61,* 401-409.

Smith, D. (1999). *Health Care Divided; Race and Healing a Nation.* Ann Arbor, MI: University of Michigan Press, 1999.

Sonenstein, F.L., Pleck, J.H., & Klu, L.C. (1991). Levels of sexual activity among adolescent males in the United States. *Family Planning Perspectives, 23,* 162-167.

Sonenstein, F.L., Pleck, J.H., & Klu, L.C. (1989). Sexual activity, condom use and AIDS awareness among adolescent males. *Family Planning Perspectives, 21,* 151-158.

Tolan, P.H., Gorman-Smith, D., Huesmann, L.R., Zelli, A. (1997). Assessment of family relationship characteristics: A measure to explain risk for antisocial behavior and depression among urban youth. *Psychological Assessment, Vol 9*(3), 212-223.

Williams, D. R. (1999). Race, socioeconomic status, and health: the added effects of racism and discrimination. *Annals of the New York Academy of Sciences, 896,* 173-88.

William, R. (2001). Opening Statement at Institute of Medicine public briefing for Crossing the Quality Chasm: a New Health System for the 21st Century. Washington, DC, March 1, 2001.

Wilson, W. J. (1987). *The truly disadvantaged: The inner city, the underclass, and public policy.* Chicago: University of Chicago Press.

doi:10.1300/J200v05n01_04

Urban African American Pre-Adolescent Social Problem Solving Skills: Family Influences and Association with Exposure to Situations of Sexual Possibility

Dorian E. Traube
Kelly Taber Chasse
Mary M. McKay
Anjali M. Bhorade
Roberta Paikoff
Stacie D. Young

Dorian E. Traube, CSW, and Kelly Taber Chasse, PhD, are affiliated with the Columbia University School of Social Work. Mary M. McKay, PhD, is Professor of Social Work in Psychiatry & Community Medicine, Mount Sinai School of Medicine. Anjali M. Bhorade, MD, and Roberta Paikoff, PhD, are affiliated with the University of Illinois at Chicago, Department of Psychiatry. Stacie D. Young, MA, is affiliated with the Community Mental Health Council, CHAMP Collaborative Board.

Address correspondence to: Mary M. McKay, PhD, Professor of Social Work in Psychiatry & Community Medicine, Mount Sinai School of Medicine, One Gustave L. Levy Place, New York, NY 10029 (E-mail: mary.mckay@mssm.edu).

The contributions of Carl C. Bell, MD, Sybil Madison-Boyd, PhD, Donna Baptiste, PhD, Doris Coleman, MSW, and CHAMP Collaborative Board members and participants are especially recognized.

Funding from the National Institutes of Mental Health (R01 MH 63662) and the W.T. Grant Foundation is gratefully acknowledged. Dorian Traube is currently a pre-doctoral fellow at the Columbia University School of Social Work supported by a training grant from the National Institutes of Mental Health (5T32MH014623-24).

[Haworth co-indexing entry note]: "Urban African American Pre-Adolescent Social Problem Solving Skills: Family Influences and Association with Exposure to Situations of Sexual Possibility." Traube, Dorian E. et al. Co-published simultaneously in *Social Work in Mental Health* (The Haworth Press, Inc.) Vol. 5, No. 1/2, 2007, pp. 101-119; and: *Community Collaborative Partnerships: The Foundation for HIV Prevention Research Efforts* (ed: Mary M. McKay, and Roberta L. Paikoff) The Haworth Press, Inc., 2007, pp. 101-119. Single or multiple copies of this article are available for a fee from The Haworth Document Delivery Service [1-800-HAWORTH, 9:00 a.m. - 5:00 p.m. (EST). E-mail address: docdelivery@haworthpress.com].

SUMMARY. The results of two studies focusing on the social problem solving skills of African American preadolescent youth are detailed. In the first study data from a sample of 150 African American children, ages 9 to 11 years, was used to examine the association between type of youth social problem solving approaches applied to hypothetical risk situations and time spent in unsupervised peer situations of sexual possibility. Findings revealed that children with more exposure to sexual possibility situations generated a wider range of social problem solving strategies, but these approaches tended to be unrealistic and ambiguous. Further, there was a positive association between the amount of time spent unsupervised and youth difficulty formulating a definitive response to hypothetical peer pressure situations. Children with less exposure to sexual possibility situations tended to be more aggressive when approaching situations of peer pressure. In the second study, data from a non-overlapping sample of 164 urban, African American adult caregivers and their 9 to 11 year old children was examined in order to explore the associations between child gender, family-level factors including family communication frequency and intensity, time spent in situations of sexual possibility, and youth social problem solving approaches. Results revealed that children were frequently using constructive problem solving and help seeking behaviors when confronted by difficult social situations and that there was a significant relationship between the frequency and intensity of parent child communication and youth help seeking social problem solving approaches. Implications for research and family-based interventions are highlighted. doi:10.1300/J200v05n01_05 *[Article copies available for a fee from The Haworth Document Delivery Service: 1-800-HAWORTH. E-mail address: <docdelivery@haworthpress.com> Website: <http:// www.HaworthPress.com> © 2007 by The Haworth Press, Inc. All rights reserved.]*

KEYWORDS. Social problem solving skills, situations of sexual possibility, family communication frequency/intensity, exposure to sexual possibility situations and problem solving approaches

Young urban African American adolescents living in poverty are at an increased risk for HIV infection (Centers for Disease Control, 2001; 2000; 1995). This may be due to the compounding effects of residing in poor, inner-city neighborhoods with higher rates of infection, significant psychosocial stressors associated with poverty, community violence, scarcity of youth-supportive resources, and limited access to health-focused preventive and treatment resources (Sikkema, Brondino, Anderson et al., 2004; Paikoff, 1995; Rotheram-Borus, Mahler & Rosario, 1995; Wilson, 1987). It is against this backdrop that youth development, particularly the transition to adolescence occurs. Cognitive changes and emotional responses, as well as the onset of puberty and early involvement in sexual activity, all take place within an urban context posing numerous threats to youth health and safety (Bell & Jenkins, 1993; Atkins et al., 1998). Given high prevalence rates of HIV infection, youth who begin sexual activity during early adolescence may be at significantly higher risk for HIV exposure as early sexual involvement has been linked with more frequent sexual encounters, as well as more frequent partners and less contraception use (Moore & Rosenthal, 1993; The Alan Gutacher Institute, 1994; Paikoff, 1995; Goldman & Goldman, 1988; Hutchinson & Cooney, 1998;).

Thus, research is needed to understand factors that contribute to the early initiation of sexual activity in order to inform youth-focused HIV prevention programs. There is a particular need to examine the social context of sexual behavior during early adolescence (Jemmott & Jemmott, 1992; Jemmott, Jemmott & Fong, 1992; Paikoff, 1995; Parfenoff, McCormick & Paikoff, 1996; Stanton, 1996). Developmentally, the peer group becomes an increasingly significant source of support, comparison and pressure to engage in sexual risk taking and other types of behavior that potentially threaten the health of the youth (Lewis & Lewis, 1984; Fuemmeler, Taylor, Metz, & Brown, 2002). However, there is also accumulated evidence that family influences, particularly those related to parental supervision and monitoring of youth activities (Romer et al., 1994; Pick & Palos, 1995; Hutchinson & Cooney, 1998) and family communication (Muller & Powers, 1990; Kafka & London, 1991; Pick & Palos, 1995; Jackson, Bijstra, & Oostra, 1998) play a critical role in delaying youth sexual involvement and reducing early adolescent sexual risk taking behaviors.

Thus, this article presents the results of two studies focused on the social problem solving approaches of African American preadolescent youth. In the first study, the association between the type of social problem solving strategies applied to hypothetical risk situations and time spent in situations of sexual possibility, periods of time spent without any adult supervision, are examined. The next study was designed to examine the association between child gender, family-level factors including family communication frequency and intensity, time spent in situations of sexual possibility, and youth social problem solving skills.

Findings are meant to inform health promotion and HIV prevention programs for urban youth entering adolescence.

RISKS ENCOUNTERED BY URBAN AFRICAN AMERICAN YOUTH: OBSTACLES TO DEVELOPMENT

African American youth approaching adolescence within inner-city communities must negotiate a myriad of risks associated with poverty, minority status and a scarcity of youth-supportive resources. African American youth are over represented among those youth living in impoverished communities, and the incidence of HIV/AIDS infection has increased significantly among these youth over the last decade (Centers for Disease Control, 2001). Urban African American youth living in poverty must confront additional risks including learning to manage pressure to use drugs and community violence exposure (Semlitz & Gold, 1986; Coombs, Paulson, & Palley, 1988; Kandel, Johnson, Bird, Camino, Goodman, Lahey et al., 1997). Yet, there is little information regarding the strategies that urban African American youth use to negotiate these risk situations (Kirby, Barth, Leland, & Fetro, 1991). Further, although there is some evidence that African American parents adapt their parenting strategies and rely on social support networks to buffer youth from peer pressure and negative urban contextual factors (see Jarrett, 1995 for examples), additional research is needed to understand the mechanisms via which preadolescents develop the necessary skills to manage risk opportunities and protect themselves from potential harm.

YOUTH SOCIAL PROBLEM SOLVING AND RISK-TAKING BEHAVIOR

Pre-adolescents' thought processes and the manner in which they perceive and responds to certain situations may influence their actions in social situations where HIV risk exposure is likely. Because problem solving involves perceiving, processing, and using information regarding self, it potentially plays an important role in behavioral health (Felton & Bartoces, 2002). Researchers have demonstrated that effective, high efficacy problem solvers use more problem-focused coping strategies, have a stronger internal locus of control, have more confidence in their decision making ability, and are less likely to be impulsive rather than ineffective, low-efficacy problem solvers (Heppner et al., 1987). Yet, the ability to think hypothetically, futuristically, and to integrate multiple aspects of a task or problem reflect formal operational thinking and are essential to reasoned decisions. Compared with adults, adolescents may make less well-reasoned decisions due to a briefer period in which to consolidate formal operational thinking skills and less opportunity to apply higher level cognitive functioning to real life situations (Haynie, Alexander, & Walters, 1997).

There is a body of research examining youth social problem solving during adolescence, while the focus on preadolescents is quite rare. The literature is clear that there are significant links between adolescent social problem solving ability and engaging in risk-taking behaviors (Hains & Herrman, 1989) with teens evidencing poorer social problem solving abilities engaging in risk-taking behavior (Caldwell & Darling, 1999; Kuperminc & Allen, 2001).

Substantial prior research has demonstrated an association between peer pressure and sexual activity, smoking, substance abuse, gang involvement, delinquent behavior, and violence among the adolescent population (Billy & Udry, 1985; Keefe, 1992; Romer et al., 1993; Dahlberg, 1998; Kung & Farrell, 2000; Walker-Barnes & Mason 2001; Fuemmeler et al., 2002). For example, Ellickson and Morton (1999) found that African American adolescents who are offered drugs at an early age are at increased risk to use hard drugs, such as cocaine and heroin, in the future, suggesting that these youth may benefit from learning how to effectively cope with peer pressure. Adolescents whose peer group engages in risk-taking behaviors tend to engage in these behaviors themselves (Kandel, 1986; Caldwell & Darling, 1999). In one of the few studies that included pre-adolescents in the examination of peer pressure, findings indicate that 10-year-olds report experiencing similar peer pressure as older adolescents to engage in certain activities, such as violence and substance use (Lewis & Lewis, 1984).

Further, in a study comparing adolescent concerns about peer pressure to other issues of significance during this developmental period, such as wanting to be popular, findings reveal that perceptions of being pressured to engage in risk behaviors is more strongly associated with engaging in risk taking behavior in comparison to the impact of wishes to be more popular (Santor, Messervey, & Kusumakar, 2000).

Deficits in addressing peer pressure effectively have also been linked with poor adolescent outcomes, including aggressive behavior, violence, delinquency, drug use, and suicide attempts (Sadowski & Kelley,

1993; Dahlberg, 1998; Kuperminc & Allen, 2001). In addition, problem solving capability has been shown to be related to sexual behavior, including contraception use (Abel, Adams, & Stevenson, 1994; Hutchinson & Cooney, 1998), and having friends who are sexually active or do not use condoms (Kalmuss et al., 2003). More specifically, in a study by Caldwell and Darling (1999) the ability to effectively social problem solve and resist peer pressure acted as a buffer against substance use even when social situations offered encouragement. Given the fact that these numerous risk opportunity and pressures to engage in risk behavior exist for African American youth within inner-city environments, and that these same youth anticipate negative consequences for not agreeing to participate in misconduct with peers (Pearl, Bryan, & Herzog, 1990), it is vital that research studies be undertaken that examine how youth develop or learn social problem solving skills and potential mechanisms for bolstering these skills be identified.

FAMILY INFLUENCES ON YOUTH
SOCIAL PROBLEM SOLVING

Research on the adolescent population indicates that parents play a role in their adolescents' development of effective social problem solving skills (Brody, Flor, Hollett-Wright, & McCoy, 1998; Hutchinson & Cooney, 1998). For example, level of parental supervision is an important familial consideration. Among low-income African American children and adolescents, a low level of parental supervision provides the opportunity for precocious sexual activity (Bakken & Winter, 2002). Parental supervision is frequently affected by the presence of a single parent due to a reduction of the number of parents in the household and the necessity for the custodial parent to work full time. Bakken and Winter (2002) found that family structure not only predicted age at sexual initiation among African American adolescents, but also continued to influence sexual behavior throughout adult life.

Adolescents who communicate with their parents about high-risk behavior have been found to more successfully negotiate peer pressure social situations and resist engaging in high-risk behavior than adolescents who do not communicate with their parents (Holtzman & Rubinson, 1995; Farrell & White, 1998; Romer et al., 1994; Pick & Palos, 1995; Hutchinson & Cooney, 1998; Somers & Paulson, 2000). In addition, in families where adolescents report open and attentive communication with their parents, the adolescents also report more satisfaction with their families and less risk taking behavior than those teens who do not communicate with their parents (Mueller & Powers, 1990; Kafka & London, 1991; Pick & Palos, 1995; Jackson, Bijstra, & Oostra, 1998).

Communicating with their adolescents may be one of the most effective ways caregivers can protect their adolescents from making poor decisions that may impact the rest of their lives (Mueller & Powers, 1990; Holtzman & Rubinson, 1995). Discussing with their adolescents possible high-risk situations that may occur and teaching them how to negotiate these situations, may result in adolescent implementing these skills outside of the family unit. This may lead to increased confidence and better decision making in social situations. Previous research has shown that adolescents who report communicating with their parents are better able to negotiate high-risk social situations (Pick & Palos, 1995; Hutchinson & Cooney, 1998; Farrell & White, 1998; Somers & Paulson, 2000).

Research examining caregiver-child communication with pre-adolescents is lacking, despite findings that indicate that the influence of caregivers decreases with increasing age of adolescents (Keefe, 1992), suggesting that caregivers have more influence during pre-adolescence, before their children are in the midst of the stressors of adolescence. One study of fourth and sixth graders conducted by Jackson (1997) found that pre-adolescents who had initiated smoking tobacco reported less communication with parents, among other factors, than pre-adolescents who were abstinent. In another study examined parent-child communication among pre-adolescents and alcohol use norms were examined (Brody, Flor, Hollett-Wright, & McCoy, 1998). Findings revealed that communication between parents and their pre-adolescents was associated with abstinent alcohol use norms for the pre-adolescents, indicating that communication during pre-adolescence may reduce risk-taking behavior for this population. In addition, research has found that pre-adolescents do not resist communicating with their parents, and may even find their parents advice helpful (Ary, James, & Biglan, 1999). Although research on the pre-adolescent population is limited, understanding the influence of caregiver communication on pre-adolescents' ability to negotiate social situations is important for all families, but particularly so for urban African American families who are raising their pre-adolescents in complex community settings.

In sum, the two studies presented within this article were undertaken to elucidate social problem solving skills of African American preadolescent youth. In the first study, the association between engaging in situations where there is a possibility of sexual activity among adolescents and the use of passive or aggressive social problem solving strategies is examined. The second study augments the first study by also examining association between time spent in situations of sexual possibility, and youth social problem solving approaches, with an added component of family communication frequency and intensity. Implications for research and family-based interventions are highlighted.

STUDY 1

Methods

As previously stated, the purpose of the first study was to investigate the association between a child's social problem solving approaches and the amount of time youth spend in situations of sexual possibility as defined by the amount of time spent with peers unsupervised by adults. The data used in this investigation was gathered from the first wave of participants in the Chicago HIV and Adolescent Mental Health Project (CHAMP) ($n = 150$), a longitudinal study of risk and protective factors associated with inner-city African American youth sexual risk taking. Pre-adolescents (9-13 years of age) were interviewed by trained research staff.

Participants

In this sample, 44% of the preadolescents were male and 56% were female. Of the primary caregivers, 39% had a total household income under $5000, 47% had no prior work experience, and approximately 53% had not completed high school. The sample was recruited from six public schools located in neighborhoods with high concentrations of urban poverty and above normal rates of HIV infection. Informed consent was obtained from all adult caregivers, assent was obtained from youth. IRB approval was also obtained.

Measures

In order to tap youth social problem solving skills, participants were presented with a variety of hypothetical social situations derived from the *Middle School Alternative Solutions Test* (Caplan, Weissberg, Bersoff, Ezekowitz & Wells, 1986) and *The Reducing the Risk: Build-*

ing Skills to Prevent Pregnancy Scale (Barth, 1989). These questions were designed to measure the child's ability to generate alternative solutions to age-relevant, hypothetical peer problems (Caplan, Weissberf, Bersoff, Ezikowitz & Wells, 1986). In the interview, youth participants were presented with a situation involving persistent teasing by peers, a second dealt with peer pressure to engage in dangerous activities, a third involved witnessing a fight, and a fourth asked for responses to pressure to engage in sexual activity. For each situation the youth were asked to generate as many responses as possible of ways they might approach the situations. The answers were recorded verbatim by a trained interviewer and coded into thirteen categories derived from a coding system presented in the Alternative Solutions Test Manual (Caplan, Weissberg, Bersoff, Ezikowitz & Wells, 1986).

In a second, separate interview, the *Youth Sexual Risk Interview* (Paikoff, 1995) was administered to assess time spent in situations of sexual possibility. Youth were questioned as to whether they had spent time in mixed sex groups and, if so, the amount of supervision present during such times. Within the total sample, 26% (n = 40) of the children had participated in at least one sexual possibility situation.

Data Analyses

Data from youth were separated by whether they had spent time in a situation of sexual possibility (yes/no) and their social problem solving responses were identified. A separate analysis was used to calculate the frequency and intensity of responses to each of the four independent problem-solving situations. T-tests were used to compare the variety and types of responses formulated by the higher risk group (yes) to those of the lower risk group (no). The strategies youth in these two groups used to solve various problems were compared to each other in order to determine problem solving factors associated with more intense and frequent exposure to situations which are hypothesized to lead to early sexual activity.

Results

Children with more intense exposure to sexual situations generated a greater variety of social problem solving methods by averaging more responses per question than those with less exposure ($t = 3.3, p < 0.05$). In addition, the higher risk children also appeared to give an overall more unrealistic response to situations ($t = 10.9, p < 0.001$), more ambiguous answers (t = 6.3, p < 0.5), and were more nonconfrontational (t = 1.2, p < 0.5) than children with lower sexual risk.

Conversely, the lower risk group appeared to respond overall more aggressively (t = 4.1, p < 0.05) than the higher risk individuals. In addition, it appears that there were more lower risk than higher risk children that did not give any type of answer to the problem solving questions (t = 4.9, p < 0.02).

STUDY 2

Methods

Again, the purpose of the second study was also to investigate the association between gender, family level processes, time spent in situations of sexual possibility, and youth social problem solving approaches. This study is also a secondary data analysis from baseline data collected as part of the CHAMP (Chicago HIV prevention and Adolescent Mental Health Project) Family Program Study, the intervention companion study to the first research project described in study #1. The CHAMP Family Program is a family-based HIV prevention project targeting 4th and 5th grade African American, low-income youth and their families in a community with a high rate of HIV infection.

The sample drawn for the current study represent the first five cohorts of youth and their families involved in the CHAMP Family Program (n = 197). This is a non-overlapping sample with study #1 presented above. All CHAMP Family program participants were chosen randomly from a roster of 550 youth and their families attending four inner-city public elementary schools. A 92% consent rate for inclusion in the random assignment process of the CHAMP Family Program study was obtained (see McKay, Baptiste, Coleman, Madison, Paikoff, & Scott, 2000, for details regarding the CHAMP Family Program study). Approximately 60% of the sample was girls, ages 9 to 11 years, and 40% were boys in the same age range. Almost 82% of parents reported a family income of less than $14,000. Three quarters of adult caregivers completed high school and 8% of parents had attended some college. Approximately 17% of the adult caregivers were between 25 and 29 years indicating that they were teenagers at the time of the target child's birth.

Data Collection Procedures

Data for the current study was derived from baseline assessment information prior to the start of the family-based intervention. All information was obtained from parents and youth separately. Each child or adult participant completed paper-pencil instruments in small groups, 6 to 8 participants, with research staff reading each item aloud.

Measures

First, parent were asked to complete the *Family Decision Making Scale* (Dornbusch et al., 1985), a 17 item instrument tapping whether discussions regarding chores, homework and other common family issues had been talked about in the last two weeks, how frequently, and their emotional tone (calm versus angry).

In a second, separate interview, the *Youth Sexual Risk Interview* (Paikoff, 1995) was administered to assess time spent in situations of sexual possibility. Youth were questioned as to whether they had spent time in mixed sex groups and, if so, the amount of supervision present during such times.

Finally, the youth were asked to complete the *Middle School Alternative Solutions Test* (Caplan, Weissberg, Bersoff, Ezekowitz & Wells, 1986) that was described in the previous study.

Data Analysis

Data from youth were separated by whether they had spent time in a situation of sexual possibility (yes/no), gender, and their social problem solving responses. T-tests were used to compare the variety and types of responses formulated by the higher risk group (time spent in situations of sexual possibility) to those of the lower risk group (no time spent in situations of sexual possibility) to determine problem solving factors which are associated with more intense and frequent exposure to situations of sexual possibility. T-tests were also used to compare social problem solving responses of males and females. Correlations and multiple regression analysis were used to determine the association between frequency and intensity of family communication on social problem solving skills.

Results

Of the 164 children and families included in the analysis, children were frequently using constructive problem solving and help seeking behaviors when confronted by difficult social situations. When being picked on by another child 50.6% ($n = 39$) said they would ignore them while 62.5% ($n = 80$) said they would seek help from a teacher or principal. When being pressured by a peer 65.4% ($n = 36$) said they would tell their peers no and 49.5% ($n = 51$) said they would tell their parent. When being touched by a peer 49.5% ($n = 52$) reported they would tell the child to stop, 52.7% ($n = 78$) said they would scream, and 43.3% ($n = 65$) said they would run away.

There was a significant difference in female social problem solving approaches versus male. Girls were more likely to have a passive response to peer pressure then boys, ($t = -2.30, p < .05$). Additionally, children who had experienced situations of sexual possibility were more likely to have aggressive social problem solving strategies, ($t = -2.40, p < .05$), but would also actively seek help from adults, ($t = -2.28, p < .05$). There was a significant relationship between the frequency of parent child communication and youth help seeking social problem solving approaches. Children who communicated infrequently with their parent were more likely to seek help from other adults in their life including their teacher or principal ($r = -.27, p < .01$), or another child's parent ($r = -.33, p < .001$). Additionally children were more likely to have aggressive responses to social situations if they engaged in conflictual conversations with their parent ($r = -.24, p < .01$).

Moreover, when controlling for frequency and exposure to sexual possibility situations, males were less likely to tell someone who was touching them to stop (B $= -.63, \beta = -.34, p < .05$). Furthermore, when controlling for frequency, exposure to sexual possibility situations, and gender, children who participated in conflictual communication with their parent were less likely to tell someone to stop touching them (B $= -.46, \beta = -.33, p < .05$).

DISCUSSION

Therefore, the majority of children within this inner-city community were reporting productive social problem solving strategies in a range of peer pressure situations. Particularly relevant for HIV/AIDS prevention, children reported they would assertively refuse to participate in sexual behavior or said they would seek help from adults in sexual pressure situations. Children who did not actively engage in conversations in their own family were turning to other adults in their life for help. Parent/child communication and level of anger expressed during communication was found to be significantly related to aggressive problem solving approaches and the inability to assertively decline sexual advances. Table 1 summarizes the outcomes of Study 2.

CONCLUSION

The results from these investigations suggest that youth exposed to situations of sexually possibility generate significantly different responses to social situations than individuals with a lower risk. Children with greater exposure tend to generate a greater variety of problem solving methods. However, these methods tend to be unrealistic, ambiguous, and non-confrontational. Children with lower exposure to sexual situations tend to respond with more aggressive solutions. In addition, a child's aggressive problem solving is augmented by the intensity of anger of parent/child communication.

An underlying assumption in both of these studies is that the strategies that a child develops towards a certain social situations may increase or decrease their risk to sexual exposure. It can be argued, however, that a child's risk to sexual exposure may influence strategies they use to make decisions in problem solving situations. In order to better understand the nature of this association, further longitudinal studies need to be conducted.

The information presented in these studies can directly enhance prevention and intervention efforts with pre- and young adolescents aimed at delaying early onset of sexual activity. Perhaps such programs can help decrease a child's risk of early sexual exposure by first presenting a series of clear rational strategies which may be used by the child in situations where sexual activity is possible. These programs may also emphasize the benefits of seeking help in such situations as well as differentiating between unrealistic and rational problem solving strategies. Implementing such social problem solving strategies in children may help decrease their exposure to situations of sexual possibility. In addition, it is important for programs to attempt to enhance the level of communication within families in order to encourage children to seek help from their parents. Family-based intervention programs should appropriately target children exhibiting aggressive responses and instruct families on alternative methods of relaying emotions when communi-

TABLE 1. Effects of Frequency of Parent-Child Communication, Intensity of Parent Child Communication, and Time Spent in Situations of Sexual Possibility

Univariate Analysis

Variable	Percent	n	Missing
When being picked on you...			
Ignore them	50.6	39	91
Tell the teacher/principal	62.5	80	40
When being peer pressured you...			
Tell them no	65.4	36	113
Tell their parent	49.5	51	65
When being touched by a peer you...			
Tell them to stop	49.5	52	63
Scream	52.7	78	20
Run away	43.3	65	18

Bivariate Analysis

T-test of Gender and Social Problem Solving Strategies

Variable	Mean of Males	Mean of Females	t(df)
Stop being their friend	1.75	2.35	−2.30(50)*

T-test of Exposure to Sexual Possibility Situations and Social Problem Solving Strategies

Variable	Mean of No Exposure to Sexual Possibility	Mean of Exposure to Sexual Possibility	t(df)
Seek help from an adult	1.75	2.17	−2.28(37)*
Pick on another child	1.71	2.48	−2.40(32)*

Correlation with Frequency of Parent-Child Communication

Variable	r
Seek help from a teacher or principal	−.266**
Seek help from another adult	−.333***
Hit the other child	−.298****
Seek help from your parent	.279**

Correlation with Conflictual Parent-Child Communication

Variable	r
Hit the other child	−.237**

Multivariate Analysis

Ordinary Least Squares Regression on "If I were being touched the first thing I would do is tell them to stop"

Variable	B	SE B	ß
Frequency of Parent-Child Communication	.06	.03	.237
Time Spent in Situations of Sexual Possibility	−.11	.31	−.05
Gender	−.63	.27	−.34*
Intensity of Parent-Child Communication	−.46	.20	−.33*

$R^2 = .21$, Adj. $R^2 = .13$, df = 46, F = 2.76, p < .05

*p < .05, **p < .01, ***p < .001, ****p < .0001

cating. This delay in onset of sexual behavior may in turn decrease the chances of preadolescents' later contraction of HIV.

REFERENCES

Abel, E., Adams, E., & Stevenson, R. (1994). Self-esteem, problem-solving, sexual risk behavior among women with and without Chlamydia. *Clinical Nursing Research, 19* (4), 353-370.

Abma, J.C., & Sonenstein, F.l. (2001). Sexual activity and contraceptive practices among teenagers in the United States, 1988 and 1995. *Vital and Health Statistics, 23* (21).

The Alan Guttmacher Institute. (1994). *Sex and America's Teenagers.* New York: The Alan Guttmacher Institute.

Ary, D.V., James, L., & Biglan, A. (1999). Parent-daughter discussions to discourage tobacco use: feasibility and content. *Adolescence, 34* (134), 275-282.

Atkins, M., McKay, M., Arvanitis, P., Madison, S., Costigan, C., Haney, P., Zevenbergen, A., Hess., Bennett, D., & Webster, D. (1998). Ecological model for school-based mental health services for urban low-income aggressive children. *Journal of Behavioral Health Services and Research, 5,* 64-75

Bakken, R.J., & Winter, M. (2002). Family characteristics and sexual risk behaviors among black men in the United States. *Perspectives on Sexual and Reproductive Health, 34*(5), 252-258.

Barber, J.G., Bolitho, F., & Bertrand, L.D. (1999). Intrapersonal versus peer group predictors of adolescent drug use. *Child and Youth Services Review, 21* (7), 565-579.

Barth, R.P. (1989) *Reducing the risk: Building skills to prevent pregnancy.* Santa Cruz, CA: Network.

Bell, C. C., & Jenkins, E. J. (1993). Community violence and children on Chicago's Southside. *Psychiatry: Interpersonal and Biological Processes, 56*(1), 46-54.

Billy, J.O.G., & Udry, J.R. (1985). The influence of male and female best friends on adolescent sexual behavior. *Adolescence, XX* (77), 21-32.

Brody, G.H., Flor, D.L., Hollett-Wright, N., & McCoy, J.K. (1998). Children's development of alcohol use norms: contributions of parent and siblings norms, children's temperaments, and parent-child discussions. *Journal of Family Psychology, 12* (2), 209-219.

Caldwell, L.L., & Darling, N. (1999). Leisure context, parental control, and resistance to peer pressure as predictors of adolescent partying and substance use: an ecological perspective. *Journal of Leisure Research, 31* (1), 57-77.

Capaldi, D., Crosby, L., & Stoolmaker, M. (1996). Predicting the timing of first sexual intercourse for at-risk adolescent males. *Child Development, 67* (2), 344-359.

Caplan, M., Weissberg, R.P., Bersoff, D., Ezsekowitz, W., & Wells, M.L. (1986). *Manual for Alternative Solutions Test for Young Adolescents.* Unpublished manuscript, Yale University Psychology Department, New Haven, CT.

Caspi, S., Lynam, D., Moffitt, T. E., & Silva, P.A. (1993). Unraveling girls' delinquency: Biological, dispositional, and contextual contributions to adolescent misbehavior. *Developmental Psychology, 29* (1), 19-30.

Centers for Disease Control (1995). *HIV/AIDS Surveillance Report.* Atlanta, GA: Center for Disease Control and Prevention.

Center for Disease Control (2000). *Tracking the hidden epidemics: Trends in STD's in the United States, 2000.* Atlanta, GA: Center for Disease Control.

Centers for Disease Control (2001). *HIV/AIDS Surveillance Report.* Atlanta, GA: Center for Disease Control and Prevention.

Coombs, R.H, Paulson, M.J., & Palley, R. (1998). The institutionalization of drug use in America: Hazardous adolescence, challenging parenthood. *Journal of Chemical Dependency Treatment, 1*(2), 9-37.

Dahlberg, L.L. (1998). Youth violence in the United States: Major trends, risk factors, and approaches. *American Journal of Prevention Medicine, 14* (4), 259-272.

Dumont, M., & Provost, M.A. (1999). Resilience in adolescents: Protective role of social support, coping strategies, self-esteem, and social activities on experience of stress and depression. *Journal of Youth and Adolescence, 28* (3) 343-363.

Farrell, A.D., & White, K.S. (1998). Peer influence and drug use among urban adolescents: Family structure and parent-adolescent relationship as protective factors. *Journal of Consulting and Clinical Psychology, 66* (2), 248-258.

Felton, G.W., & Bartoces, M. (2002). Predictors of Initiation of Early Sex in Black and White Adolescent Females. *Public Health Nursing, 19* (1), 59-68.

Fuemmeler, B.F., Taylor, L.A., Metz, A.E.J., & Brown, R.T. (2002). Risk-taking and smoking tendency among primarily African American school children: Moderating influences of peer susceptibility. *Journal of Clinical Psychology and Medical Settings, 9* (4), 323-330.

Giordano, P.C., Cernkovich, S.A., & DeMaris, A. (1993), The family and peer relations of Black adolescents. *Journal of Marriage & the Family, 55* (2), 277-287.

Goldman, R. J., & Goldman, J. D. G. (1988). *Show Me Yours: Understanding Children's Sexuality.* Ringwood: Penguin.

Hains A.A., & Herrman L.P. (1989) Social cognitive skills and behavioral adjustment of delinquent adolescents in treatment. *Journal of Adolescence, 12* (3), 323-328.

Haynie, D.L., Alexander, C., & Walters, S.R. (1997). Considering a decision-making approach to youth violence prevention programs. *The Journal of School Health, 67* (5), 165-170.

Heppner, P.P., Kampa, M., & Brunning, L. (1987). The relationship between problem-solving, self-appraisal and indices of physical and psychological health. *Cognitive Therapy and Research, 19* (2), 155-168.

Holtzman, D., & Rubinson, R. (1995). Parent and peer communication effects on AIDS-related behavior among U.S. high school students. *Family Planning Perspectives, 27* (6), 235-247.

Hutchinson, M.K., & Cooney, T.M. (1998). Patterns of parent-teen sexual risk communication: Implications for intervention. *Family Relations, 47* (2), 185-194.

Illinois 9th Grade Adolescent Health Survey, 1991: A Collaborative Project of the Illinois Department of Public Health, Illinois Department of Alcoholism and Substance Abuse, and Illinois State Board of Education. (1992, Summer). *Prevention Forum,* 21-29.

Jackson, C. (1997). Initial and experimental stages of tobacco and alcohol use during late childhood: Relation to peer, parent, and personal risk factors. *Addictive Behaviors, 22* (5), 685-698.

Jackson, S., Bijstra, J., & Oostra, L (1998). Adolescents' perceptions of communication with parents relative to specific aspects of relationships with parents and personal development. *Journal of Adolescence, 21,* 305-322.

Jarrett, R. L. (1995). Growing up poor: the family experiences of socially mobile youth in low-income African American neighborhoods. *Journal of Adolescent Research, 10,* 111-135.

Jemmott, J. B., Jemmott, L. S., & Fong, G. T. (1998). Reductions in HIV risk associations sexual behaviors among Black male adolescents. Effects of an AIDS prevention intervention. *American Journal of Public Health, 82,* 372-377.

Jemmott, J. B., Jemmott, L.S., & Fong, G. T. (1992). Reduction in HIV risk associations sexual Behaviors among Black male adolescents. Effects of an AIDS prevention intervention. *American Journal of Public Health, 82,* 372-377.

Kafka, R.R., & London, P. (1991). Communication in relationships and adolescent substance use: the influence of parents and friends. *Adolescence, 26* (103), 587-598.

Kalmuss, D., Davidson, A., Cohall, A., Laraque, D., & Cassell, C. (2003). Preventing sexual risk behaviors and pregnancy among teenagers: Linking Research and programs. *Perspectives on Sexual and Reproductive Health, 35* (2), 87-93.

Kandel, D.B., Johnson, J.G., Bird, H.R., Canino, G., Goodman, S.H., Lahey, B.B., Regier, D.A., & Schwab-Stone, M. (1997). Psychiatric disorders associated with substance use among children and adolescents: Findings from the methods for the epidemiology of child and adolescent mental disorders (MECA) study. *Journal of Abnormal Child Psychology, 25* (2), 121-132.

Keefe, K. (1992). Perceptions of normative social pressure and attitudes toward alcohol use: changes during adolescence. *Journal of Studies on Alcohol,* January, 46-54.

Keller, S.E., Bartlett, J.A., Schleifer, S.J., Johnston, R.L., Pinner, E., & Delaney, B. (1991). HIV-relevant sexual behavior among a healthy inner-city heterosexual adolescent population in an endemic area of HIV. *Journal of Adolescent Health, 12,* 44-48.

Kirby, D., Barth, R.P., Leland, N., & Fetro, J.V. (1991). Reducing the risk: Impact of a new curriculum on sexual risk-taking. *Family Planning Perspectives, 23* (6), 253-263.

Kuperminc, G.P., & Allen, J.P. (2001). Social Orientation: Problem behavior and motivations toward interpersonal problem solving among high risk adolescents. *Journal of Youth and Adolescence, 30* (5), 597-622.

Kung, E.M., & Farrell, A.D. (2000). The role of parents and peers in early adolescent substance use: an examination of mediating and moderating effects. *Journal of Child and Family Studies, 9* (4), 509-528.

Levy, S.R. Lampman, C., Handler, A., Flay, B.R., & Weeks, K. (1993). Young adolescent attitudes towards sex and substance use: Implications for AIDS prevention. *AIDS Education and Prevention, 5,* 340-351.

Lewis, C.E., & Lewis, M.A. (1984). Peer pressure and risk-taking behaviors in children. *American Journal of Public Health, 74* (6), 172-194.

Moore, S.M., & Rosenthal, D. A. (1993). Venturesomeness, impulsivity, and risky behavior among older adolescents. *Perceptual & Motor Skills, 76*(1), 98.

Mueller, K.E., & Powers, W.G. (1990). Parent-child sexual discussion: perceived communicator style and subsequent behavior. *Adolescence, XXV* (98), 469-482.

Okwumabua, J.O., Okwumabua, T.M., Hayes, A., & Stovall, K. (1994) Cognitive level and health decision making in children: a preliminary study. *Journal of Primary Prevention, 14* (4), 279-287.

Paikoff, R.L. (1995). Early heterosexual debut: Situations of sexual possibility during the transition to adolescence. *American Journal of Orthopsychiatry, 65,* 389-401.

Parfenoff, S. H., McCormick, A., & Paikoff, R. L. (1996). *Parents' communication with preadolescents about HIV/AIDS: Implications for prevention.* Poster presented at the XI International Conference on AIDS: Role of Families in Preventing and Adapting to HIV/AIDS, Vancouver, British Columbia, Canada.

Pearl, R., Bryan, T., & Herzog, A. (1990). Resisting or acquiescing to peer pressure to engage in misconduct: adolescents' expectations of probable consequences. *Journal of Youth and Adolescence, 19* (1) 43-55.

Pick, S., & Palos, P.A. (1995). Impact of the family on the sex lives of adolescents. *Adolescence, 30* (119), 667-675.

Pleydon, A.P., & Schner, J.G. (2001). Female adolescent friendship and delinquent behavior. *Adolescence, 36* (143), 189-205.

Pretorius, J.W.M., Ferreira, G.V., & Edwards, D.N. (1999). Crisis phenomena among African American adolescents. *Adolescence, 34* (133), 139-146.

Ramirez-Valles, J., Zimmerman, M., & Juarez, L. (2002). Gender differences of neighborhood and social control processes: a study of the timing of first intercourse among low-achieving, urban, African American youth. *Youth and Society, 33* (3), 418-441.

Romer, D., Black, M., Ricardo, I., Feigelman, S., Kalijee, L., Galbraith, J. et al. (1994). Social influences on the sexual behavior of youth at risk for HIV exposure. *American Journal of Public Health, 84* (6), 977-985.

Rotheram-Borus, M.J., Mahler, K.A., & Rosario M., (1995). AIDS prevention with adolescents families. AIDS *Education and Prevention, 7* (4), 320-336.

Sadowski, C., & Kelley, M.L. (1993). Social problem solving in suicidal adolescents. *Journal of Consulting and Clinical Psychology, 61* (1), 121-127.

Santor, D.A., Messervey, D., & Kusumakar, V. (2000). Measuring peer pressure, popularity, and conformity in adolescent boys and girls: predicting school performance, sexual attitudes, and substance abuse. *Journal of Youth and Adolescence, 29* (2), 163-182.

Semlitz L., & Gold M.S. (1986). Adolescent drug abuse: Diagnosis, treatment, and prevention. *Psychiatric Clinics of North America, 9*(3), 455-73.

Sikkema, K.J., Brondino, M.J., Anderson, E.S., Gore-Felton, C., Kelly, J.A., Winett, R.A. et al. (2004). HIV risk behavior among ethnically diverse adolescents living in low-income housing developments. *Journal of Adolescent Health, 35*(2), 141-150.

Somers, C.L., & Paulson, S.E. (2000). Students' perceptions of parent-adolescent closeness and communication about sexuality: relations with sexual knowledge, attitudes, and behaviors. *Journal of Adolescence, 35* (137), 167-180.

Stanton, B. (1996). Longitudinal evaluation of AIDS prevention intervention. In *Adolescent and HIV/AIDS Research: A Developmental Perspective.* Rockville, MD.

Walker-Barnes, C.J., & Mason, C.A. (2001). Perceptions of risk factors for female gang involvement among African American and Hispanic women. *Youth and Society, 32* (3), 303-326.

Weissberg, R.P., Ayerst, T., Barone, C. & Schwab-Stone, M. (1992). The prevention and co-occurrence of high-risk problem behavior in urban adolescence. Unpublished manuscript, Department of Psychology, Yale University: New Haven, CT.

Wilson, W. J. (1987). *The truly disadvantaged: The inner city, the underclass, and public policy.* Chicago: University of Chicago Press.

doi:10.1300/J200v05n01_05

Social Support for African American Low-Income Parents: The Influence of Preadolescents' Risk Behavior and Support Role on Parental Monitoring and Child Outcomes

Scott Miller
Mary M. McKay
Donna Baptiste

SUMMARY. Urban parents, particularly single mothers living within inner-city communities, often struggle to obtain sufficient social support for themselves and for parenting. Support for these parents is particu-

Scott Miller, PhD, and Mary M. McKay, PhD, are affiliated with the Mount Sinai School of Medicine, Department of Psychiatry. Donna Baptiste, PhD, is affiliated with the University of Illinois, Chicago, CHAMP Collaborative Board, New York and Chicago.

Address correspondence to: Mary M. McKay, PhD, Professor of Psychiatry & Community Medicine, Mount Sinai School of Medicine, One Gustave L. Levy Place, New York, NY 10029.

The significant contributions of Drs. Roberta Paikoff, Carl Bell, Donna Baptiste, Sybil Madison-Boyd and the CHAMP Collaborative Boards in Chicago and New York and CHAMP participants and staff are acknowledged.

Funding from the National Institute of Mental Health (R01 MH 63662) and the W.T. Grant Foundation is gratefully recognized.

[Haworth co-indexing entry note]: "Social Support for African American Low-Income Parents: The Influence of Preadolescents' Risk Behavior and Support Role on Parental Monitoring and Child Outcomes." Miller, Scott, Mary M. McKay, and Donna Baptiste. Co-published simultaneously in *Social Work in Mental Health* (The Haworth Press, Inc.) Vol. 5, No. 1/2, 2007, pp. 121-145; and: *Community Collaborative Partnerships: The Foundation for HIV Prevention Research Efforts* (ed: Mary M. McKay, and Roberta L. Paikoff) The Haworth Press, Inc., 2007, pp. 121-145. Single or multiple copies of this article are available for a fee from The Haworth Document Delivery Service [1-800-HAWORTH, 9:00 a.m. - 5:00 p.m. (EST). E-mail address: docdelivery@haworthpress.com].

larly important given the prevalence of risk-taking behaviors among youth in these communities, which necessitates vigilant monitoring of these youth. The current study explored from whom low-income mothers obtain social support, the influence of child externalizing on source of social support, and how social support and child behavior interrelate with parental monitoring and supervision. Contrary to expectations, parental monitoring at time 1 did not predict child externalizing at time 2, but, as expected, a significant negative association was noted at time 1 between these constructs. Higher time 1 child externalizing did predict lower time 2 maternal monitoring, suggesting frustrated efforts by mothers to monitor high externalizing children. Mothers reporting strong support networks, however, showed higher levels of monitoring, and mothers who turned to children for social support also showed a tendency to monitor more closely. Although mothers of high externalizing children reported poor support quality, mothers did not discriminate between high and low externalizing children when choosing source of social support. These findings suggest the importance of monitoring prior to child initiation into risk-taking behavior, and the possible role of children in strengthening support networks. doi:10.1300/J200v05n01_06

[Article copies available for a fee from The Haworth Document Delivery Service: 1-800-HAWORTH. E-mail address: <docdelivery@haworthpress.com> Website: <http://www.HaworthPress.com> © 2007 by The Haworth Press, Inc. All rights reserved.]

KEYWORDS. Single urban mothers, parental support, child externalizing, monitoring prior to initiation of risk-taking behavior

Parents rearing children within urban, low income communities must offer support and protection to youth against a contextual backdrop that can include unprecedented community-level violence, poverty, substance abuse, high prevalence rates of HIV infection, and sparse youth-supportive resources, including a serious shortage of mental health services (Attar et al., 1995; Bell & Jenkins, 1993; Black & Krishnakumar, 1998). These features of the urban environment have been linked with serious consequences for youth, necessitating HIV prevention programming to focus on factors operating at the level of the family, child, and community to provide protection for youth and foster health-promoting behaviors (Flay, 2002).

Nationwide, it has been estimated that between 5% and 10% of children between the ages of 8 and 16 evidence disruptive behavioral difficulties

(Angold & Costello, 2001). Yet, in urban, low-income communities, prevalence rates for youth externalizing behavioral difficulties may be up to four times national estimates (Gorman-Smith, Tolan, & Henry, 2000). Thus, HIV prevention programs must be prepared to assist in addressing elevated mental health needs. In addition, parents are in the unenviable position of simultaneously dealing with the impact of urban psychosocial stressors on themselves, attempting to protect their children from the potentially negative consequences of growing up within an inner-city context, reducing risk behaviors, and addressing the resulting mental health issues experienced by their children.

Yet, there is accumulating evidence to suggest that urban parents, particularly single mothers living within inner-city communities, do not have sufficient social support for themselves as individuals or for parenting (Wilson, 1995). A primary target for several family-based HIV prevention programs is to enhance parenting, particularly parental supervision and monitoring of youths' whereabouts and activities in order to delay onset of sexual activity and decrease risk-taking. Thus, the current study is meant to inform HIV prevention programming for urban youth and their families by exploring how low-income mothers attempt to obtain needed social support, the influence of child characteristics, such as child externalizing behaviors, on the choice of social support, and associations with parenting practices, specifically maternal monitoring and supervision. Implications for family-based HIV prevention programming and research are discussed.

CHILDHOOD DISRUPTIVE BEHAVIORAL DIFFICULTIES

Each year, billions of dollars are spent responding to the legal, correctional, educational and psychological needs of risk-taking youth (Burke, Loeber & Birmaher, 2002; Loeber, Burke, Lahey, Winderts & Zera, 2000). Nationwide, conduct difficulties and related risk-taking behaviors account for one third to one half of all child and adolescent mental health referrals (Loeber et al., 2000). A particularly salient factor associated with child externalizing and risk-taking outcomes is sociocultural context (Hammond & Yung, 1994), which includes neighborhood characteristics that may increase risk for poor child outcomes. Urban neighborhoods characterized by poverty, low employment rates, and a large percentage of families headed by single mothers may be especially prone to elevated psychosocial stressors, such as violence exposure (Wilson, 1995), and high rates of substance abuse and HIV infection (Osby, 1993), which may have serious consequences for children growing up in urban neighborhoods. According to Osby (1993), crime, drug use, and gang-related violence are among the most serious problems facing families in poor urban neighborhoods. About a quarter of mothers surveyed in a Washington D.C. housing project, for example, considered guns an ever-present danger in their neighborhood. Children in these neighborhoods may find it especially challenging to resist the strong pull of the peer culture, which may lead to their initiation into high-risk behaviors (Osby, 1993; Wilson, 1995).

PARENTING PRACTICES
AND DECREASING YOUTH RISK BEHAVIOR

Prospective studies have identified a robust set of risk factors for the occurrence and persistence of serious risk-taking behaviors during childhood. More specifically, poor parental discipline and monitoring (Dishion, French & Patterson, 1995; Klein & Forehand, 2000; Romer et al., 1994), within-family support (McCabe, Clark, & Barnett, 1999), and low level family interactions (Loeber & Stouthamer-Loeber, 1987; Tolan, Gorman-Smith, Huesmann, & Zelli, 1997; Biglan et al., 1990; Katchadourin, 1990) have all been empirically linked to the development of serious childhood conduct difficulties and sexual risk-taking behaviors. In addition, children may develop behavioral difficulties in the presence of family conflict (Brody, Stoneman, & Flor, 1996; Black et al., 1997), lack of parent-child bonding, stressors, inadequate behavioral limits and family disorganization (Kumpfer and Alvarado, 2003). There is also evidence to suggest that some parenting practices, such as poor parental monitoring and low acceptance and involvement with the child, are associated with disruptive behavior across cultures (Feldman, Rosenthal, Mont-Reynaud, Leung, & Lau, 1991) and ethnic groups (Steinberg, Darling, Fletcher, Brown, & Dornbusch, 1995).

Kazdin and Whitley (2003) emphasize specific family factors tied particularly to urban living, such as socioeconomic disadvantage, social isolation, poor living conditions, violence exposure, high levels of stress, and lack of social support that may undermine parenting and contribute to the development of childhood risk-taking behavior. African American mothers living in high-risk contexts, however, often tailor their parenting practices to lessen the likelihood of their children's involvement in high-risk behaviors (Mason, Cauce, Gonzales, & Hiraga, 1996). This style of parenting, sometimes called "no nonsense parenting" (Brody, Flor, & Gibson, 1999), features moderate levels of parental warmth and high levels of parental monitoring, control, and vigilance (Murry, Bynum, Brody, Willert, & Stephens, 2001). Furstenberg (1993) has noted a positive association between parental monitoring and youth who tend to steer clear of risk-taking behavior in the inner city. Also, high levels of behavioral control, which includes strict monitoring, has been found to be especially effective in reducing Black adolescents' risk-taking behavior when risk-taking behavior among peers was high (Mason et al., 1996). In this high-risk neighborhood context, strict monitoring of children's activities and whereabouts may prevent their involvement in dangerous situations that are often close at hand (Garbarino, Kostelny, & Dubrow, 1991).

Urban parents, therefore, play an important role in protecting youth from negative experiences within the urban environment, particularly by limiting negative experiences or buffering the influence of risk-taking peers. Furthermore, emerging evidence indicates that parents, typically mothers, rearing children in inner-city environments can adapt their parenting strategies in order to limit the influence of the neighborhood on their children and enhance developmental outcomes (Jarrett, 1995). For example, in addition to increasing supervision and monitoring efforts, urban mothers might foster connections with churches and youth programs in an effort to minimize violence exposure (Jarret, 1995). Further, a growing body of literature (Jarret, 1990; Jarret, 1992; Osby, 1993) suggests that minority families living in poor neighborhoods often utilize creative strategies for enhancing positive outcomes for their youth. These strategies serve to limit dangerous extrafamilial influences, thereby minimizing neighborhood dangers and setting up developmental trajectories characterized by reduced risk taking. For example, mothers may protectively seclude their children from dangerous influences (Osby, 1993), form strategic alliances with positive institutions (Jarret, 1995), or seek support from extended family (Jackson, 1998; Jarret, 1995) in order to improve their monitoring capacity and the safety of their children. Brody and Flor (1998), for example, found community organizations, religious institutions, and schools to provide enhanced monitoring for single African American mothers.

SOCIAL SUPPORT FOR LOW-INCOME AFRICAN AMERICAN MOTHERS

African American mothers provide opportunities for their youth through their own supportive adult networks, particularly family members who help to monitor youth, and make connections to other resources (e.g., churches and schools). Networks of extended family and friends who support these mothers are one of most direct influences on parenting practices (Cochran & Nieglo, 1995). According to this body of research, supportive networks are a source of instrumental, emotional, and informational support for mothers, all of which may strengthen mothers' efforts to monitor and supervise their children (Crockenberg, 1988). For example, supportive individuals may reduce mothers' stress, thereby providing additional psychosocial resources for monitoring (Jarret, 1994). Furthermore, supportive networks provide emotional support that helps mothers see themselves as capable being a good parent in the midst of a challenging environment (Boyd-Franklin, 1989). The benefits of a supportive network may also spill over into child outcomes. In a sample of sixth grade children of single African American mothers, for example, social support from extended family members was associated with lower levels of child externalizing behaviors (McCabe et al., 1999). Furthermore, Taylor (2000) reported that African American mothers in high crime areas who reported more neighborhood resources tended to have adolescents with lower levels of risk-taking behavior.

CHILDREN AS SOCIAL SUPPORT RESOURCES

A much less studied area is the consideration of children as sources of social support for single African American mothers, and how children's instrumental and emotional support of single mothers influences children's and mothers' psychological well-being and behavioral health outcomes. Elevated levels of instrumental caregiving have been observed in African American families (Jurkovic, Morrell, & Casey, 2001), as children may be a valuable resource to single mothers living in poverty. Others (Wells & Jones, 2000), however, have warned that parents who have unrealistic caregiving expectations for their children may rob their children of developmentally appropriate experiences that are important for adjustment to adulthood. This type of excessive caregiving has been termed "parentification" (Boszormeny-Nagy & Spark, 1973) and has been found to forecast adjustment problems in adulthood (Hetherington, 1990). Jurkovic and colleagues (2001), however, found that African American children who performed more instrumental caregiving did not perceive this as unfair. Because other family members can serve as an important source of social support for single-parent mothers living in poverty (Jarret, 1992), it is important to know how social support from children, which may be culturally normative for African American families (Harrison, Wilson, Pine, Chan, & Buriel, 1990), affects the psychological adjustment of these children. Furthermore, because maternal monitoring can serve as a key deterrent against children's behavior problems (e.g., Furstenberg, 1993; Klein & Forehand, 2000), it is important to learn the extent to which children's support of single mothers enables mothers to devote more resources to monitoring their children. Finally, given the high levels of need present in inner-city children, it is important to learn the extent to which mothers discriminate between youth at risk and less affected youth when seeking social support.

Based on the preceding considerations, the present study sought to answer the following research questions:

1. What is the relationship between maternal monitoring and child externalizing behavior both concurrently and over a two-month period?
2. To what extent is mothers' reliance on her children for social support associated with maternal monitoring both concurrently and over a two-month period?
3. To what extent is quality of social support associated with maternal monitoring both concurrently and over a two-month period?
4. To what extent are mothers likely to choose children with high levels of externalizing behavior as sources of social support?
5. To what extent do mothers of high externalizing children receive quality social support from their support networks?

METHOD

Participants

The sample involved in the present study was recruited to be part of the CHAMP (Chicago HIV prevention and Adolescent Mental Health Project) Family Program Study (McKay, Baptiste, Coleman, Madison,

Paikoff, & Scott, 2000). CHAMP is a family-based HIV prevention program whose primary targets are 4th and 5th grade African American children from low-income families living in a community with high rates of HIV. Data were collected at two time points approximately two months apart from the children and their mothers. All children were randomly selected from a roster of 550 children who attended four inner-city schools in a large midwestern city. Research staff made presentations to these classrooms, met with parents at the schools, and made phone calls or home visits in order to secure consent from parents for the children to participate in the study (McCormick, McKernan-McKay, Wilson, McKinney, Paikoff, Bell et al., 2000). A total of 209 children provided data across time points.

All children in the sample were 9 to 11 years of age, and approximately 52% were female. About 89% of mothers were teenagers at the time of their first child's birth, and about 74% were unmarried at the time of assessment. Approximately 93% of mothers had finished high school. Almost three-quarters of the families were exclusively on public assistance, and all participants lived in federally subsidized housing indicative of poverty status. Thus, the children in the present study were primarily living in poverty, and most had unmarried mothers with at least a high school education.

Data Collection

Three of the measures used for the present study were collected prior to the CHAMP family-based intervention that sought to decrease sexual risk-taking and reduce risk of HIV exposure. These measures included (1) parent and child reports of mothers' monitoring, (2) parent report of children's externalizing behaviors, and (3) parent report of social support. Monitoring and CBCL were also examined two months later after the intervention was completed. At both baseline and post-intervention assessments, the child or caregiver completed paper and pencil measures in small groups with research staff reading each item aloud. Families were paid $25 for their participation.

Measures

Child Behavior Checklist (CBCL; Achenbach & Edelbrock, 1983). Mothers completed the externalizing disorders subscale from this common measure of childhood mental health symptomatology for children and youth aged 4 to 18. Mothers completed this measure both at baseline and approximately two months after baseline assessment. The excellent internal consistency of this subscale ($\alpha = .90$) has been noted in past research (Schiff & McKay, 2003) using data from the same general sample of youth. Mothers responded "not true (1)," "sometimes (2)," or "very true (3)" to 37 statements indicative of externalizing behavior. A composite score was computed by summing across all items with higher scores indicating higher externalizing symptoms.

Mother's monitoring. Mothers completed the House Rules–Parent Version subscale of the Family Assessment Measure (Gorman-Smith, Tolan, Zelli, & Huesman, 1996) at both baseline and follow-up assessments. This subscale served as a measure of maternal monitoring of the child's behavior. Previous research (Schiff & McKay, 2003) using the same general sample found adequate internal consistency ($\alpha = .78$) for this subscale. Mothers responded "always true (1)," "usually true (2)," "usually false (3), or "always false (4)" to statements indicative of maternal monitoring behavior. Five of the seventeen items were reverse coded (e.g., "My child is allowed to have friends over to my house when I am not home"), and therefore required recoding of values for analyses. A composite score was computed by summing across all items with higher scores indicating higher levels of monitoring.

Youth completed the House Rules–Child Version subscale of the Family Assessment Measure (Gorman-Smith et al., 1996) at both baseline and follow-up assessments. As with the parent version, youth responded "always true (1)," "usually true (2)," "usually false (3), or "always false (4)" to statements indicative of maternal monitoring behavior. Again, five of the seventeen items were reverse coded, but there was a total of only fourteen items. Again, a composite score was computed by summing across all items with higher scores indicating higher levels of monitoring.

Social support of mother. Mothers were asked to list the three most important adults in their lives, and were also asked to respond to 11 questions about each individual to determine the extent to which each of these individuals supported the mother. Mothers responded "always (1)," "most of the time (2)," "sometimes (3), "hardly ever (4)," or "never (5)" to statements indicative of supportive behavior. Support was examined in multiple areas, such as being available to the mother, providing practical help, taking time to listen, and not causing problems for the mother. Scores were summed across the 11 items and averaged to obtain an average support score across the three individuals chosen. Therefore, summary scores ranged from 11-55, with a score of 55 indicating the individual was optimally supportive. Two of the eleven items were reverse coded (e.g., "This person often criticizes me"), and were transformed before computing original summary scores.

In the present study, the extent to which the target child supported the mother was of primary interest. Therefore, a "child reliance" variable was created by summing the number of children that the mother chose as one of the three most important sources of social support. Forty- seven mothers chose at least one of their children as one of the three most supportive individuals in their lives, 25 mothers named two or more children, and 7 mothers named three children as comprising the most supportive individuals in their lives. Mothers who chose all adults, such as a spouse or sibling, as the three most important support persons were assigned a score of zero on the "child reliance" variable, indicating that adults were the primary means of social support for these mothers. Therefore, child reliance scores ranged from 0-3 depending on the number of children chosen as important by the mother. Analyses addressing total number of children as a factor that might artificially inflate the number of children chosen as social support resources showed no significant relationship ($r = -.13, p > .05$) between total number of children and number of children chosen as an important source of social support.

Data Analysis

Analyses involved bivariate correlations for all study variables, analysis of variance (ANOVA), and structural equation modeling via LISREL 8.54 (Joreskog & Sorbom, 2003). This version of LISREL is especially beneficial due to its ability to compensate for missing data via the full information maximum likelihood (FiML) feature. Although approximately 45% of the data was missing due to attrition over time, FiML used a likelihood function at the individual level to predict model parameters from all available data and from parameter estimates computed from existing data. The overall estimates were obtained by summing the likelihood functions related to each case. This procedure maximizes the use of available data, as opposed to other methods, such as listwise deletion, which may eliminate important information associated with individual cases missing large portions of data. Reliable missing data tools, such as FiML, are especially important in studies of urban children where neighborhood conditions make it difficult to retain participants over time.

Testing of Hypotheses

Testing of all hypotheses for the present study involved using structural equation modeling to test a series of nested models (Widamon, 1985). Specifically, this approach begins with testing the fit of a baseline model in which none of the parameters corresponding to hypothesized paths are freely estimated. Parameters corresponding to hypothesized paths are then freed one at a time to test both the improvement in the fit of the model and the strength of the hypothesized relationship. The difference in chi-squared values with the associated difference in degrees of freedom can be plotted on a standard chi-squared distribution table to assess whether freeing the path of interest resulted in a statistically significant improvement in fit. Both the statistical significance of path coefficients and statistically significant improvements in fit were used to test the present study's hypotheses.

Low chi-squared values indicate that the specified model has accounted for the majority of the covariation present among relevant variables. In other words, a chi-squared value of zero indicates a perfect fit of the specified model to the true model that exists in the population. However, because this statistic measures discrepancies from a perfectly fitting model, it tends to be an overly strict test of model fit. Furthermore, the chi-square statistic is highly sensitive to sample size, which is evident from the equation $\chi^2 = (N-1) F_{min}$, where F_{min} represents the minimum fit function. In order to obtain a broader measure of model fit, Hu and Bentler (1999) have recommended the root mean square error of approximation (RMSEA). The RMSEA represents the discrepancy per degree of freedom between the population data and the proposed model. Hu and Bentler (1999) recommend a cutoff close to .06, but Vandenberg and Lance (2000) have commented that values up to .08 may be accepted as indicating adequate fit.

The magnitude of path coefficients corresponding to hypothesized relationships were also used to test hypotheses. Because all study variables and LISREL output were standardized in the present analyses, these path coefficients may also be referred to as standardized beta coefficients. Because these coefficients are standardized, their value represents the amount of change in the predicted variable per unit change in the predictor variable.

The model depicting all hypothesized relationships is shown in Figure 1. The only parameters estimated in the baseline model, however, were the six latent variable variances, the eight observed variable vari-

FIGURE 1. Hypothesized Model

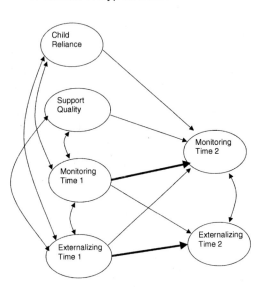

ances, and the causal paths from time 1 to time 2 maternal monitoring, and time 1 to time 2 child externalizing. Testing this model provided a baseline chi-squared value to which the chi-squared values of less restrictive models were compared. The first hypothesis addressed the relationship between maternal monitoring and child externalizing. Consistent with past studies (Klein & Forehand, 2000, Pettit, Bates, & Dodge, 1997), higher levels of maternal monitoring were expected to be negatively associated with child externalizing both concurrently and across time. To test this hypothesis, the path from time 1 maternal monitoring to time 2 child externalizing was freely estimated in the second model, and the improvement in fit via chi-squared was noted. Similarly, in the third model the path from time 1 externalizing to time 2 monitoring was freely estimated to assess possible bidirectional effects and improvement in fit was noted. Finally, to test the contemporaneous relationship of these constructs, their covariance at time 1 and 2 was freely estimated in the fourth and fifth models respectively.

The second and third hypotheses addressed the relationship of time 1 support variables to time 2 maternal monitoring. The second hypothesis addressed the extent to which mothers' reliance on their children was associated with mothers' monitoring of their children. Mothers who relied on their children for social support were expected to monitor their children more closely. To test this hypothesis, the path from child reliance to time 2 maternal monitoring was freed and the improvement in fit over the previous model was assessed. The quality of social support, whether from children or other adults, was also expected to positively predict more monitoring at time 2, so this path was also freely estimated and the decrease in chi-square was noted. Finally, the covariance of each of the support variables with time 1 monitoring was freely estimated to assess the contemporaneous relationships among these variables.

The final two hypotheses addressed the extent to which mothers of children with high levels of externalizing relied on their children for social support, and also the quality of support these mothers received from their children and other sources. Given the expectation that a mother's reliance on her child would be positively associated with her monitoring of that child, child reliance was expected to be associated with less child externalizing. Similarly, mothers who received quality support were expected to have children with fewer externalizing problems. Therefore, the covariance of each of these support variables with time 1 externalizing was freely estimated to assess the improvement in the fit of the model. Also, to provide additional evidence to inform these final two hypotheses, high and low externalizing groups were formed with a median split, and a one-way analysis of variance (ANOVA) examined whether a mother's reliance on her child and the quality of support were the same or significantly different across externalizing groups.

Therefore, in summary, the following five hypotheses were proposed:

1. Higher levels of maternal monitoring at baseline will be negatively associated with child externalizing at both baseline and two months later.
2. Mothers' reliance on their children for social support will be positively associated with mothers' monitoring of their children.
3. Social support quality at baseline from children and other adults will be positively associated with mothers' monitoring at both baseline and two months later.
4. Mothers' reliance on their children for social support will be associated with less child externalizing behavior at baseline.
5. Mothers' social support quality will be negatively associated with child externalizing behavior at baseline.

RESULTS

Data for all study variables showed no elevated skewness or kurtosis, and no outliers were noted. Intercorrelations, mean, and standard deviation for all study variables are shown in Table 1.

Child report of maternal monitoring ($r = .32$, $p < .02$), mothers' self-report of monitoring ($r = .36$, $p < .02$) and child externalizing ($r = .73$, $p < .001$) showed continuity across time, which is not surprising given the short two-month interval between assessments. The relatively weak association between mother's report and child's report on time 1 monitoring ($r = -.04$, $p > .10$) and time 2 monitoring ($r = .05$, $p > .10$), however, was surprising. Quality of support was marginally associated with mothers' self report of monitoring ($r = .17$, $p < .10$), but not child's report of mothers' monitoring ($r = -.04$, $p > .10$). Also, time 2 externalizing was marginally associated with child's report of time 1 maternal monitoring ($r = -.23$, $p < .10$), but not with mothers' self-reports of monitoring behavior ($r = -.01$, $p > .10$).

Nested Models Results

The baseline model estimated the six latent variable variances, the eight observed variable variances, the path from time 1 to time 2 mater-

TABLE 1. Intercorrelations, Means, and Standard Deviations for all Variables (N = 209)

Variable	1	2	3	4	5	6	7	M	SD
1. Monitoring (T1-Mother rep.)	-							60.55	5.62
2. Externalizing (T1-Mother rep.	−.09	-						53.02	11.16
3. Monitoring (T1-Child rep.)	−.04	−.09	-					47.15	4.82
4. Support quality (T1-Mother rep.)	.17+	−.12	−.04	-				42.59	5.78
5. Externalizing (T2-Mother rep.)	-.01	.73**	−.23+	−.19	-			52.98	9.45
6. Monitoring (T2-Mother rep.)	.36**	−.10	.16	.11	−.14	-		56.90	5.32
7. Monitoring (T2-Child rep.)	.17	.02	.32*	.15	.01	.05	-	48.26	5.15
8. Child reliance (T1-Mother rep.)	.04	.05	.12	−.13	.09	.12	.21	0.73	0.96

Note: Values rounded to 2 decimal places. + = p < .10, * = p < .05, ** = p < .01.

nal monitoring, and the path from time 1 to time 2 child externalizing. This model, as expected, showed poor fit: $\chi^2 = 195.26$, $df = 24$, $p < .05$), indicating a statistically significant difference between the proposed model and the model implied by the data. The root mean square error of approximation was .19, also indicating poor fit. Both monitoring ($B = .55$, $t = 4.10$, $p < .01$) and child externalizing ($B = .82$, $t = 9.00$, $p < .001$), however, showed expected continuity across time.

The first set of analyses addressed both the contemporaneous and longitudinal relationship of maternal monitoring and child externalizing. Freeing the path from time 1 maternal monitoring to time 2 child externalizing ($B = .01$, $t = 0.15$, $p > .10$), resulted in a negligible improvement in the fit of the model $\Delta\chi^2$ (1, N = 209) = 0.02, $p > .10$). Although freeing the path from time 1 externalizing to time 2 monitoring also resulted in a non-significant improvement in fit $\Delta\chi^2$ (1, N = 209) = 2.61, $p > .10$), time 1 externalizing did result in a significant residual decrease in maternal monitoring across time ($B = -.19$, $t = -1.79$, $p < .05$), indicating that mothers with lower levels of monitoring at time 2 tended to have children with high levels of externalizing behavior at time 1. Freeing the covariance between time 1 monitoring and externalizing ($\Phi = -.20$, $t = -1.75$, $p < .05$) resulted in a marginal improvement in the fit of the model $\Delta\chi^2$ (1, N = 209) = 2.81, $p < .10$), but freeing the time 2 covariance between these variables ($\Phi = .07$, $t = 0.78$, $p > .10$) did not improve model fit. In sum, as expected, child externalizing was negatively associated with maternal monitoring at time 1, and also predicted less time 2 monitoring, but, contrary to expectations, time 1 monitoring did not predict time 2 externalizing, nor were these variables associated at time 2.

The second hypothesis asserted that mothers who relied on their children for social support would monitor them more. Similarly, the third hypothesis asserted that mothers who received higher support quality would monitor their children more. Although child reliance was not associated with time 2 monitoring ($B = .03$, $t = 1.20$, $p > .10$), it showed marginally significant covariance with time 1 monitoring ($\Phi = .10$, $t = 1.43$, $p < .10$). Support quality, however, was associated both contemporaneously with maternal monitoring ($\Phi = .29$, $t = 1.77$, $p < .05$), and also predicted positive residual change in monitoring over time ($B = .35$, $t = 1.97$, $p < .05$). There was marginally significant improvement in model fit when child reliance and support quality were added as predictors of time 2 monitoring $\Delta\chi^2$ (2, N = 209) = 4.80, $p < .10$). Furthermore, mothers who chose their child as a source of social support did not differ in support quality from mothers who chose only adults as sources of social support, $F(2, 105) = 0.901, p > .05$). More specifically, mothers reported mean levels of support quality indicative of adequate support whether they chose their children or adults as sources of social support.

The final two sets of analyses addressed the association between child externalizing behavior and the social support variables. The extant literature is unclear regarding which factors influence which individuals mothers choose for social support. A rational choice model, however, would suggest that if mothers do choose children as sources of social support, they would be most likely to gain reliable support from children with fewer externalizing problems. Results, however, showed no relationship between mothers' reliance on children and children's externalizing behavior ($\Phi = .03, t = 0.33, p > .10$). The literature is more clear concerning the relationship of support quality and children's externalizing (McCabe et al., 1999); therefore, it was expected that greater support quality would be associated with less externalizing behavior. Indeed, freeing the covariance between support quality and children's externalizing revealed a significant negative association ($\Phi = -.25, t = -1.75, p < .05$), and was associated with a marginally significant improvement in the fit of the model $\Delta\chi^2 (1, N = 209) = 3.10, p < .10$). In sum, the final two sets of analyses suggested that although the extent of children's externalizing behavior may not be associated with whether mothers seek support from their children, the quality of support, whether from children or adults, tends to be negatively associated with the extent of children's externalizing behaviors.

For all of the preceding LISREL analyses the covariance of mother's and child's reports of maternal monitoring was not freely estimated due to the negligible zero-order correlations between these variables. Zero-order correlations, however, do not partial out other influences that affect the relationship between variables. Because the fit of the final model after freeing all hypothesized paths was still poor, $\chi^2 = 175.48, df = 14, p < .05$, the covariance of mother's and child's reports at both time 1 and time 2 was freed, which resulted in a drastic improvement in the fit of the model, $\Delta\chi^2 (2, N = 209) = 140.30, p < .001$. A significant negative association between mother's and child's reports of monitoring was found at time 1, ($\Phi = -.74, t = -10.37, p < .001$), and a significant positive association between mother's and child's reports was found at time 2 ($\Phi = .37, t = 10.16, p < .001$). Therefore, mothers and their children significantly disagreed about maternal monitoring behavior at time 1, but were much more in agreement about maternal monitoring behavior post-intervention at time 2. The final model, shown in Figure 2, showed reasonable fit, $\chi^2 = 35.48$, $df = 12$, $p > .05$. Although the RMSEA (.097) was slightly above the .08 cutoff suggested by Vandenberg and Lance (2000), the χ^2 to degrees of freedom ratio was between 1-3, which, according to Arbuckle and Wothke (1999) indicates a good fit of the hypothesized model to the data.

DISCUSSION

The present study evaluated the relationship between maternal monitoring and child externalizing and how each of these factors relates to social support from children and other sources of social support. Of particular interest were the direction of effects regarding whether maternal monitoring would predict less child externalizing over a two month pe-

FIGURE 2. Results for Hypothesized Paths. + p < .10, * p < .05, **p < .01. Only Bolded Paths Estimated in Baseline Model. With All Hypothesezed Paths Estimated, $\chi^2 = 35.48$, $df = 12$, $p > .05$, RMSEA = .097

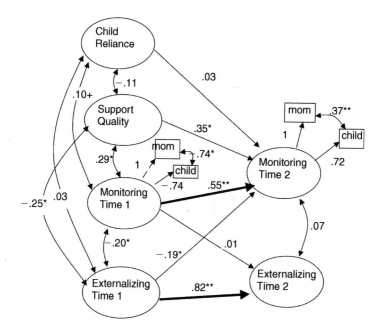

riod, or whether children with more externalizing behavior would evoke more or less monitoring from their mothers. Also of particular interest was whether a mother's reliance on her children for social support would be associated with increased monitoring, and whether overall quality of social support would bolster maternal resources such that maternal monitoring would be enhanced. Finally, the source of social support and the quality of support for mothers of high externalizing children was of interest. Specifically, we were interested in learning whether mothers are more likely to choose better behaved children as a source of support, and, given the challenge of parenting children with elevated problem behavior, whether mothers of these children were receiving quality social support from family and other sources.

Past studies (Klein & Forehand, 2000; Pettit et al., 1997) have indicated maternal monitoring as an effective deterrent against child externalizing behavior. Therefore, it was expected that more monitoring would be associated with less child externalizing both concurrently and across time. Because the research is more equivocal concerning whether children's problem behaviors evoke more or less maternal monitoring over time, analyses regarding this direction of effects were strictly exploratory. Regarding social support, mothers who relied on their children for support were expected to monitor their children more closely. It is not uncommon for African American children to provide instrumental support to parents, which may enhance the psychological resources available to these mothers (Jurkovic et al., 2001). Furthermore, consistent with past studies (Crockenberg, 1988; Jarret, 1994), the quality of social support from friends and family was expected to be positively associated with maternal monitoring. Finally, given that reliance on one's children and quality of support were expected to enhance maternal monitoring, and that monitoring was expected to be negatively associated with less child externalizing, both the extent of child reliance and the quality of support were expected to be associated with less child externalizing.

Maternal Monitoring and Child Externalizing

Contrary to expectations, baseline maternal monitoring did not account for a residual decrease in child externalizing over a two month period. There was a significant negative association between these variables at baseline, but, unexpectedly, these constructs were not associated with one another two months later.

However, although not specifically hypothesized, child externalizing at baseline was associated with a negative residual change in maternal monitoring. Monitoring showed moderate consistency across time points with baseline monitoring accounting for about 32% of the variance in maternal monitoring two months later. Baseline externalizing, however, explained an additional 4% of the variance in monitoring two months later such that mothers of high externalizing kids tended to monitor children less over time, and mothers of low externalizing kids tended to monitor children more over time. Therefore, it appears that although high levels of monitoring were not able to effect a change in child externalizing behavior across time points, mothers who were already engaging in high levels of monitoring behavior at time 1 tended to have kids who were staying out of trouble.

Social Support and Maternal Monitoring

Given that monitoring was expected to be associated with lower child externalizing, the second and third hypotheses addressed social support factors that may be associated with maternal monitoring. Mothers showed a moderate tendency to monitor more closely those children who they chose as social support resources, but showed even more stringent monitoring with their children when mothers reported quality social support from friends and family. Support quality was not only contemporaneously associated with elevated monitoring, but also accounted for 12% of the variance in monitoring two months later over and above the effects of baseline monitoring. Furthermore, mothers appeared to be receiving quality social support not only from other adults, but also from their children.

Social Support and Child Externalizing

The final two hypotheses addressed whether mothers of high externalizing children felt they could rely on these children, and whether these mothers were receiving adequate social support from friends and family. Mothers appeared to be relying on low and high externalizing children fairly equally for social support, which is consistent with Jurkovic and colleagues' (2001) observation of elevated levels of instrumental caregiving from children in African American families. Also, consistent with recent findings (McCabe et al., 1999; Taylor, 2000), mothers reporting greater support quality had children with lower levels of externalizing behavior. Furthermore, if one considers both the direct association of support quality with externalizing, and the indirect association via each of these construct's significant association with mother's monitoring, support quality accounts for almost 10% of the variance in child externalizing at baseline. In other words, mothers receiving quality support tended to monitor more, and mothers who monitored more tended to have children with fewer externalizing behaviors.

Auxiliary Results

A particular strength of the present study was the use of both mothers' and children's reports of maternal monitoring. The loadings of each informant's report on the latent maternal monitoring variable are similar to factor analytic loadings in which one is interested in how each observed variable contributes to the latent construct. At baseline, when a one-to-one relationship (for reference purposes) was set between mother's self-report of monitoring and the latent monitoring construct, children's report of monitoring showed a significant negative loading, revealing high disagreement between mothers and children concerning mothers' monitoring behaviors. Two months later, however, which as post-intervention, children's report of monitoring showed a significant positive loading, and mothers' and children's reports were significantly positively associated. Indeed, helping children and parents communicate more effectively was a goal of the intervention, so this finding is not surprising. Studies that focus more specifically on parent-child agreement concerning parenting behaviors may shed additional light on this issue.

Implications for HIV Prevention Programming

Results from the present study suggest several conclusions regarding how mothers, their support networks, and children can work together to optimize children's behavioral health and HIV prevention outcomes. Children growing up in dangerous urban neighborhoods are exposed to risky behaviors at a very early age (Osby, 1993; Wilson, 1995), which accentuates the importance of parental monitoring of these children. Indeed, the 4th and 5th grade children in this study were very persistent in their levels of problem behavior and risk taking. This was evidenced by the inability of maternal monitoring to effect any change in child externalizing across time. Children who were exhibiting high levels of problem behavior in 4th or 5th grade (at time 1), however, tended to have mothers who showed low levels of monitoring behavior at both time points. Therefore, it may be wise to intervene at an earlier stage so that mothers can establish consistent monitoring of their children, even as early as grades 1 or 2 in dangerous contexts such as the inner city.

Mothers in these neighborhoods cannot manage the task of monitoring on their own. Indeed, networks of family and friends are a primary source of instrumental, emotional, and informational support for mothers, and may enhance mothers' monitoring efforts (Crockenberg, 1988; Cochran & Nieglo, 1995). Therefore, HIV preventative interventions should seek to rally neighborhood support for mothers and teach family members how they can help in mothers' attempts to protect and educate children. Furthermore, results from the present study suggest that children as young as 4th or 5th grade may possibly serve as a support for parents, as overall support quality was only slightly lower when children were chosen as a primary source of social support, and monitoring was marginally enhanced when mothers turned to their children for support. Therefore, mothers may be wise to not only consider adults when seeking support for parenting, but also seek support from children from whom they feel they can obtain quality social support.

Limitations and Future Directions

Although results from the present study shed light on the interrelationship of support, monitoring, and children's behavior among Blacks in urban contexts, there are issues not addressed in the present study that are worth attending to in future studies in this area. First, a significant number of participants who participated in the study at time 1 were not able to be retained for assessment at time 2. This necessitated the use of sophisticated missing data techniques that, although powerful in estimating relationships in which sizeable portions of data are missing, always fall short of having available data. Future studies should consider ways in which young participants and their mothers can be retained across time points. Second, the children in this study were not originally intended to be potential social support resources for mothers. In other words, the child reliance variable was created by accident. Future studies should be more intentional in fine tuning this variable in order to further clarify the extent to which quality social support from children influences both maternal monitoring and children's externalizing behaviors.

Young children as a source of social support for African American mothers in poverty is not a new idea (Harrison et al., 1990). However, the examination of what types of children are sought for support and how children's support may possibly enhance parenting in these households is a relatively new area of research. It has become increasingly evident that extended family (Jackson, 1998; Jarret, 1995), and key community institutions (Brody & Flor, 1998; Jarret, 1995) enhance the monitoring capacity of mothers in African American families, which is often associated with better behavioral outcomes for children. We may be only just beginning, however, to learn the role that children themselves play in this process.

REFERENCES

Achenbach, T.M., & Edelbrock, C.S. (1983). *Manual for the Child Behavior Checklist and Revised Child Behavior Profile.* Burlington, VT: Department of Psychiatry, University of Vermont.

Angold, A., & Costello, J.E. (2001). The epidemiology of disorders of conduct: Nosological issues and comorbidity. In J. Hill and B. Maughan (Eds), *Conduct disorders in childhood and adolescence* (pp. 126-168). New York, NY, US: Cambridge University Press.

Attar, B.K., Guerra, N.G., & Tolan, O.H. (1994). Neighborhood disadvantage, stressful life events, and adjustment in urban elementary-school children. *Journal of Clinical Child Psychology, 23,* 391-400.

Bell, C., & Jenkins, E.J. (1993). Community violence and children on Chicago's southside. *Psychiatry: Interpersonal and Biological Processes, 56,* 46-54.

Biglan, A., Matzler, C. W., Wirt, R., Ary, D., Noell, J., Ochs, L., L., French, C., and Hood D. (1990). Social and behavioral factors associated with high-risk sexual behavior among adolescents. *Journal of Behavioral Medicine, 13,* 245-261.

Black, M.M., & Krishnakumar, A. (1998). Children in low-income, urban settings: Interventions to promote mental health and well-being. *American Psychologist, 53,* 635-646.

Black, M. M., Ricardo, I. B., and Stanton, B. (1997). Social and psychological factors associated with AIDS risk behaviors among low-income, urban, African American adolescents. *Journal of Research on Adolescent, 7*(2), 173-195.

Boszormenyi-Nagy, I., & Spark, G. (1973). *Invisible loyalties: Reciprocity in intergenerational family therapy.* New York: Harper & Row.

Boyd-Franklyn, N. (1989). *Black families in therapy: A multisystems approach.* New York: Guilford.

Brody, G. H., & Flor, D. L. (1998). Maternal resources, parenting practices, and child competence in rural, single-parent African American families. *Child Development, 69,* 803-816.

Brody, G. H., Flor, D. L., & Gibson, N. M. (1999). Linking maternal efficacy beliefs, developmental goals, parenting practices, and child competence in rural single parent African American families. *Child Development, 70,* 1197-1208.

Brody, G.H., Stoneman, Z., & Flor, D. (1996). Parental religiosity, family processes, and youth competence in rural, two-parent African American families. *Developmental Psychology, 32*, 696-706.

Burke, J.D., Loeber, R., & Birmaher, B. (2002). Oppositional defiant disorder and conduct disorder: A review of the past 10 years, part II. *Journal of the American Academy of Child and Adolescent Psychiatry, 41*, 1275-1293.

Cochran, M., & Nieglo, S. (1995). Parenting and social networks. In M. Bornstein (Ed.), *Handbook of parenting: Vol. 3, Status and social conditions of parenting* (pp. 393-418). Hillsdale, NJ: Lawrence Erlbaum.

Crockenberg, S. (1988). Social support and parenting. In W. Fitzgerald, B. Lester, & M. Yogman (Eds.), *Research on support for parents and infants in the postnatal period* (pp. 67-92). New York: Ablex.

Dishion, T. J., French, D. C., & Patterson, G. R. (1995). The development and ecology of antisocial behavior. (In D. Cicchetti & D. J. Cohen (Eds.), Developmental psychopathology (pp. 421-471). New York: Wiley.).

Feldman, S., Rosenthal, D.A., Mont-Reynaud, R., Leung, K., & Lau, S. (1991) Ain't misbehavin': Adolescent values and family environments as correlates of misconduct in Australia, Hong Kong, and the United States. *Journal of Research on Adolescence, 1.2*, 109-134.

Flay, B.R. (2002). Positive youth development requires comprehensive health promotion programs. *American Journal of Health Behavior, 26*, 407-424.

Furstenburg, F. J., Jr. (1993). How families manage risk and opportunity in dangerous neighborhoods. In W. J. Wilson (Ed.), *Sociology and the public agenda* (pp. 231-258). Newbury Park, CA: Sage.

Garbarino, J., Kostelny, K., & Dubrow, N. (1991). *No place to be a child: Growing up in war zone.* Lexington, MA: Lexington.

Gorman-Smith, D., Tolan, P.H., & Henry, D.B. (2000). A developmental-ecological model of the relation of family functioning to patterns of delinquency. *Journal of Quantitative Criminology, 16*, 169-198.

Gorman-Smith, D., Tolan, P. H., Zelli, A., & Huesman, L. R. (1996). The relation of family functioning to violence among inner-city minority youth. *Journal of Family Psychology, 10*, 115-129.

Hammond, W. R., & Yung, B. R. (1994). Preventing violence in at-risk African American youth. *Journal of Health Care for the Poor and Underserved, 2*, 1-16.

Harrison, A. O., Wilson, M. N., Pine, C. J., Chan, S. Q., & Buriel, R. (1990). Family ecologies of ethnic minority children. *Child Development, 61*, 347-363.

Hetherington, M.E. (1990). Coping with family transitions: Winners, losers, and survivors. *Annual Progress in Child Psychiatry and Child Development*, 221-241.

Hu, L., & Bentler, P.M. (1999). Cutoff criteria for fit indexes in covariance structure analysis: Conventional criteria versus new alternatives. *Structural Equation Modeling, 6*, 1-55.

Jackson, A. (1998). The role of social support in parenting for low-income, single African American mothers. *Social Service Review, 72*, 365-379.

Jarret. R. L. (1990). *A comparative examination of socialization patterns among low-income African Americans, Chicanos, Puerto Ricans, and Whites: A review of the ethnographic literature.* New York: Social Science Research Council.

Jarret, R. L. (1992). A family case study: An examination of the underclass debate. In G. K. Gilgun, G. Handel, & K. Dill (Eds.), *Qualitative methods In family research* (pp. 172-197). Newbury Park, CA: Sage.

Jarret, R. L. (1994). Living poor: Family life among single-parent, African American women. *Social Problems, 41,* 30-39.

Jarret, R. L. (1995). Growing up poor: The family experiences of socially mobile youth In low-income African American neighborhoods. *Journal of Adolescent Research, 10,* 111-135.

Joreskog, K., & Sorbom, D. (2003). *Lisrel 8 (Version 8.54) [Computer software].* Chicago: SSI, Inc.

Kazdin, A.E., & Whitley, M.K. (2003). Treatment of parental stress to enhance therapeutic change among children referred for aggressive and antisocial behavior. *Journal of Consulting and Clinical Psychology, 71,* 504-515.

Klein, K., & Forehand, R. (2000). Family processes as resources for African American children exposed to a constellation of sociodemographic risk factors. *Journal of Clinical Child Psychology, 29,* 53-65.

Kumpfer, K.A., & Alvarado, R. (2003). Family-strengthening approaches for the prevention of youth problem behaviors. *American Psychologist, 58,* 457-465.

Loeber, R., Burke, J.D., Lahey, B.B., Winderts, A., & Zera, M. (2000). Oppositional defiant and conduct disorder: A review of the past 10 years, Part I. *Journal of the American Academy of Child and Adolescent Psychiatry, 39,* 1468-1484.

Loeber, R., & Stouthamer-Loeber, M. (1987). Prediction. In H.C. Quay (Ed)., *Handbook of juvenile delinquency* (pp. 325-382). Oxford, England: John Wiley & Sons.

Mason, C. A., Cauce, A. M., Gonzales, N., & Hiraga, Y. (1996). Neither too sweet nor too sour: Problem peers, maternal control, and problem behavior in African American Adolescents. *Child Development, 67,* 2115-2130.

McCabe, K., Clark, R.,& Barnett, D. (1999). Family protective factors among urban African American youth. *Journal of Clinical Psychology, 28,* 137-150.

McCormick, A., McKernan-McKay, M., Wilson, M., McKinney, L., Paikoff, R., Bell, C., et al. (2000). Involving families in an urban HIV preventive intervention: How community collaboration addresses barriers to participation. *AIDS Education and Prevention, 12,* 299-307.

McKay, M., Baptiste, D., Coleman, D., Madison, S., Paikoff, R., & Scott, R. (2000). Preventing HIV risk exposure in urban communities: The CHAMP Family Program. In W. Pequegnat & J. Szapocznic (Eds.), *Working with families in the era of HIV/AIDS* (pp. 67-87). Thousand Oaks, CA: Sage.

Murry, V.M., Bynum, M.S., Brody, G.H., Willert, A., & Stephens, D. (2001). African American single mothers and children in context: A review of studies on risk and resilience. *Clinical Child and Family Psychology Review, 4,* 133-155.

Osby, O. (1993). *World views and child rearing behaviors of African American women in public housing.* Unpublished doctoral dissertation, Howard University, Washington, DC.

Pettit, G.S., Bates, J.E., & Dodge, K.A. (1997). Supportive parenting, ecological context, and children's adjustment. *Child Development, 68,* 908-923.

Romer, D., Black, M., Ricardo, I., Feigelman, S., Kalijee, L., Galbraith, J. et al. (1994).m Social influences on the sexual behavior of youth at risk for HIV exposure. *American Journal of Public Health, 84* (6), 977-985.

Schiff, M., & McKay, M. (2003). Urban youth disruptive behavior difficulties: Exploring association with parenting and gender. *Family Process*, *42*, 517-529.

Steinberg, L. Darling, N.E., Fletcher, A.C., Brown, B.B., & Dornbusch, S.M. (1995). Authoritative parenting and adolescent adjustment: An ecological journey. In P. Moen, G.H. Elder, & K. Luescher (Eds.), *Examining lives in context: Perspectives on the ecology of human development* (pp. 423-466). Washington, DC, US: American Psychological Association.

Taylor, R.D. (2000). An examination of the association of African American mothers' perceptions of their neighborhoods with their parenting and adolescent adjustment. *Journal of Black Psychology*, *26*, 267-287.

Tolan, P.H., Gorman-Smith, D., Huesmann, L., & Zelli, A. (1997). Assessment of family relationship characteristics: A measure to explain risk for antisocial behavior and depression among urban youth. *Psychological Assessment*, *9*, 212-223.

Vandenberg, R. J., & Lance, C. E. (2000). A review and synthesis of the measurement invariance literature: Suggestions, practices, and recommendations for organizational research. *Organizational Research Methods*, *3*, 4-70.

Wells, M., & Jones, R. (2000). Childhood parentification and shame-proneness: A preliminary study. *The American Journal of Family Therapy*, *28*, 19-27.

Widamon, K. (1985). Hierarchically tested covariance structure models for multitrait-multimethod data. *Applied Psychological Measurement*, *9*, 1-26.

Wilson, W.J. (1995). Jobless ghettos and the social outcome of youngsters. In P. Moen, G. Elder, K. Luscher (Eds.), *Examining lives in context: Perspectives on the ecology of human development* (pp. 527-544). Washington, DC: American Psychological Association.

doi:10.1300/J200v05n01_06

Creating Mechanisms for Meaningful Collaboration Between Members of Urban Communities and University-Based HIV Prevention Researchers

Mary M. McKay
Richard Hibbert
Rita Lawrence
Ana Miranda
Roberta Paikoff
Carl C. Bell

Sybil Madison-Boyd
Donna Baptiste
Doris Coleman
Rogério M. Pinto
William M. Bannon, Jr.

Mary M. McKay, PhD, Richard Hibbert, CSW, Rita Lawrence, BA, and Ana Miranda are affiliated with the Mount Sinai School of Medicine. Roberta Paikoff, PhD, Carl C. Bell, MD, Sybil Madison-Boyd, PhD, Donna Baptiste, PhD, and Doris Coleman, LCSW are affiliated with the University of Illinois at Chicago. Rogério M. Pinto, PhD is affiliated with the HIV Center for Clinical and Behavioral Studies. William M. Bannon, Jr., MSW, is affiliated with Columbia University, CHAMP Collaborative Boards in New York and Chicago.

Address correspondence to: Mary M. McKay, PhD, Professor of Social Work in Psychiatry & Community Medicine, Mount Sinai School of Medicine, One Gustave L. Levy Lane, New York, NY 10029 (E-mail: mary.mckay@mssm.edu).

Without the contributions of CHAMP Collaborative Board members and participants, this work would not have been possible.

Funding from the National Institute of Mental Health (R01 MH 63662) and the W. T. Grant Foundation is gratefully acknowledged. Dr. Pinto is a post-doctoral fellow at the HIV Center for Clinical and Behavioral Studies (New York State Psychiatric Institute and Columbia University) supported by a training grant from the NIMH (T32 MH19139 Behavioral Sciences Research in HIV Infection). The HIV Center is supported by a center grant from NIMH (P30 MH43520). William Bannon is currently a pre-doctoral fellow at the Columbia University School of Social Work supported by a training grant from the National Institutes of Mental Health (5T32MH014623-24).

[Haworth co-indexing entry note]: "Creating Mechanisms for Meaningful Collaboration Between Members of Urban Communities and University-Based HIV Prevention Researchers." McKay, Mary M. et al. Co-published simultaneously in *Social Work in Mental Health* (The Haworth Press, Inc.) Vol. 5, No. 1/2, 2007, pp. 147-168; and: *Community Collaborative Partnerships: The Foundation for HIV Prevention Research Efforts* (ed: Mary M. McKay, and Roberta L. Paikoff) The Haworth Press, Inc., 2007, pp. 147-168. Single or multiple copies of this article are available for a fee from The Haworth Document Delivery Service [1-800-HAWORTH, 9:00 a.m. - 5:00 p.m. (EST). E-mail address: docdelivery@haworthpress.com].

SUMMARY. This article provides a description of a Community/University Collaborative Board, a formalized partnership between representatives from an inner-city community and university-based researchers. This Collaborative Board oversees a number of research projects focused on designing, delivering and testing family-based HIV prevention and mental health focused programs to elementary and junior high school age youth and their families. The Collaborative Board consists of urban parents, school staff members, representatives from community-based agencies and university-based researchers. One research project, the CHAMP (Collaborative HIV prevention and Adolescent Mental health Project) Family Program Study, an urban, family-based HIV prevention project will be used to illustrate how the Collaborative Board oversees a community-based research study. The process of establishing a Collaborative Board, recruiting members and developing subcommittees is described within this article. Examples of specific issues addressed by the Collaborative Board within its subcommittees, Implementation, Finance, Welcome, Research, Grant writing, Curriculum, and Leadership, are detailed in this article along with lessons learned. doi:10.1300/J200v05n01_07 *[Article copies available for a fee from The Haworth Document Delivery Service: 1-800-HAWORTH. E-mail address: <docdelivery@haworthpress.com> Website: <http://www.HaworthPress.com> © 2007 by The Haworth Press, Inc. All rights reserved.]*

KEYWORDS. Community collaborative board, family-based HIV prevention and mental health, community board recruitment and development, elementary and junior high school age youth and their families

Collaboration with key community constituents has been described as necessary to: (1) enhance relevance of research questions; (2) develop research procedures that are acceptable to potential participants; (3) address obstacles to conducting community-based research activities; (4) maximize usefulness of research findings; and (5) expand community-level resources to sustain youth-focused intervention and prevention programs beyond research or demonstration funding (Israel, Schulz, Parker & Becker, 1998; Institute of Medicine, 1998; Schensul, 1999; Trickett, Hoagwood & Jensen, 1999; Wandersman, 2003). The urgency to increase collaborative participatory research efforts has been logically associated with pressing public health epidemics (National Institute of Mental Health, 1998). The AIDS epidemic, now entering its third decade, is an example of a serious public health issue which has mobilized prevention scientists, health and mental health care providers and community members to come together and collaborate in an effort to decrease rates of infection.

Over the last three decades, the focus of HIV prevention collaborations has shifted. This shift has followed the demographic changes of the epidemic as it began to penetrate ethnic minority communities and particularly impact young people. This article, therefore, focuses on adolescent HIV preventative research efforts as teenagers, particularly urban youth of color, are among the fastest growing populations at risk for HIV infection (Center for Disease Control, 2001; 2000; 1998).

Adolescents now account for more than 25% of all sexually transmitted diseases reported annually. Young females and minority youth are disproportionately affected by STDs and HIV infections (Centers for Disease Control, 2000; 1998; DiLorenzo & Hein, 1993; Jemmott & Jemmott, 1992). Over the last ten years, the incidence of HIV infection has raised dramatically in low income, ethnic minority neighborhoods. African American and Latino youth are over represented among those living in urban, poor neighborhoods, which increase their likelihood of exposure to HIV and other sexual transmitted disease. The likelihood of exposure for sexually active youth relates to higher overall rates of neighborhood HIV prevalence, along with poorer access to preventive health care, early detection and treatment services (Centers for Disease Control, 2001; Institute of Medicine, 1997; Miller, Clark, & Moore, 1997; Minnis & Padian, 2001; Rotheram-Borus, Mahler & Rosario, 1995; Wilson, 1987).

Prevention scientists have developed and tested a number of sexual risk reduction and STD and HIV prevention programs targeting urban minority youth (Forehand, Miller, Armistead, Kotchick, & Long, 2003; Kirby, Short, Collins, Rugg, Kolbe, Howard, Miller, Sonenstein, & Zahan, 1994; Jemmott, Jemmott & Fong, 1997). The Centers for Disease Control has published a compendium of such evidence-based programs in an attempt to more widely disseminate needed prevention services to urban youth (Centers for Disease Control, 2001). However, efforts to transport empirically supported prevention programs have encountered numerous obstacles, including insufficient school-based resources, poor community participation and tensions or suspicions between community residents and outside researchers (Dalton, 1989;

Galbraith, Stanton, Feigelman, Ricardo, Black & Kalijee, 1996; Thomas & Quinn, 1991).

As a result, it is becoming clear that community-based HIV prevention programs targeting urban youth of color are likely to fail if they attempt to provide interventions in a non-collaborative manner (Aponte, 1988; Boyd-Franklin, 1993; Fullilove & Fullilove, 1993; Secrest, Lassiter, Armistead, Wychoff, Johnson, Williams, & Kotchick, 2004; Fullilove, Green, & Fulliove, 2000; Schensul, 1999) or neglect to design and implement programs that do not take into account the stressors, scarce contextual resources or target groups' core values (Boyd-Franklin, 1993; McLoyd, 1990; Sanstad, Stall, Goldstein, Everett, & Brousseau, 1999). Therefore, the establishment of strong community partnerships to support health prevention efforts is critical. Meaningful community participation enhances the chances that: (1) effective adolescent sexual risk prevention programs will be well received within urban communities; (2) programs can be sustained after federal funding and research has ended; and (3) greater efficacy might be achieved if target communities are involved in all phases of development and delivery of the program.

Below we provide a description a Community/University Collaborative Board, a formalized partnership between representatives from inner-city communities and university-based researchers currently in operation in Chicago and New York. These Collaborative Boards oversee a number of research projects focused on designing, delivering and testing family-based prevention and intervention services for elementary and junior high school age urban youth and their families. Each Collaborative Board consists of urban parents, school staff members, representatives from community-based agencies and university-based researchers. One research project overseen by the Board, the CHAMP (Collaborative HIV prevention and Adolescent Mental health Project) Family Program Study will be used as an example of how key stakeholders in the community are involved in every step of the research process, thereby, building further capacity for future prevention research oriented collaborations and community-level leadership (for a description see Paikoff, McKay & Bell, 1994; McKay, Paikoff, Bell, Madison & Baptiste, 2000).

In addition, we describe the role of the Collaborative Board in seeking additional funding for youth and family-focused programs and research studies, implementing the family-based program, overseeing research activities and disseminating findings. The process of establishing a Collaborative Board, recruiting Board members and developing task-oriented subcommittees is also described below. Examples of specific issues addressed by the Collaborative Board subcommittees (which are: Implementation, Finance, Welcome, Research, Grant writing, Curriculum and Leadership) are detailed in this article along with lessons learned.

ROLE OF COMMUNITY COLLABORATION IN HIV/AIDS PREVENTION RESEARCH

Prevention programs designed to increase health protective behavior in adolescents must be culturally sensitive (Weeks, Schensul, Williams, Singer, 1995) and also address developmental processes, specific reinforcers of risk behavior, relevant contextual factors, and a population's unique risk-profile (Brown & DiClemente, 1992). Given the nature of the behavioral changes that need to be made to avoid HIV infection, HIV prevention programs are often controversial. Minority communities, and in particular the African American community, have histories of mistrust regarding involvement with outsiders representing the government in research or programs aimed at improving health. Experience with projects such as the Tuskegee Syphilis Study, which deliberately misled African Americans in order to continue to study naturalistically a health problem for which a cure was available, have fueled misgiving regarding health promotion and prevention projects within communities of color (Madison, Bell et al.,; Stevenson et al., 1995; Thomas & Quinn, 1991; Dalton, 1989).

Given this history of mistrust, the importance of working with community members in the design, delivery and testing of youth-focused prevention research efforts has been stressed, especially those directed at reducing HIV risk behaviors. (Hatch, Moss, Saran, Presley-Cantrell, & Mallory, 1993; Eccles, 1996; Farhall, Webster et al., 1998; Stevenson & White, 1994). In order to guide prevention research efforts, a theoretical paradigm has been proposed. This model identifies four models of community collaboration ranging from community members involved as: (1) advice or consent givers; (2) gate keepers and endorsers of the research; (3) deliverers of research or programs (e.g., front line staff); and (4) active participants in the direction and focus of the research (Hatch et al.,

1993). This fourth level has been considered ideal for research and program delivery in under-served, low-income minority communities. Over time, through constitution of the Collaborative Board, the degree of collaboration around the design, delivery and testing of the CHAMP Family Program has increased to this fourth level, reflected in the significant role key community members play in the direction, leadership and testing and dissemination of findings discussed below (Madison, Bell et al., in press; Madison, McKay et al., 2000; McKay, Baptiste et al., 2000; McKay, Chase et al., 2004).

THE CHAMP FAMILY PROGRAM

The CHAMP Family Program, funded by the National Institute of Mental Health since 1995, was designed to impact three interrelated outcomes for pre and early adolescent youth: (1) decrease time spent in situations of sexual possibility; (2) delay initiation of sexual activity; and (3) reduce sexual risk taking behavior. The program was designed specifically to address the prevention needs of urban youth of color living in communities with high rates of HIV infection (see McKay, Baptiste et al., 2000; Madison, McKay et al., 2000; McKay, Chase et al., 2004 for a detailed descriptions of this program).

More specifically, the CHAMP Family program targets 4th and 5th grade youth (9 to 11 years of age) and their families. The program is developmentally timed to involve youth prior to the onset of sexual activity, but close to the beginning of early adolescence when initiation of sexual activity occurs for many youth. CHAMP also has adopted a family-based approach to support families, enhance family protective processes and bolster parenting skills as urban families attempt to rear children in urban environments where risks and psychosocial stressors are often elevated. The CHAMP Family Program study was also designed to address some of the serious difficulties that prior HIV prevention research efforts had encountered within urban communities, particularly low rates of participation, community misgivings about the appropriateness of HIV prevention programs for children and mistrust of program and project staff. Thus, a strong community collaborative research method was employed by investigators of the CHAMP Family Program study that draws upon key elements of participatory research paradigms (Israel et al., 1998).

COMMUNITY PARTICIPATORY RESEARCH

A range of descriptions and definitions of participatory or community collaborative research have been offered (Altman, 1995; Arnstein, 1969; Chavis, Stucky, & Wandersman, 1983; Singer, 1993; Israel et al., 1998). There is agreement on some central themes and core foundational principles of participatory research efforts. On the most basic level, participatory research has been described as "providing direct benefit to participants either through direct intervention or by using the results to inform action for change" (Israel, Schulz, Parker, & Becker, 1998, p. 175). Further, what distinguishes community collaborative research from other investigative approaches is the emphasis on the intensive and ongoing participation and influence of community members in building knowledge (Israel et al., 1998). Research questions that result from collaboration between researchers and community members tend to reflect the pressing concerns of community members, acknowledge the importance of indigenous knowledge and resources, rather than over relying on expertise brought by the university partner (Institute of Medicine, 1998; Minkler & Wallerstein, 2003; Secrest et al., 2004; Schensul, 1999; Stringer, 1996).

In sum, community collaborative research activities are defined by: (1) a recognition that community development must be a focus of research activities; (2) a commitment to build upon the strengths and resources of individual communities; (3) ongoing attention to involvement of all members of the collaborative partnership across phases of a research project; (4) an integration of knowledge and action for mutual benefit of all partners; (5) the promotion of a process that actively addresses social inequalities; (6) opportunities for feedback; (7) a commitment to addressing health problems from both a strength and an ecological perspectives and; (8) dissemination of findings and knowledge gained to all partners" (Israel et al., 1998; pp. 178-179). The CHAMP Family Program Study was guided by these principles of community participatory research and translated them into action via steps detailed next. A summary of these principles in action is provided (on page 158). Each phase of the research process from the design of the intervention, to the development of research procedures including data collection and recruitment/retention strategies, was viewed as an opportunity to identify mechanisms for maximum participation by community members.

OPPORTUNITIES FOR COLLABORATION
ACROSS THE RESEARCH PROCESS

Although one of the core tenants of community participatory research is the involvement of key community stakeholders in *every* aspect of the research process, there have been few systematic attempts to identify the choices available to community/research partnerships throughout a given research project that would make this recommendation a reality. McKay and colleagues (Madison, McKay et al., 2000; McKay, in press) have identified a range of concrete opportunities to collaborate and conceptualized possible levels of intensity during each research phase based upon prior work of Hatch et al. (1993). This model of collaboration across the research process is represented in Figure 1 and incorporates key aspects of a paradigm conceptualize by Hatch et al., 1993.

Low-intensity collaborations. Hatch and colleagues propose that initial collaborative efforts often begin with a relatively less intense form of collaboration whereby researchers consult with persons, either for advice or consent, representing agencies or institutions within a specific community. At the next stage of collaboration, researchers identify key informants from the community (e.g., representatives from churches, business, etc.) and seek acceptance of the research project. Although this group of key informants is considered to be representative of community stakeholders, the research agenda and therefore, the decision-making power remains with the researcher. As collaboration proceeds, influential community leaders might be sought out by investigators to provide advice and guidance at a particular point in a research study. Often they are asked to sit on ongoing advisory boards. Further, their assistance is actively sought so that community members can be hired by the project as paid staff and fill positions, such as interviewers or recruiters.

Moderate to high intensity collaboration characterizes the current CHAMP Community Collaborative Board structure. Hatch and colleagues (1993) indicate that although additional input is sought as collaborative efforts intensify, key decisions regarding who has ultimate control about research questions and decisions regarding research methods, procedures and interpretation of study results are critical. At the highest level of collaboration, the research partners, from both the university and community, work together to develop the focus of the research and an action agenda. Then, all partners are responsible for pursuing these shared goals. At the most intense level of collaboration, there is true partnership between community and university. The decision-making process is therefore a shared enterprise that recognizes the specific talents of both university and community members.

As indicated in Figure 1, researchers and community members can collaborate during all phases of the research process. For example, collaborative partnerships meant to increase *recruitment and retention* in youth-focused prevention research projects might develop strategies such as incorporating consumers as paid staff or community members as interviewers or recruiters. These community representatives can fulfill liaison roles between youth and families in need and prevention programs (Elliott et al., 1998; Koroloff et al., 1994; McCormick et al., 2000). In some cases, consumers are the first contact that a youth or adult caregiver has with a specific prevention project. This is the case within the CHAMP Family Program where community parent facilitators are trained to reach out to their neighbors and invite them to learn more about the program. As part of the training of CHAMP parent facilitators, they and their children have actually participated in the program. Thus, in addition to being able to provide information about the program to potential participants, CHAMP parent facilitators are also able to use personal, first hand experience to answer any questions that participants may have or address any concerns raised (see McCormick, McKay et al., for a detailed description of CHAMP parent facilitator recruitment efforts).

As one moves to the right in Figure 1, community/university partnerships can also focus on facilitating the *implementation* of prevention approaches. For example, preventative interventions can be delivered by "naturally existing community resources," such as teachers (Atkins, McKay et al., 1998) and/or parents (McKay et al., 2000). In the case of the CHAMP Family Program, each of the intervention sessions is co-facilitated by a mental health intern/parent facilitator team. All CHAMP facilitators, those with a mental health background and community parents, receive weekly joint training in the content of the CHAMP Family Program, in skills related to facilitation of child, parent and multiple family groups, in issues related to prevention research efforts and in protection of human subjects, including confidentiality and addressing mandated safety issues.

PROCESS OF ESTABLISHING A COMMUNITY/UNIVERSITY COLLABORATIVE BOARD

In 1995, the National Institute of Mental Health supported the development of the first Collaborative Board to guide the development, delivery and testing of a family-based HIV prevention program in an inner-city community with high rates of HIV infection. Thus, the first Collaborative Board was initially organized to consist of 15 to 25 members representing key stakeholders, parent community, partner schools, community-based youth-serving agencies and university-based researchers. This first Collaborative Board was initially organized to meet once per month, however, as the project evolved over time, some of the Boards in other sites began to meet two times per month. Each Collaborative Board member is compensated for their time either via stipends for each meeting attended or by employment as a staff member as part of the CHAMP Family Program study. Through the workings of the first Collaborative Board, the following conceptual model of Board development was defined and fine tuned (for additional details see Madison et al., 1995; Madison, McKay et al., 2000). Figure 2 summarizes the steps taken to formalize the partnership among members of the community, urban parents, school and community-based agency staff and university-based researchers.

First, the development of relationships between university-based researchers and community partners is based upon the building of trust. A major task in the initial stage of collaboration is the establishment of a mission statement that addresses all parties' visions for the collaborative work and serves as a guide for future work. The mission statement of the first Collaborative Board organized in Chicago is provided in Table 1 (Madison, McKay et al., 2000; McKay, Baptiste et al., 2000).

The second stage of collaboration concerns the exchange of information. A major task in this phase of the partnership is the development of a common language that facilitates communication between university and community partners. For community members, immersion in the project helps further their understanding of the research, while for university members, immersion in the community aids in their understanding of the context of the work. The third stage of partnership involves shared decision making. In this stage, the task is to share influence, such that multiple stakeholders are involved in determining the direction of the work.

Organizationally, the use of committees facilitates the sharing of decision-making and power. The following committees exist within the current Community Collaborative Board: Implementation, Finance, Welcome, Research, Grant writing, Curriculum and Leadership. More specifically, the *Implementation Committee* consists of representatives from the community, youth serving agencies, members of the university-based research team and the Principal Investigator of the CHAMP

FIGURE 1. Collaborating Across the Research Process

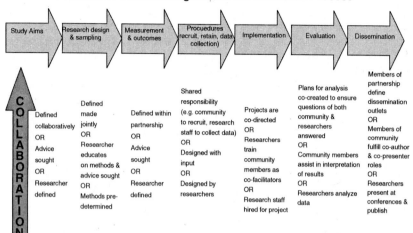

FIGURE 2. A Model of the Development of Collaborative Partnerships: Stages and Tasks

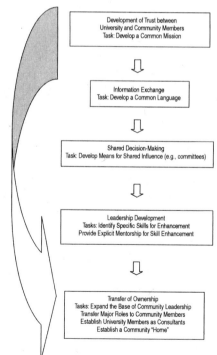

TABLE 1. CHAMP Family Program Mission Statement

(1)   We are committed to preventing families and children from getting HIV/AIDS.

(2)   We will not exploit communities in the process. We are doing research with and for communities, not to communities.

(3)   We want to increase communities' understanding of how research can be used against them so that they can protect themselves.

(4)   We want to increase communities' understanding of the strengths within their communities.

(5)   If a community likes the program, the research staff will help the community find ways to continue the program on its own.

Family Program Study. The Implementation Committee functions similar to that of a personnel committee or an overarching policy and procedures committee for the project. For example, this is the committee that interviews all candidates for employment as staff for the project. Committee members have developed a standard set of interview questions, application procedures and criteria for selection to ensure that suitable candidates are hired as project directors, research assistants and program facilitators. On the rare occasion that an employee is not performing tasks appropriately, it is also this Implementation Committee that meets with the employee and makes a decision as to whether to develop a remedial plan or terminate employment. The key to the success of the Implementation Committee in collaborative research projects is that community representatives are an important part of this decision making, thus increasing the perception of sensitivity and fairness by all.

The *Welcome Committee* was organized somewhat later in the process of establishing the Collaborative Board. Its primary responsibilities focus on orienting new members joining the Board. The Welcome Committee has developed a set of standard procedures and materials to assist new Board members in learning about: (1) the project; (2) HIV prevention; (3) organization of the Board; (4) mission of the Board; and (5) Board by-laws and CHAMP Family Program study policy and procedure manual. In addition, a member of the Welcome Committee serves as a mentor to a new Board member for the first six months of the new persons' involvement. The mentor provides opportunities to answer ongoing questions and support the integration of the new member into the social fabric of the Collaborative Board.

The *Research Committee* was organized to review: (1) research procedure used throughout the project, including recruitment or data collection procedures, and selection of measures; (2) progress of data collection and entry; (3) preliminary analyses; and (4) proposed presentations and publications of findings. The Research Committee also reviews all manuscripts, including this one, and approves each paper for presentation at a full Board meeting.

In preparation for involvement in the Research Committee, each member took an introductory research methods seminar that was that was facilitated by one of the University-based staff members over an 8-week period. This research seminar focused on: (1) formulating research questions; (2) generating testable hypotheses; (3) reading and reviewing the literature; (4) strengths/challenges of research designs; (5) available sampling strategies; and (6) conceptual description of data analytic approaches.

The Grant Writing Committee was established to seek research and services funding in order to plan for sustainability of innovations focused on youth and families within the community. During the initial phase of formation, members reviewed all aspects of funding process, from development of proposal narratives, to preparation of budgets, to the process of submission. Over time, committee members accepted increasing levels of responsibility, including reviewing literature, writing text, preparing draft budgets, obtaining letters of support and making contact with potential funders. This process lead to the successful funding of additional tests of family-based interventions, including those focused on substance abuse prevention, reduction of community violence exposure and child mental health.

Next, the *Curriculum committee*, again consisting of representatives from the parent community, agency and school representatives and university-based research staff, is responsible for developing the content of the family-based interventions and preparing intervention protocols to be used in training program facilitators and guiding program delivery. The development of curriculum is conducted in the following steps: (1) existing literature and programs are reviewed by the Curriculum committee; (2) an outline of key intervention targets are identified; (3) each session of the program is then written; (4) a first pilot test with families recruited from the community involved as both program participants and also consultants to the Curriculum committee is conducted; (5) revisions to the program are made based upon feedback obtained from the first pilot test; (6) a second pilot test of the program is conducted with new participants recruited from the community; and finally (7) members of the Curriculum committee and their preadolescent children participate in the final pilot test of the program to experience, first hand, the process and impact of the program and provide the opportunity to give the program a "community stamp of approval."

Another example of a Collaborative Board subcommittee is the *Finance Committee*. This subset of Collaborative Board members are responsible for three primary tasks: (1) overseeing and managing grant funding throughout the course of the project; (2) planning future expenditures and targets for fund raising; and (3) preparing and planning of budgets for new proposals. The Finance Committee is comprised of the Principal Investigator, the financial officer from one of the community-based organizations, the community coordinator and five community parent representatives. Early in the formation of the Finance Committee, the community-based finance officer organized a series of seminars for the committee members that focused on bolstering necessary skills. These seminars focused on: (1) reading financial statements; (2) understanding direct and indirect costs, fringe benefits, personnel and other than personnel expenses; (3) creating spread sheets to track expenditures; and (4) budget planning and completion of budget forms.

Finally, the *Leadership Committee* is responsible for the training and skill development of the Collaborative Board members. The main tasks of the Leadership Committee include: (1) identifying the skills needed to deliver the intervention and explicitly enhancing those skills through mentoring and training; and (2) supporting the personal development of Board members via identifying needed job training or educational opportunities. In addition, the Leadership Committee developed their own workshops or hired resources from the community to provide seminars. An example of one of the workshops organized is based on the book titled, *Who Moved My Cheese?*, by Spencer Johnson, M.D., which focused on helping Board members incorporate change at work and in life.

It is through these subcommittees that authentic decision making power and direction of the research project are shared among researchers and community members. Further, experiences within these subcommittees are meant to provide the opportunity for skill advancement and learning in order to prepare urban community representatives for future prevention oriented research projects and for ensuring the sustainability of programs like the CHAMP Family Program once research funding has ended. These set of opportunities is meant to prepare Collaborative Board members for the ultimate model of collaboration identified by Hatch and colleagues (1993).

Finally, the penultimate stage of university-community collaborative partnerships concerns leadership development (which is being en-

TABLE 2. Participatory Research Principles to Action in CHAMP

(1) Community development is a focus	Leadership Committee of Board; regular content training (e.g., information about HIV/AIDS, prevention research) and consistent opportunities for personal/professional development (e.g., communication and conflict resolution skill building).
(2) Builds on strengths of community	The entire project is guided by the premise that youth are at contextual risk for HIV exposure (e.g., living in a high HIV infection rate community) rather than youth or families being presumed to evidence specific individual risk factors, thus a strength-presumed, primary prevention approach has been adapted.
(3) Involvement of all members in each phase of the project	Board members are involved in defining project goals and research procedures; overseeing implementation; and dissemination of findings.
(4) Providing direct benefits to participants	Training, opportunities for skill and personal development for Board members.
(5) Promotion of a process that actively addresses social inequalities	Care has been taken to achieve salary equity in key project staff roles (e.g., project is co-directed by a university-trained staff member and talented community member, co-facilitators, parents and mental health interns, are paid exactly the same).
(6) Opportunities for feedback	The full CHAMP Collaborative Board meets one or two times per month, subcommittees meet frequently across each week, all members participate in a full day-day retreat at least once a year.
(7) Commitment to addressing heath problems from an ecological perspective	The CHAMP Family Program Study targets individual child and adult caregiver skills, family-level processes and community resources to meet the prevention needs of inner-city youth.
(8) Disseminating findings and knowledge gained to all partners.	CHAMP academic and community partners are responsible for co-presenting findings at research meetings, provider and community-oriented forums, community partners serve as co-authors on peer reviewed, newsletters and book chapter publications.

hanced by larger Board meetings and the committee work described in the preceding paragraph). The outcome of this stage of collaboration is the planning for sustaining of the program within a community-based organization once research or demonstration funding has ended. This planning for community transfer began several years prior to the ending of federal funding (see Madison et al., in press for a description of issues related to transfer of the CHAMP Family Program to community leadership). In sum, the organizational structure of the Board via regular full Board meetings and subcommittee work are key to putting participatory research principles into action (see summary in Table 2).

RECRUITING COLLABORATIVE BOARD MEMBERS

Recruitment of Collaborative Board members takes place in distinct phases with the goal of achieving representation of different segments of the target community, particularly underrepresented portions of the community. More specifically, in each city that a Collaborative Board was formed, urban parents who were involved in school related activities or who were employed at the school were likely to be tapped as initial members. For example, representatives of elementary or junior high schools' Parent Association were approached to become members of the Board. In addition, key youth-service agencies in the community were identified. Meetings with the executive director of these community-based organizations generally yielded the identification of a representative to attend Collaborative Board meetings. Once a core group of Board members had been identified, then a question posed at a Collaborative Board meeting was, "who is in this community that is not represented here?" For example, within the New York Collaborative Board, initially identified members were 60% African American and 40% Latino. Yet, the community targeted for the CHAMP Family Program was estimated to include at Latino population that made up 67% of the neighborhood. Thus, recruitment of additional Latino representatives was prioritized.

In addition, within the New York community, an influx of immigrants from Africa were arriving. Efforts to reach out and find representatives for these newly arriving groups of families was also made a priority for the Collaborative Board. Thus, in each of the sites, recruitment of a full complement of Board members took place over time, as long as 12 months, and increasingly was guided by identifying all segments of the community, not just those represented by parents who were easily accessible.

LESSONS LEARNED AND IMPLICATIONS
FOR FUTURE COLLABORATIVE EFFORT

The formation and ongoing attention to a collaborative partnership between researchers and community members requires significant time, attention and care by all partners. If the partnership is to be genuine in that consensus is strived for, decisions are shared and input is sought at every phase of research activities, then continual opportunities for communication, forums for discussions and mechanisms to solve differences must be available.

In order to accomplish a true partnership among university-based researchers and community constituents, both researchers and community members must consider change in their attitudes and behavior. For example, community stakeholders must have some willingness to overcome negative attitudes about research, as well as to bring an interest in learning more about research activities. To accomplish this, community members must be afforded opportunities to learn about the advantages and limitations of specific research designs and methods. Concepts such as random assignment and standardization must become familiar, along with the advantages and limitations of validated instruments.

Collaboration requires community constituents to take risks and share honest information with researchers regarding community needs, perceptions of research, ideas regarding cultural values and contextual norms. It must be understood that this is a risk given the serious concern that vulnerable communities often hold that researchers will use this information to reinforce negative stereotypes about the community and its' members (Stevenson & White, 1996). Finally, community partners must be willing to ask questions and seek clarification to ensure understanding. This is necessary in order to work productively and resolve conflicts and to ensure joint decision-making (McKay, in press). Not only must community partners accommodate to collaborative research projects, so too, must university-based researchers. University partners need to begin with a willingness to share information with community partners. Necessary information includes sharing knowledge regarding a research study's specific aims, primary hypotheses, advantages and limitations of research procedures and budgets. Further, in addition to the sharing of information, researchers need to have a level of openness to sharing control over decision making process. It is only when joint decision-making and consensus becomes the norm that trust can be established. In order to build a critical level of trust, researchers must proceed more slowly to ensure community participation and under- standing. This often requires the researcher to build in a longer period of start-up in order to ensure that community participation has been accomplished prior to the beginning of research activities. Finally, researchers need to accept substantial responsibility to provide ongoing training and support as constituents advance in their research skill development (Madison et al., 2000; Madison, Bell et al., in press)

CONCLUSIONS AND IMPLICATIONS

Increasingly, there have been calls to maximize community/prevention scientist collaboration in order to design relevant risk reduction programs for youth living within high risk urban contexts (Trickett, 1998). Concerns regarding the consequences of early and high risk sexual behavior for urban minority youth have been constant over the past several decades. HIV infection rates continue to rise in young people, with youth of color disproportionately affected. Programs designed specifically for these youth are critically needed (Center for Disease Control, 2001; 2000). Though collaboration with communities has been emphasized as a necessary component of building successful interventions, there are still too few models regarding how to develop and sustain such critically needed partnerships focused on HIV prevention programming and research activities. The Collaborative Board mechanism, described here, offers some encouragement that such structures can succeed in urban communities and be replicated across sites.

REFERENCES

Altman, D.G. (1995). Sustaining interventions in community systems: On the relationship between researchers and communities. *Health Psychology*, 14(6), 526-536.
Aponte, H.J., Zarskl, J., Bixenstene, C., & Cibik, P. (1991). Home/community based services: A two-trier approach. *American Journal of Orthopsychiatry*, 61(3), 403-408. 224.
Arnstein, S. (1969). The ladder of citizen participation. *Journal of American Institute Planners*, 35(4), 216-224.
Atkins, M., McKay, M., Arvanitis, P., Madison, S., Costigan, C., Haney, P., Zevenbergen, A., Hess., Bennett, D., & Webster, D. (1998). Ecological model for school-based mental health services for urban low-income aggressive children. *Journal of Behavioral Health Services and Research*, 25(1), 64-75.
Bourdieu, P. (1996). *The forms of capital.* In J.G. Richardson (Ed.). *Handbook of theory and research for the sociology of education.* New York: Greenwood Press.
Boyd-Franklin, N. (1993). *Black Families.* In F. Walsh (Ed.), *Normal Family Process.* New York: Guilford Press.

Brown, L. K. & DiClemente, R. J., & Park, T. (1992). Predictors of condom use in sexually active adolescents. *Journal of Adolescent Health,* 13(8), 651-657

Centers for Disease Control and Prevention (1998). *HIV/AIDS Surveillance Report, 9,* 1-43.

Centers for Disease Control and Prevention (2000). *HIV/AIDS Surveillance Report, 12* (2).

Centers for Disease Control and Prevention (2001). *Compendium of HIV Prevention Interventions with Evidence of Effectiveness.* Atlanta, GA: Author.

Chavis, D. M., Stucky, P. E. & Wandersman, A. (1983). Returning basic research to the community: The relationship between scientist and citizen. *American Psychologist, 38*(4), 424-434.

Dalton, H.L. (1989). AIDS in blackface. *Daedalus, 118* (3), 205-227.

DiLorenzo, T. & Hein, K. (1993). Adolescents: The leading edge of the next wave of the HIV epidemic. In J. L. Wallender, L. J. Siegel (Eds.), *Adolescent Health Problems: Behavioral Perspectives* (pp. 117-140). Advances in Pediatric Psychology. New York: Guilford Press.

Eccles, J.S. (1996). The power and difficulty of university-community collaboration. *Journal of Research on Adolescence,* 6(1), 81-86.

Elliott, D., Koroloff, N., Koren, P., & Friesen, B. (1998). Improving access to children's mental health services: The Family Associate approach. In Epstein, M. & Kutash, K. (Eds.), *Outcomes for children and youth with emotional and behavioral disorders and their families: Programs and evaluation best practices* (pp. 581-609). Austin, TX: PRO-ED.

Farhall, J., Webster, B., Hocking, B., Leggatt, M., Riess, C., & Young, J. (1998). Training to enhance partnerships between mental health professionals and family caregivers: A comparative study. *Psychiatric Services,* 49(11), 1488-1490.

Forehand, R., Miller, K. S., Armistead, L., Kotchick, B. A., & Long, N. (2003). The Parents Matter! Program: An introduction. *Journal of Child & Family Studies, 13,* 1-3.

Fullilove, M. T. & Fullilove, R. E., III. (1993). Understanding sexual behaviors and drug use among African Americans: A case study of issues for survey research. In D. G. Ostrow & R. C. Kessler (Eds.), *Methodological Issues in AIDS Behavioral Research* (pp. 117-132). New York: Plenum Press.

Fullilove, R. E, Green, L., & Fullilove, M. T. (2000). The Family to Family program: A structural intervention with implications for the prevention of HIV/AIDS and other community epidemics. *AIDS, 14* (Suppl 1), S63-S67.

Galbraith, J., Stanton, B., Feigelman, S., Ricardo, I., Black, M., & Kalijee, L. (1996). Challenges and rewards of involving community in research: An overview of the "Focus on Kids" HIV-risk reduction program. To be published in *Health Education Quarterly, 23* (3), 383-94.

Hatch, J., Moss, N., Saran, A., Presley-Cantrell, L., & Mallory, C. (1993). Community research: Partnership in black communities. *American Journal of Preventive Medicine, 9* (6, Suppl) 27-31.

Institute of Medicine (1997). *The Hidden Epidemic: Confronting Sexually Transmitted Diseases.* Washington, DC: National Academy Press.

Institute of Medicine (1998). *Bridging the Gap Between Practice and Research: Forging Partnerships with Community-Based Drug and Alcohol Treatment.* Washington, DC: National Academy Press.

Israel, B. A., Schulz A. J., Parker E. A., & Becker, A. B. (1998). Review of community-based research: assessing partnership approaches to improve public health. *Annual Review of Public Health*, 19, 173-202.

Jemmott, J.B., Jemmott, L. S., & Fong, G. T. (1998). Abstinence and safer sex HIV risk-reduction interventions for African American adolescents: a randomized controlled trial. *JAMA*, 279(19), 1529-36.

Jemmott, L. S. & Jemmott, J. B. (1992). Increasing condom-use intentions among sexually active Black adolescent women. *Nursing Research*, 41(5), 273-279.

Jensen, P. S., Hoagwood, K., & Trickett, E. J. (1999). Ivory towers or earthen trenches? Community collaborations to foster real-world research. *Applied Developmental Science*, 3, 206-212.

Kirby, D., Short, L., Collins, J., Rugg, D., Kolbe, L., Howard, M., Miller B., Sonenstein, F., & Zabin, L. S. (1994). School-based programs to reduce sexual risk behaviors: a review of effectiveness. *Public Health Reports*, 109(3), 339-60.

Koroloff, N. M., Elliott, D. J., Koren, P. E., & Friesen, B. J. (1994). Connecting low-income families to mental health services: The role of the family associate. *Journal of Emotional & Behavioral Disorders*, 2(4), 240-246.

Madison, S., Bell, C., Sewell, S., Nash, G., McKay, M., & Paikoff, R. (in press). True community/academic partnerships. *Psychiatric Services*.

Madison, S. & CHAMP Collaborative Board (1996, July). *Creating the conditions for meaningful university-community partnerships*. Paper presented at the NIMH Role of Families in Preventing and Adapting to HIV/AIDS, an official satellite conference for the XI International conference on AIDS, Vancouver, Canada.

Madison, S., McKay, M., Paikoff, R.L., & Bell, C. (2000). Community collaboration and basic research: Necessary ingredients for the development of a family-based HIV prevention program. *AIDS Education and Prevention*, 12, 281-298.

McCormick, A., McKay, M., Marla, Wilson, McKinnwy, L., Paikoff, R., Bell, C., Baptiste, D., Coleman, D., Gillming, G., Madison, S., & Scott, R. (2000). Involving families in an urban HIV preventive intervention: How community collaboration addresses barriers to participation. *AIDS Education and Prevention*, 12(4), 299-307.

McKay, M. (in press). "Collaborative child mental health services research: Theoretical perspectives and practical guidelines." In K. Hoagwood (Ed.). *Collaborative research to improve child mental health services*.

McKay, M., Baptiste, D., Coleman, D., Madison, S., Paikoff, R., & Scott, R. (2000). Preventing HIV risk exposure in urban communities: The CHAMP Family Program in W. Pequegnat & Jose Szapocznik (Eds). In *Working with families in the era of HIV/AIDS*. California: Sage Publications.

McKay, M., Chasse, K., Paikoff, R., McKinney, L., Baptiste, D., Coleman, D., Madison, S., Bell, C., & CHAMP Collaborative Board (2004). Family-level impact of the CHAMP Family Program: A community collaborative effort to support urban families and reduce youth HIV risk exposure. *Family Process*, 43(1) 77-91.

McLoyd, V. C. (1990). The impact of economic hardship on Black families and children: Psychological distress, parenting, and socioemotional development. *Child Development*, 61(2), 311-345.

McNeal, R. B. (1999). Parental involvement as social capital: Differential effectiveness on science achievement, truancy, and dropping out. *Social Forces*, 78(1), 117-144.

Miller, K. S., Clark, L. F., & Moore, J. S. (1997). Sexual initiation with older male partners and subsequent HIV risk behavior among female adolescents. *Family Planning Perspectives*, 29(5), 212-4.

Minkler, M. & Wallerstein, N. (2003). *Community based participatory research for health*. San Francisco, CA: Jossey-Bass.

Minnis, A. M. & Padian, N. S. (2001). Choice of female-controlled barrier methods among young women and their male sexual partners. *Family Planning Perspectives*, 33(1), 28-34.

National Institute of Mental Health (1998). *Priorities for Prevention Research at NIMH*. National Institute of Mental Health, National Institutes of Health. Available at: http://www.nimh.nih.gov/publist/984321.htm.

Paikoff, R., McKay, M. M., & Bell, C. (1994). *Collaborative HIV prevention and Adolescent Mental health Project (CHAMP)* grant proposal submitted to the National Institute of Mental Health.

Puttman, R.D. (2000). *Bowling Alone: The collapse and revival of American community*. New York: Simon and Schuster.

Rotheram-Borus, M. J., Mahler, K. A., & Rosario, M. (1995). AIDS prevention with adolescents families. *AIDS Education and Prevention*, 7 (4), 320-336.

Sanstad, K. H., Stall, R., Goldstein, E., Everett, W., & Brousseau, R. (1999). Collaborative community research consortium: A model for HIV prevention. *Health Education & Behavior*, 26(2), 171-184.

Schensul, J. J. (1999). Organizing community research partnerships in the struggle against AIDS. *Health Education & Behavior*, 26(2), 266-83.

Secrest, L. A., Lassiter, S. L., Armistead, L. P., Wyckoff, S. C., Johnson, J., Williams, W. B., & Kotchick, B. A. (2004). The Parents Matter! Program: Building a successful investigator-community partnership. *Journal of Child & Family Studies*, 13, 35-45.

Singer, M. (1993). Knowledge for use: Anthropology and community-centered substance abuse. *Social Science Medicine*, 37, 1, 15-25.

Stanton, B. (1996). Longitudinal evaluation of AIDS prevention intervention. In *Adolescent and HIV/AIDS Research: A Developmental Perspective*. Rockville, MD.

Stevenson, H. C., Davis, G., Weber, E., Weiman, D. et al. (1995). HIV prevention beliefs among urban African American youth. *Journal of Adolescent Health*, 16(4), 316-323.

Stevenson, H. C. & White, J. J. (1994). AIDS prevention struggles in ethnocultural neighborhoods: Why research partnerships with community based organizations can't wait. *AIDS Education & Prevention*, 6, 126-139.

Stringer, E. T. (1996). *Action research: A handbook for practitioners*. Thousand Oaks, CA: Sage Publications.

Thomas, S.B. & Quinn, S.C. (1991). The Tuskegee syphilis study, 1932 to 1972: Implications for HIV education and AIDS risk education programs in the black community. *American Journal of Public Health*, 81, 1498-1505.

Trickett, E. J. (1998). Toward a framework for defining and resolving ethical issues in the protection of communities involved in primary prevention projects. *Ethics & Behavior*, 8, 321-337.

Wandersman, A. (2003). Community science: bridging the gap between science and practice with community-centered models. *American Journal of Community Psychology, 31*, 227-42.

Weeks, M. R., Schensul, J. J., Williams, S. S., Singer, M. et al. (1995). AIDS prevention for African American and Latina women: Building culturally and gender-appropriate intervention. *AIDS Education & Prevention, 7*, 251-264.

Wilson, W. J. (1987). The truly disadvantaged: The inner city, the underclass, and public policy. Chicago: University of Chicago Press.

doi:10.1300/J200v05n01_07

Understanding Motivators and Challenges to Involving Urban Parents as Collaborators in HIV Prevention Research Efforts

Mary M. McKay
Rogério M. Pinto
William M. Bannon, Jr.
Vincent Guilamo-Ramos

Mary M. McKay, PhD, is Professor of Psychiatry & Community Medicine, Mount Sinai School of Medicine. Rogério M. Pinto, PhD, is affiliated with the New York State Psychiatric Institute. William M. Bannon, Jr., MSW, and Vincent Guilamo-Ramos, PhD, are affiliated with Columbia University, CHAMP Collaborative Board-New York.

Address correspondence to: Mary M. McKay, PhD, Professor of Psychiatry & Community Medicine, Mount Sinai School of Medicine, One Gustave L. Levy Place, New York, NY 10029 (E-mail: mary.mckay@mssm.edu).

This work would not have been possible without the significant contributions of the Collaborative Board members, CHAMP participants and Roberta Paikoff, PhD, Carl C. Bell, MD, Donna Baptiste, PhD, Sybil Madison-Boyd, PhD and Doris Coleman, LCSW.

Funding from the National Institute of Mental Health (R01 MH 63662) and the W.T. Grant Foundation is gratefully acknowledged. William M. Bannon, MSW is currently a pre-doctoral fellow at the Columbia University School of Social Work supported by a training grant from the National Institutes of Mental Health (5T32MH014623-24). Dr. Pinto is a post-doctoral fellow at the HIV Center for Clinical and Behavioral Studies (New York State Psychiatric Institute and Columbia University) supported by a training grant from the NIMH (T32 MH19139 Behavioral Sciences Research in HIV Infection). The HIV Center is supported by a center grant from NIMH (P30 MH43520).

[Haworth co-indexing entry note]: "Understanding Motivators and Challenges to Involving Urban Parents as Collaborators in HIV Prevention Research Efforts." McKay, Mary M. et al. Co-published simultaneously in *Social Work in Mental Health* (The Haworth Press, Inc.) Vol. 5, No. 1/2, 2007, pp. 169-185; and: *Community Collaborative Partnerships: The Foundation for HIV Prevention Research Efforts* (ed: Mary M. McKay, and Roberta L. Paikoff) The Haworth Press, Inc., 2007, pp. 169-185. Single or multiple copies of this article are available for a fee from The Haworth Document Delivery Service [1-800-HAWORTH, 9:00 a.m. - 5:00 p.m. (EST). E-mail address: docdelivery@ haworthpress.com].

SUMMARY. This study was designed to explore the experiences of urban parents in their role as Collaborative Board members as part of the CHAMP (Collaborative HIV prevention and Adolescent Mental health Project) Family Program Study. The CHAMP Collaborative Board is comprised of urban parents, representatives from schools and community-based agencies and university-based researchers and is charged with overseeing the design, delivery and testing of a family-based HIV prevention program for pre and early adolescent youth. The current qualitative study, guided by the Theory of Unified Behavior Change, is meant to elucidate: (1) pathways to involvement by urban parents; (2) benefits and costs of participating in this collaborative HIV prevention research effort; and (3) the role of social relationships in influencing initial and ongoing participation by parent participants. Twenty-nine parent Collaborative Board members were interviewed for this study. In-depth interviews were audio recorded and ranged from 30 to 90 minutes in length. Transcripts were coded and analyzed using NUD*IST, computerized software used for examining narratives. Findings include community parent members identifying social support and learning opportunities as major reasons for involvement with the Collaborative Board. Prior involvement with other community-based projects and knowledge of at least one other person on the Board also influenced members to join the Board and remain involved over time. Further, recommendations for future collaborative partnerships are made. Findings have direct implication for participatory HIV prevention research activities. doi:10.1300/J200v05n01_08 *[Article copies available for a fee from The Haworth Document Delivery Service: 1-800-HAWORTH. E-mail address: <docdelivery@haworthpress.com> Website: <http://www.HaworthPress.com> © 2007 by The Haworth Press, Inc. All rights reserved.]*

KEYWORDS. Pathways to involvement by urban parents, family-based HIV prevention, programming, influential social relationships, community narratives, urban pre and early adolescent youth

As the HIV epidemic enters its third decade, the demographic characteristics of those most likely to be infected and affected by the disease have also changed. Rates of new infections are climbing for urban minority youth and low-income women of color (Centers for Disease Control, 2001; 2000; 1998). Factors associated with living in urban, low-income neighborhoods, including higher overall rates of neighborhood prevalence, along with poorer access to preventive health care, early detection and treatment services appear to be fueling rates of HIV infection in these emerging risk groups (Centers for Disease Control, 2001; Institute of Medicine, 1997; Miller, Clark, & Moore, 1997; Minnis & Padian, 2001; Rotheram-Borus, Mahler & Rosario, 1995; Wilson, 1987).

Over the last decade, a number of HIV prevention programs have demonstrated efficacy in reducing HIV risk behavior among women or adolescents (Centers for Disease Control, 2001). However, efforts to transport empirically supported prevention programs to a larger number of urban communities have encountered numerous obstacles, including, insufficient school and community-based resources, poor community participation or tensions and suspicions between community residents and outside researchers (Dalton, 1989; Galbraith, Parcel et al., 1989; Galbraith, Stanton, Feigelman, Ricardo, Black & Kalijee, 1996; Thomas & Quinn, 1991). As a result, it is becoming clear that community-based HIV prevention programs targeting urban minority youth or low-income women are likely to fail if they attempt to provide interventions in a non-collaborative manner (Aponte, 1988; Boyd-Franklin, 1993; Fullilove & Fullilove, 1993; Secrest, Lassiter, Armistead, Wychoff, Johnson, Williams, & Kotchick, 2004; Fullilove, Green, & Fullilove, 2000; Schensul, 1999) or neglect to design and implement programs which do not appreciate stressors, scarce contextual resources or target groups' core values (Boyd-Franklin, 1993; McLoyd, 1990; Sanstad, Stall, Goldstein, Everett, & Brousseau, 1999).

One model for maximizing community participation within a HIV prevention research project has been offered, that of a Collaborative Board structure that is responsible for overseeing all aspects of a HIV prevention research project (McKay, Hibbert et al., 2004; Madison, McKay et al., 2000; McKay, Chasse et al., 2004; McKay, Baptiste et al., 2000). More specifically, a Collaborative Board, consisting of urban parents, representatives from community schools and youth-service agencies and university-based researchers, has been funded by that National Institute of Mental Health and charged with overseeing all aspects of the design, delivery and testing of the CHAMP Family Program.

The CHAMP Family Program is intended to impact three interrelated outcomes for pre and early adolescent youth: (1) time spent in situations of sexual possibility; (2) initiation of sexual activity and; (3) sexual risk taking behavior. The program was designed specifically to address the prevention needs of urban youth of color living in communities with high rates of HIV infection (see McKay, Baptiste et al., 2000; Madison, McKay et al., 2000; McKay, Chase et al., in press for a detailed descriptions of this program).

In addition, the CHAMP Family Program study was designed to address some of the serious difficulties that prior HIV prevention research efforts had encountered within urban communities, particularly low rates of participation, community misgivings about the appropriateness of HIV prevention programs for children and mistrust of program and project staff. Thus, a strong community collaborative research method was employed by investigators of the CHAMP Family Program study that draws upon key elements of participatory research paradigms (Israel et al., 1998). However, as the investigative team was organizing this community/research partnership and developing the Collaborative Board structure, little guidance was available to understand mechanisms to involve community members in this effort. In addition, little knowledge was available regarding the experiences of urban community members in prevention research partnerships, specifically reasons behind choice of participation, barriers to involvement, perceptions of ongoing community/research collaboration and recommendations for future collaborative arrangements.

Thus, this article presents the results of a study designed to explore the participation of urban parents as Collaborative Board members as part of the CHAMP (Collaborative HIV prevention and Adolescent Mental health Project) Family Program Study. The current qualitative study, guided by the Unified Theory of Behavior Change, is meant to elucidate: (1) pathways to involvement by urban parents; (2) benefits and costs of participating in the collaborative HIV prevention research efforts; and (3) the role of social relationships in influencing initial and ongoing participation by parent participants.

THEORETICAL UNDERSTANDING OF INVOLVEMENT IN COMMUNITY COLLABORATIVE PREVENTION RESEARCH EFFORTS

In order to guide the current study, a framework for understanding collaborative behavior, referred to as the Unified Theory of Behavior Change, was employed to offer guidance regarding potential motivators and challenges to involving urban parents in a collaborative HIV prevention research effort and specifically to participating as members of a Collaborative Board. By way of background, in 2001, the National Institute of Mental Health (NIMH) convened a meeting focused on relevant theories of behavior change, including the Theory of Reasoned Action (Ajzen & Fishbein, 1975; 1981), Social Learning Theory (Bandura, 1975, 1986), the Health Belief Model (Janz & Becker, 1984; Rosenstock, Strecher, & Becker, 1988) and Triandis' (1972) Theory of Subjective Culture, and Self-Regulation Theories of Behavior (e.g., Kanfer, 1987). The primary architects of each of these theories (Bandura, Becker, Fishbein, Kanfer, and Triandis) met for intensive interactions to develop a common theoretical framework that integrated the core constructs of each approach (Fishbein, Triandis, Kanfer, Becker, Middlestadt, & Eichler et al. 2001). A general framework emerged, the Unified Theory of Behavior Change, (Jaccard et al. 1999), forming the basis for the conceptual framework guiding the current study.

The core variables of the model are organized into two sequences. The first sequence focuses on the immediate determinants of behavior and is illustrated in Figure 1.

Behavior is hypothesized to be influenced by five core variables. First, an individual must be *willing to perform or intend to perform the behavior* in question in order for behavior to occur. Second, the individual must have the requisite *knowledge and skills* to enact the behavior. Third, there must be no *environmental constraints* that render behavioral performance impossible. Fourth, the behavior must be *salient* to the individual so that the person does not forget to enact it. Finally, *habitual and automatic processes* may influence behavior.

These five variables are believed to interact in complex ways to determine behavior. For example, a positive behavioral intention will generally be a necessary, but not a sufficient condition, for behavioral performance to occur. Behavior is most likely to occur when each of the variables coalesce toward behavioral performance. For example, for community/university collaboration to occur, an individual will be most likely to collaborate if he/she intends to collaborate, if he/she has the skills to do so, if the environmental constraints against doing so are absent (e.g., meetings take place at convenient times and familiar community locations), if he/she remembers to do so, and if he has done so in the past. To understand a given behavior, it is important to consider and explicate each of these facets of the theory, namely collaborators' intentions to engage in partnerships, their skill levels relative to collaboration, features of the environment that are constraining (or facilitating) collaborative efforts, the salience of prevention oriented collaboration, and relevant habitual and automatic processes (Jaccard et al., 1999).

FIGURE 1. Determinants of Behavior

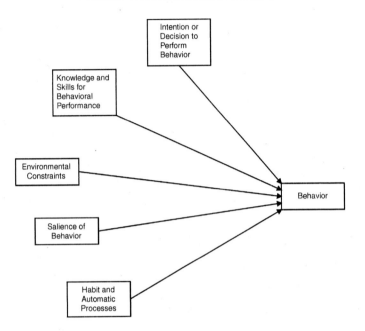

The second aspect of the theoretical framework focuses on the determinants of an individual's willingness, intention, or decision to perform a behavior (summarized in Figure 2).

There are six major factors that serve as the immediate psychological determinants of one's decision to perform a behavior. The construct of *attitude* refers to how favorable or unfavorable the individual feels about performing the behavior. *Normative beliefs* reflect the idea that the more pressures an individual feels to perform a behavior, the more likely it is that he will decide to perform the behavior. *Expectancies* refer to an individual's perceived advantages and disadvantages of performing the behavior. *Self-concept* refers to an individual's conception of self and whether performing the behavior is consistent with that self-image. *Affect* refers to fundamental affective and emotional reactions to behavioral performance. Theories of emotion emphasize two core facets, the degree of arousal and the affective direction of that arousal, positive or negative (Ekman & Davidson, 1994). In general, individuals who have a strong negative emotional reaction to a behavior will be less inclined to perform it and those who have a strong positive

FIGURE 2. Determinants of Intentions to Perform a Specific Behavior

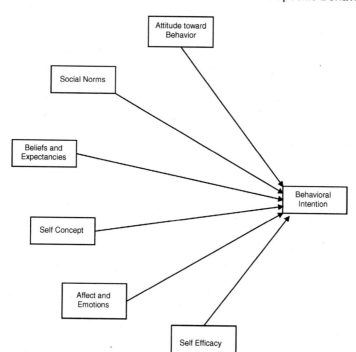

emotional reaction will be more inclined to perform it. *Self-efficacy* is derived from Bandura's social learning theory and refers to one's perceived confidence that he or she can perform the behavior.

To understand community parents' intentions to engage in key leadership roles as Collaborative Board members, we considered attitudes about becoming involved with university-based partners, expectancies about the advantages and disadvantages of prevention oriented collaborations, the normative pressures and social support influences that were brought to bear on parent members with respect to becoming community leaders, their emotional and affective reactions to the prospects of being a deliverer of HIV prevention programming, and their perceptions of their abilities to become an effective collaborator. Within the current study, we hypothesized that attention to these factors would potentially yield large returns in terms of explaining in urban parents collaborative behavior.

METHODS

The current qualitative study, guided by the Theory of Unified Behavior Change, is meant to elucidate: (1) pathways to involvement as Collaborative Board members by urban parents; (2) benefits and costs of participating in this collaborative HIV prevention research effort; and (3) the role of social relationships in influencing initial and ongoing participation by parent participants.

PARTICIPANTS

Twenty nine parent Collaborative Board members were interviewed for this study. These participants were urban parents serving as part of the oversight Collaborative Board of the CHAMP Family Program study. This study is set within a low-income, inner-city community with high rates of poverty and overlapping psychosocial stressors, including high rates of poverty, community violence, substance abuse and HIV infection.

Demographic characteristics of study participants are summarized in Table 1.

The average age of parent Collaborative Board members is 42 years (s.d. = 10.02). Approximately 41% ($n = 12$) of participants were Latino and 41% ($n = 12$) were African American. Finally, the vast majority of participants were female with five male Collaborative Board members also represented in the current study. The average length of time as a Collaborative Board member was 3.5 years (s.d. = 0.9).

DATA COLLECTION PROCEDURES

The first author of this article presented the purpose of the current study at a Collaborative Board meeting. The Board reviewed the general interview questions, data collection procedures and met the research assistants who would conduct the interviews. Informed consent was obtained along with Institutional Review Board approval.

Next, research assistants contacted each parent member of the Collaborative Board to schedule an interview. All interviews were scheduled at the convenience of the participant and generally took place at community-based sites, although a few occurred at the university or over the telephone. Every parent Board members agreed to participate

TABLE 1. Summary of demographic characteristics of study participants

	Mean	Standard Deviation	n
Age	42	10.02	29
Length of time on Board	3.5	0.9	29

	Latino	African American
Ethnicity	41% (n = 12)	41% (n = 12)
Gender	Male	Female
	17% (n = 5)	83% (n =24)

in the study. At the start of each interview, the procedures and goals of the study were re-explained by research staff. Interviewers reminded participants that involvement in the study was entirely voluntary and offered to answer any questions that participants had. Interviews ranged in length from 30 to 90 minutes.

Interviews were semi-structured, consisting of open-ended questions meant to elicit narrative responses. Each question was followed by prompts in order to elicit further information and clarifications when necessary. Six general content areas were covered in each interview: (1) history of involvement with the CHAMP Family Program study and the Collaborative Board; (2) perceptions of the Board and its' work including, sources of motivation and challenges to initial and ongoing participation; (3) social support and network among Board members; (4) social support and network outside the Collaborative Board, including support and discouragement offered by family and members of formal and informal social support networks related to participation in the collaborative research effort; (5) consistency and conflicts between commitments and priorities in participants' lives and involvement with the Collaborative Board; and (6) advice or recommendations for researchers about collaborating with communities on future prevention research studies.

Interviewers attempted to elicit self-generated accounts of participants' experiences as part of the Collaborative Board and their opinions about their work as part of the Board. For example, during the part of the interview that related to history of involvement with the CHAMP Family Program Study and the Collaborative Board, interviewers specifically asked participants to "tell me the story about how you became involved in the Collaborative Board." This question was followed by several prompts, such as "Is HIV/AIDS what inspired you? Could you tell me more about that?" and Is there a person who may have influenced you to join the Board?"

All interviews were audio taped and transcribed verbatim. Total transcribed qualitative data approximated 900 double-spaced pages of text. Interview data were analyzed to explore the appropriateness of applying the Unified Theory of Behavior Change (Jaccard et al., 1999) to understanding community collaborative behavior. First, using a ground theoretical approach, in-depth qualitative interviews were coded based upon key constructs identified in Figures 1 and 2. These interviews were next analyzed using the QSR NUD*IST software package (QSR NUD*IST 4.0, 1999). The use of NUD*IST (Non-numerical Unstructured Data Indexing Searching and Theorizing) software package was chosen in the current data analysis for two primary reasons. First, the NUD*IST software facilitates the effective organization and analysis of large amounts of textual data. Second, this software package is considered particularly adept in the analysis of theories through the manner in which textual data may be structured (Gahan & Hannibal, 1997). More specifically, the NUD*IST program allows the researcher to create an outline or a coding structure of primary and secondary fixed headings to which participants' comments may be copied and categorized. Primary fixed headings, called index nodes, represent the central outcome under analysis that the applicable theory proposes to explain. The secondary fixed headings, called sub-nodes, are a series of smaller categories that are ascribed to each index node and reflect salient aspects of the index node construct.

Data analysis proceeded using standard NUD*IST software protocol, where each individual interview was prepared as an electronic rich text document file and then imported into the NUD*IST database (QSR NUD*IST 4.0, 1999). Two index nodes were created. The first index node was named "behavior" and the second "behavior intention," which reflected the two primary outcomes of the Unified Theory of Behavior Change (Fishbein et al., 2001; Jaccard, Dittus, & Litardo, 1999; Jaccard, Dodge, & Dittus, 2001). The first index node was ascribed five sub-nodes reflecting the constructs (i.e., willing to perform or intend to perform the behavior, knowledge and skills, environmental constraints, salient and habitual and automatic processes) that are theoretically believed to influence behavior. The second index node was ascribed six sub-nodes reflecting the constructs (attitude, normative beliefs, expectancies, self-concept, affect, self-efficacy) that are theoretically believed to influence behavioral intention. In analyzing the data, partic-ipant responses were broken down into individual phrases that reflected a single aspect of the Theory of Unified Behavioral Change. Each phrase was then copied into the applicable sub-node of the theoretical dimension that the participants' comment reflected. A single phrase could be coded in multiple sub-nodes, if it were relevant to more than one theoretical construct.

Coding reliability was established by having transcripts coded by multiple coders and comparing the codes. Two individuals were in-volved in coding the transcripts and a conservative approach was taken to establishing agreement. Any code for which there was not agreement by both coders was discussed; if agreement could not be reached, the code was not assigned. Once reliability was established, as indicated by consistent agreement among the coders (> 85%), transcripts were coded by individual coders. Reliability checks were then conducted periodi-cally to ensure that reliability was maintained.

RESULTS

Community parents identified several key factors that served as the foundation for their intention to begin involvement and stay involved with the community/research partnership. For example, in relation to *intention* to continue involvement in the collaboration, strong endorse-ments were revealed.

> *Every little bit I could give to this community, I will.*
> *There's a lot of drugs, gangs, murders, and rapes (in the commu-nity). If I have anything to give to help the community, I would like to share it with them.*

Salience of involvement with CHAMP, normative social pressure and supports created within the partnership and *emotional response* to involvement were consistently identified as prime motivators to remain actively engaged in the community/research partnership. For example, for community parent partners, *salience* was described in these ways:

> *My brother and sister died of AIDS and I need to teach my 13 year old daughter about disease and pregnancy.*
> *I lost a nephew and a couple of friends to HIV . . . I figured if I could help someone else, I would be doing something for the peo-ple I lost.*

> *Programs are needed to help parents deal with their children and make them more aware of what's going on.*
> *There are a lot of people that I know (in the community) that do unprotected sex . . . and I liked to let them know and try to inform them . . . so that they learn to protect themselves a little better.*
> *When I learned that a lot of kids don't know information about STDs, HIV and AIDS, I realized that we had to get the word out.*
> *I wanted to sit in the same room and work together with people of all nationalities from my community.*

Further, community partners described other members of the partnership as providing additional encouragement to remain involved and social support when faced with obstacles to involvement. For example, community partners described *normative social pressures and supports* in these ways:

> *The Board has become like a family . . . anything goes wrong and we call each other.*
> *. . . recently, I had a girlfriend who committed suicide. She was pregnant and I spoke to (one of the Board members) about this and she kind of made me feel a little better.*
> *(another Board member) helps me with things sometimes, like if I don't have money, uh, she'll loan me money or she'll treat me to breakfast or lunch.*
> *I really like working with our university partner . . . she gets so animated and when you are working with a person like that, it makes you want to give more of yourself.*

Social support outside the collaborative partnership also was cited as an important influence on ongoing collaborative involvement.

> *My husband looks after the baby when I attend meetings . . . if he did not, I would not be able to go.*
> *My wife and the boy are the exact same, pushing me and giving me confidence in what I could do (in CHAMP).*

Finally, members of the Board described their *emotional response* to HIV prevention research efforts in these ways:

> *I noticed the commitment and seriousness of the board coming together to help the community . . . I really loved it and was happy to be there.*

CHAMP is an amazing program. . . . how families reach out to each other and I am excited to see everyone connecting well.
The program made me a believer of the need to educate children on the issues of HIV prevention and sex education.

Feelings of *personal self esteem* and respect for other Collaborative Board members were also noted.

I like the feeling CHAMP gives me, you know, helping other people, and helping where you live at, it feels good.
People in CHAMP are down-to-earth, they're friendly, and they really dedicate themselves to doing wonderful things.

Many Collaborative Board members described their participation in the research partnership as feeling natural to them (*habitual or automatic response*) because they had prior experience with community-based projects.

I was involved in my kid's school . . . volunteering to help kids read or helping the teachers.
All my life, I've volunteered to counsel or do anything I can to help children.

In addition, participants identified the building of knowledge and skills (*self efficacy*) in key areas as being highly influential in their decision to remain involved with the Collaborative Board. For example, benefits to self included development of personal attributes.

CHAMP has helped me to be a little more patient, and they offer workshops, like for listening skills.
CHAMP helped me to be more open when I'm around a lot of people.

In addition, participants identified involvement in the collaborative partnership as assisting in the acquisition of HIV/AIDS knowledge.

I knew certain things about HIV, but there was more stuff that I didn't know . . . so CHAMP was another opportunity for me to learn more about HIV/AIDS.

Despite so many positive endorsements to participation in the collaborative partnerships, some costs (*environmental constraints*) to members were also identified.

> *My little girl says, 'Ma, you're not home no more,' but, I take her to meetings with me . . . and she stays with her father . . . it makes me feel bad because she's used to me being there all the time . . . and I love being around my kids . . . but, the Board is only until 7 . . . but, she says that she's used to seeing me home all the time.*

DISCUSSION AND IMPLICATIONS

Results indicate that the Unified Theory of Behavior Change (Jaccard et al., 1999) did help identify key factors that influenced urban parents to decide to join and remain as members of the Collaborative Board, thereby, supporting a community-wide HIV prevention research partnership. Given that concerns regarding the consequences of early and high risk sexual behavior for urban minority youth have been constant over the past several decades and infection rates continue to rise in young people and women of color, prevention programs designed specifically for urban youth and women are critically needed (Centers for Disease Control, 2000). Though collaboration with communities has been emphasized as a necessary component of building successful preventative interventions, not much is known about the factors critical to the development of such partnerships. We believe that the current study contributes to the field by defining specific factors that motivate urban community members to collaborate with HIV prevention researchers.

Implications of the current findings include the possibility that if consideration is specifically given to the factors that motivate and retain community participants in collaborative prevention efforts, then recruitment of community partners could be facilitated. Further, future research might focus on ways that bolstering these factors could enhance rates of ongoing involvement, satisfaction and productivity of community/university prevention partnerships. Finally, the current study may shed light on the foundation of effective community-based prevention oriented groups.

REFERENCES

Ajzen, I. & Fishbein, M. (1981). *Understanding attitudes and predicting social behavior.* Englewood Cliffs, N.J.: Prentice-Hall.

Aponte, H.J., Zarskl, J., Bixenstene, C., & Cibik, P. (1991). Home/community based services: A two-trier approach. *American Journal of Orthopsychiatry, 61,* 3, 403-408. 224.

Bandura, A. (1975). *Social learning theory.* Englewood Cliffs, New Jersey: Prentice-Hall.

Bandura, A. (1986). *Social foundations of thought and action: A social cognitive theory.* Englewood Cliffs, N.J.: Prentice-Hall.

Boyd-Franklin, N. (1993). *Black Families.* In F. Walsh (Ed.), *Normal Family Process.* New York: Guilford Press.

Centers for Disease Control and Prevention (1998). *HIV/AIDS Surveillance Report, 9,* 1- 43.

Centers for Disease Control and Prevention (2000). *HIV/AIDS Surveillance Report, 12* (2).

Centers for Disease Control and Prevention (2001). *Compendium of HIV Prevention Interventions with Evidence of Effectiveness.* Atlanta, GA: Author.

Dalton, H.L. (1989). AIDS in blackface. *Daedalus, 118* (3), 205-227.

Ekman, P. & Davidson, R.J. (1994). *The nature of emotion: Fundamental questions.* New York: Oxford University Press.

Fishbein, M. & Ajzen, I. (1975). *Belief, attitude, intention, and behavior: An introduction to theory and research.* Reading, MA: Addison-Wesley.

Fishbein, M., Triandis, H. C., Kanfer, F. H., Becker, M., Middlestadt, S. E., Eichler, A., Leventhal, H., Leventhal, E. A. et al. (2001). Part I. Basic Processes. In A. Baum & T. Revenson (Eds); et al. *Handbook of health psychology,* 3-318. Mahwah, N.J.: Lawrence Erlbaum Associates.

Fullilove, M. T. & Fullilove, R. E., III. (1993). Understanding sexual behaviors and drug use among African Americans: A case study of issues for survey research. In D. G. Ostrow & R. C. Kessler (Eds.), *Methodological Issues in AIDS Behavioral Research,* (pp. 117-132). New York: Plenum Press.

Fullilove, R. E, Green, L., & Fullilove, M. T. (2000). The Family to Family program: A structural intervention with implications for the prevention of HIV/AIDS and other community epidemics. *AIDS, 14* (Suppl 1), S63-S67.

Galbraith, J., Stanton, B., Feigelman, S., Ricardo, I., Black, M., & Kalijee, L. (1996). Challenges and rewards of involving community in research: An overview of the "Focus on Kids" HIV-risk reduction program. To be published in *Health Education Quarterly.*

Gahan, C. & Hannibal, M. (1997). *Doing Qualitative Research Using QSR NUD*IST.* Thousand Oaks, CA: Sage publications.

Institute of Medicine (1997). *The Hidden Epidemic: Confronting Sexually Transmitted Diseases.* Washington, DC: National Academy Press.

Israel, B. A., Schulz A. J., Parker E. A., & Becker, A. B. (1998). Review of community-based research: assessing partnership approaches to improve public health. *Annual Review of Public Health, 19,* 173-202.

Jaccard, J., Dodge, T., & Dittus, P. (2001). Parent-adolescent communication about sex and birth control: A conceptual framework. In S. Feldman, S. Shirley, & D. A. Rosenthal (Eds). *Talking sexuality: Parent-adolescent communication. New directions for child and adolescent development.* San Francisco, CA, US: Jossey- Bass.

Jaccard, J., Dittus, P., & Litardo, H. (1999). Parent-adolescent communication about birth control: implications for parent based interventions to reduce unintended adolescent pregnancy. In W. Miller & L. Severly (Eds), *Advances in population research: Psychosocial perspectives.* London, England: Kingsley.

Janz, N. & Becker, M. (1984). The Health Belief Model: A decade later. *Health Education Quarterly, H,* 1-47.

Kanfer, R. (1987). Task-specific motivation: An integrative approach to issues of measurement, mechanisms, processes, and determinants. *Journal of Social & Clinical Psychology, 5,* 237-264.

Madison, S., McKay, M., Paikoff, R.L. & Bell, C. (2000). Community collaboration and basic research: Necessary ingredients for the development of a family-based HIV prevention program. *AIDS Education and Prevention, 12,* 281-298.

McCormick, A., McKay, M., Gilling, G., & Paikoff, R. (2000). Involving families in an urban HIV preventive intervention: How community collaboration addresses barriers to participation. *AIDS Education and Prevention, 12,* 299-307.

McKay, M. (in press). "Collaborative child mental health services research: Theoretical perspectives and practical guidelines." In K. Hoagwood (Ed.). *Collaborative research to improve child mental health services.*

McKay, M., Baptiste, D., Coleman, D., Madison, S., Paikoff, R. & Scott, R. (2000). Preventing HIV risk exposure in urban communities: The CHAMP Family Program in W. Pequegnat & Jose Szapocznik (Eds). *Working with families in the era of HIV/AIDS.* California: Sage Publications.

McKay, M., Chase, K., Baptiste, D., Bell, C., Coleman, D., Madison, S., McKinney, L., & CHAMP Collaborative Board (2004). Family-level impact of the CHAMP Family Program: A community collaborative effort to support urban families and reduce youth HIV risk exposure. *Family Process, 43(1),* 77-91.

McKay, M., Hibbert, R., Lawrence, R., Miranda, A., Paikoff, R., Bell, C., Madison, S., Baptiste, D., & Coleman, D. (under review). Creating mechanisms for meaningful collaboration between members of urban, minority communities and university-based researchers. *Journal of Child & Family Studies.*

McLoyd, V. C. (1990). The impact of economic hardship on Black families and children: Psychological distress, parenting, and socioemotional development. *Child Development, 61,* 311-345.

Miller, K. S., Clark, L. F., & Moore, J. S. (1997). Sexual initiation with older male partners and subsequent HIV risk behavior among female adolescents. *Family Planning Perspectives, 29,* 212-4.

Minnis, A. M. & Padian, N. S. (2001). Choice of female-controlled barrier methods among young women and their male sexual partners. *Family Planning Perspectives, 33,* 28-34.

QSR NUD*IST 4.0 [computer software]. (1999). Thousand Oaks, CA: Sage publications.

Rosenstock, I., Strecher, V. & Becker, H. (1988), Social learning theory and the Health Belief Model. *Health Education Quarterly, 15,* 175-183.

Rotheram-Borus, M. J., Mahler, K. A., & Rosario, M. (1995). AIDS prevention with adolescents families. *AIDS Education and Prevention, 7*(4), 320-336.

Sanstad, K. H., Stall, R., Goldstein, E., Everett, W., & Brousseau, R. (1999). Collaborative community research consortium: A model for HIV prevention. *Health Education & Behavior, 26*, 171-184.

Schensul, J. J. (1999). Organizing community research partnerships in the struggle against AIDS. *Health Education & Behavior, 26*, 266-83.

Secrest, L. A., Lassiter, S. L., Armistead, L. P., Wyckoff, S. C., Johnson, J., Williams, W. B., & Kotchick, B. A. (2004). The Parents Matter! Program: Building a successful investigator-community partnership. *Journal of Child & Family Studies, 13*, 35-45.

Stanton, B. (1996). Longitudinal evaluation of AIDS prevention intervention. In *Adolescent and HIV/AIDS Research: A Developmental Perspective.* Rockville, MD.

Thomas, S.B. & Quinn, S.C. (1991). The Tuskegee syphilis study, 1932 to 1972: Implications for HIV education and AIDS risk education programs in the black community. *American Journal of Public Health, 81*, 1498-1505.

Triandis, H.C. (1972). *The Analysis of Subjective Culture,* N.Y.: John Wiley and Sons.

Wilson, W. J. (1987). *The truly disadvantaged: The inner city, the underclass, and public policy.* Chicago: University of Chicago Press.

doi:10.1300/J200v05n01_08

Motivators and Barriers to Participation of Ethnic Minority Families in a Family-Based HIV Prevention Program

Rogério M. Pinto
Mary M. McKay
Donna Baptiste
Carl C. Bell
Sybil Madison-Boyd
Roberta Paikoff
Marla Wilson
Daisy Phillips

Rogério M. Pinto, PhD, is affiliated with the HIV Center for Clinical and Behavioral Studies, New York State Psychiatric Institute/Columbia University. Mary M. McKay, PhD, is affiliated with the Mount Sinai School of Medicine. Donna Baptiste, PhD, Carl C. Bell, MD, Sybil Madison-Boyd, PhD, Roberta Paikoff, PhD, Marla Wilson, BA, and Daisy Phillips are affiliated with the University of Illinois, Chicago, CHAMP Collaborative Board-New York.

Address correspondence to: Rogério M. Pinto, PhD, CSW, New York State Psychiatric Institute, HIV Center for Clinical and Behavioral Studies, Unit 15, 1051 Riverside Drive, New York, NY 10032 (E-mail: RMP98@columbia.edu).

The authors thank CHAMP staff and participant families.

This study was supported by grants from NIMH (R01 MH 63662) and the W. T. Grant Foundation. Dr. Pinto is currently post-doctoral fellow at the HIV Center for Clinical and Behavioral Studies supported by training grant from NIMH (T32 MH19139, Behavioral Sciences Research in HIV Infection).

[Haworth co-indexing entry note]: "Motivators and Barriers to Participation of Ethnic Minority Families in a Family-Based HIV Prevention Program." Pinto, Rogério M. et al. Co-published simultaneously in *Social Work in Mental Health* (The Haworth Press, Inc.) Vol. 5, No. 1/2, 2007, pp. 187-201; and: *Community Collaborative Partnerships: The Foundation for HIV Prevention Research Efforts* (ed: Mary M. McKay, and Roberta L. Paikoff) The Haworth Press, Inc., 2005, pp. 187-201. Single or multiple copies of this article are available for a fee from The Haworth Document Delivery Service [1-800-HAWORTH, 9:00 a.m. - 5:00 p.m. (EST). E-mail address: docdelivery@haworthpress.com].

187

SUMMARY. Involving low-income, ethnic minority families in lengthy HIV prevention programs can be challenging. Understanding the motivators and barriers to involvement may help researchers and practitioners design programs that can be used by populations most at risk for HIV exposure. The present study discusses motivators and barriers to involvement in the Collaborative HIV Prevention and Adolescent Mental Health Project (CHAMP), using data from a sample of 118 families that participated at varying levels in the twelve sessions of the program. Most participants chose motivators that reflect their perceptions of individual and/or family needs ("CHAMP might help me, mine, and other families"), and of characteristics of the program, such as CHAMP staff were friendly, CHAMP was fun. Among barriers to involvement, respondents expressed concerns about confidentiality, and about being judged by program staff. Respondents also reported experiencing many stressful events in their families (e.g., death and violence in the family) that may have been barriers to their involvement. Knowing these motivators and barriers, researchers and practitioners can enhance involvement in HIV prevention programs. doi:10.1300/J200v05n01_09 *[Article copies available for a fee from The Haworth Document Delivery Service: 1-800-HAWORTH. E-mail address: <docdelivery@haworthpress.com> Website: <http://www.HaworthPress.com> © 2007 by The Haworth Press, Inc. All rights reserved.]*

KEYWORDS. Involvement, motivators, barriers, HIV prevention program, African American families

Ethnic minority adolescents comprise the group at highest risk for contracting STDs (DiLorenzo & Hein, 1993; Jemmott & Jemmott, 1992), including HIV (CDC, 2002a), and economically vulnerable young females have the highest rates of pregnancy (Children's Defense Fund, 2000), further evidence of unprotected sex and risk for HIV exposure. This adverse picture has prompted behavioral scientists to develop a range of prevention research programs to target populations at highest risk for HIV infection, including adolescents, women, and families of color (CDC, 2002b; Pequegnat and Szapocznik, 2000). In general, these programs aim to increase protective knowledge and behavior, and to decrease both risk behavior and exposure to HIV.

The available research indicates that family relationships and processes are significantly associated with sexual behavior in adolescence (Biglan, Matzler, Wirt, Ary, Noell, Ochs, French, & Hood 1990; Black,

Ricardo, & Stanton, 1997; Romer, Black, Ricardo, Feigelman, Kaljee, Galbraith, Nesbit, Homik, & Stanton 1994); however, programs that can reach adolescents in the context of their own families are still scarce (Pequegnat & Szapocznik, 2000). Therefore, building on the strength of ethnic families as a protective factor against high-risk sexual behavior, CHAMP represents an HIV prevention intervention that targets simultaneously the prevention needs of the entire family, while focusing on pre-adolescent youth.

Given the socioeconomic context in which many adolescents of color live, effective HIV prevention interventions usually require lengthy approaches, including multiple individual and group sessions (McCormick, McKay, Wilson, McKinney, Paikoff, Bell, Baptiste, Coleman, Gillming, Madison, & Scott, 2000; Pinto, 200, Pinto, 2000). Family-based interventions may require extended participation as urban families may have experienced significant life stressors, have fewer resources, and are less likely to be served by responsive providers and culturally relevant interventions (Boyd-Franklin, 1993; Flaskerud, 1986; Gary, 1982, Wahler & Dumas, 1989; Webster-Stratton, 1985).

Nonetheless, it may be difficult to attract, engage and retain low-income, ethnic minority families precisely for these reasons. Indeed, the literature on service utilization reveals that involvement of highly stressed families is low and that not enough is known about the factors that influence minority families to become involved (Bui & Takeuchi, 1992; Miller & Priz, 1991) and that not enough is known about the factors that influence minority families to become involved in preventative interventions (Pinto, 2003). Understanding the motivators and barriers to involvement in HIV prevention programs may help researchers and health practitioners design programs that can be used by the minority populations most at risk for HIV exposure.

THEORETICAL FRAMEWORK

The literature on service utilization consistently indicates that myriad motivators and barriers in the service system may influence involvement of individuals and families in medical and social services, including HIV prevention programs. Extensively used frameworks suggest that health-related behaviors, such as involvement in HIV prevention programs, is a social process managed within social networks, including families and services systems (see, for example, Pescosolido, 1991, 1992). Others indicate that enabling factors, such as the characteristics of a service or program, may facilitate or hinder the use of social and medical services (Andersen, 1968; Andersen & Newman, 1973).

Given the high risk context in which low-income families reside in neighborhoods with high HIV prevalence, McCormick et al. (2000) have proposed that separately or in combination multiple conditions may influence involvement in family-based prevention programs like CHAMP. These include both motivators and barriers. Program level motivators (e.g., monetary incentive), as well as individual and family level barriers–concerns about program content and life stressors–have been hypothesized as influencing family involvement.

Beyond factors that influence individual families to participate in HIV prevention programs, program level characteristics may be important influences on involvement. Therefore, the present study focuses on program level characteristics of CHAMP, and reports motivators and barriers reported by a sample of families that participated at varying levels in the twelve sessions of the program. This information may prove to be crucial to researchers and practitioners developing HIV prevention programs, and could inform strategies for addressing barriers and for enhancing motivators to participation in their programs.

MOTIVATORS TO INVOLVEMENT

In an attempt to clarify some of the motivators to participation in preventative programs, including CHAMP, a series of studies, using data collected from both program participants and program staff, have been conducted to identify motivators to involvement (Lynn, 2002; McKay, 1995; McKay, McCadam, & Gonzales, 1996; McKay, Nudelman, & McCadam, 1996; McKay, Stoewe, McCadam, & Gonzales, 1998; Pinto, 2003). These authors found that involvement was related to participants' understanding of the program's purposes, and their perceptions about the program staff. Participants also identified program logistics, scheduling, transportation to program site, commitment to their children, and concerns about HIV infection as critical issues related to their involvement.

Other studies also suggest that recruitment and service delivery strategies (Prochaska, Redding, Evers, 1997), and reminders from services providers (Larson, 1982) may also facilitate involvement in prevention programs. Monetary incentives have been also shown to be positively associated with recruitment and retention in HIV prevention programs. For example, Greenberg, Lifshay, Van Devanter, Gonzales, and Celentano

(1998) found that the average number of paid sessions women participants attended was greater than the average of unpaid sessions attended.

Other concrete conditions that appear to facilitate involvement include health coaching, vouchers for medical office visits, materials resources, scheduling, time of year and to program sites (Montaño, Kasprzyk, & Taplin, 1997; Yen, Edington, McDonald, Hischl, & Edington, 2001). These findings suggest that these factors may also facilitate participation in HIV prevention programs and are explored in the current study.

BARRIERS TO INVOLVEMENT

The literature on service utilization covers barriers to participation that relate to both the characteristics of a program, and the stressors within a family system (McCormick et al., 2000; Pinto, 2003).

Program characteristics. These authors have suggested that concerns related to community skepticisms and HIV/AIDS stigma may deter involvement. The sensitive content of the program material and its duration also may be regarded as barriers (Stevenson & White, 1994). Other barriers found in the literature on service utilization relate to concrete obstacles, such as hard-to-reach locations and lack of information about the services rendered (Acosta, 1980; Baekeland & Lundwall, 1975; Boyd-Franklin, 1993, Windle, 1980) have been shown to influence negatively rates of utilization of mental health services. This literature also reveals that attitudes about professionals (as opposed to informal helpers) have been identified as important factors that influence engagement of minority families (Leaf, Bruce, Tischler, & Holzner, 1985; Snow, 1983). Moreover, receptivity to services and previous experiences with unresponsive service providers have been shown to be associated with attrition (Muecke, 1983).

Life stressors. A range of life stressors may affect minority families in urban areas. These stressors have been described as distributed across three key domains (Tolan, Miller, & Thomas, 1987) are hypothesized as barriers to involvement in prevention programs. Induced transition stressors include situations that change the patterns of family behavior (e.g., mental illness). Developmental transition stressors refer to expected life changes that prompt reorganization of family structure (e.g., pregnancy). Circumscribed life events can be either short- or long-term, and include life events such being robbed and being arrested.

Since many urban, low income, families experience huge numbers of stressors from each of these domains, this has raised the question of whether or not the presence of multiple stressors is a barrier to participation in CHAMP. The knowledge that family stressors create difficulties in retaining participants in mental health services (Bui & Takeuchi, 1992; Cohen & Hesselbart, 1993; Kazdin, 1993) supports exploring family stressors as possible barriers to involvement in prevention programs, including CHAMP.

METHODS

All research procedures described below have been approved by Institutional Review Boards at Columbia University and the University of Illinois at Chicago.

Sample and Data Sources

The current study examines data from a cohort of 118 African American mothers who participated in both CHAMP (Collaborative HIV Prevention and Adolescent Mental Health Project), *and* another NIMH-funded study, KAARE (Knowledge About the African American Research Experience). Of all families that participated in CHAMP, a sample of adult women caregivers were randomly selected to participate in a more in-depth interview in the KAARE study. KAARE re-interviewed this sample of women regarding issues related to their perceptions about research, including motivators and barriers to their participation in CHAMP.

The mean age of participants was 33.3 years (SD = 7.7). More than half (54%) were between 19 and 35 years old. Seventy-three percent of respondents were not married at the time of interview; 92% were single and never married; and 8% were separated, divorced or widowed. Approximately 34% of respondents reported that their total income for the year prior to the interviews was less than $5,000. All had completed either high school (90%) or some college (10%). More than half of all respondents (54%) were working outside the home. Even though the majority of respondents had a high school education, and worked for pay, 74% of all respondents reported that they were receiving public assistance at the time of their interviews.

Of the 118 African American mothers invited to participate in the CHAMP Family Program, 92 attended at least one session. Forty percent of mothers brought their children to nine each of the twelve CHAMP scheduled sessions. Eighty-nine percent attended at least half of the scheduled CHAMP sessions.

Data Collection Procedures

The women in this study were identified when they gave consent for their pre-adolescent children to participate in a study carried out in four inner-city public schools in the Midwest. Five hundred and fifty eligible youths were identified as eligible from the 4th and 5th grades. Research staff recruited the adolescents' mothers through personal contacts, telephone calls and home visits.

Trained community interviewers conducted individual interviews lasting approximately 90 minutes. Each participant received $25.00. Research staff assisted participants by reading instrument items aloud. Data collection occurred at community sites. To ensure readability and cultural relevance, instruments were pilot-tested.

Using a cross-section research design, data were drawn from both CHAMP and KAARE. Four instruments were used to collect data for the current study: (1) Demographic Characteristics Questionnaire; (2) Program Motivators; (3) Program Barriers; and (4) the Family Stress Scale (Tolan, Miller, & Thomas, 1987).

Measures

In order to arrive at a fuller understanding of specific conditions that influenced involvement in CHAMP, the mothers in this sample were asked about both motivators and barriers to their involvement in CHAMP. These measures were derived from separate listings of motivators, and barriers–concerns about participation and major life stressors.

Motivators. Interviewers presented respondents a list of potential motivators for their involvement in CHAMP, such as "Money," "Friends were in it," "It seemed like fun." They were asked to mark those motivators that might have made them want to be in CHAMP.

Barriers. Barriers in this study have been conceptualized as including two separate categories. *Concerns about participation* in research projects refers to participants apprehensions and unease in the context of an HIV prevention program, and which might have hindered their involvement. *Major life stressor*, another category, refers to major events that might disrupt family life and thus may also have impeded, and/or made participation more difficult.

Concerns about participation. Respondents were presented a list of potential concerns about their involvement in CHAMP, e.g., "People would know my business," "Don't know anyone in CHAMP." They were asked to mark those concerns that might have made them not want to be in CHAMP.

Major life stressor. This variable was measured by using the Family Stress Scale (Tolan, Miller, & Thomas, 1987). This 21-item scale was used to identify major life stressors that might have occurred within the families attending CHAMP, such as "Had a family member die," "Had a new baby come into the family." Descriptive statistics were used to describe these motivators and barriers to involvement in CHAMP.

RESULTS

Table 1 summarizes the motivators to participation in CHAMP.

Many participants identified program characteristics as motivating their involvement. A total of 82 respondents (70%) marked "CHAMP might help me, mine, and other families" as an important motivator for their involvement in the program. Seventy six respondents (65%) found that CHAMP staff were nice and friendly, and 67 (57%) found CHAMP to be a fun program with which to get involved. Others found that the food served during the program sessions ($n = 38$; 32%), as well as the monetary incentive ($n = 33$; 28%) were important motivators.

Many participants also found that personal and/or family needs were important motivators. Sixty five respondents reported that they wanted "to stop AIDS," 48 participants (41%) reported wanting their children to be in an after-school program like CHAMP, and 28 (24%) found that having friends in CHAMP was also a motivator to their involvement. Overall, participants perceived each factor listed as a motivator.

Table 2 summarizes the results for concerns about participation.

Thirty (25%) respondents marked "other people would know my business" as a concern that may have made them not to want to be in CHAMP. Nineteen (16%) respondents who did not know anyone in CHAMP, and 14 (12%) who did not want their children to participate in an after-school program, all indicated these as concerns for not getting involved. Most other concerns referred to program characteristics as follows. Nineteen (16%) respondents marked that CHAMP staff were strangers to them, 17 (14%) did not need CHAMP, 15 (13%) seemed to

TABLE 1. Motivators for Participation in CHAMP

Motivator (n = 118)	N	%
CHAMP might help me, my family and other families	82	70
CHAMP people are nice and friendly	76	65
CHAMP seemed like fun	67	57
To stop HIV/AIDS	65	56
Wanted to be in an after-school program	48	41
They give you food	38	32
Money	33	28
Friends were in CHAMP	28	24

Note:
n = number of respondents choosing that motivator

TABLE 2. Concerns About Participation in CHAMP

Concern (n = 118)	N	%
Other people would know my business	30	25
Don't know anyone in CHAMP	19	16
CHAMP people were strangers	19	16
Didn't need CHAMP	17	14
CHAMP is about HIV/AIDS	15	13
Didn't want to stay after school	14	12
CHAMP people might think I'm bad	13	11
CHAMP seemed boring	13	11
CHAMP people might think my family is bad	11	9

Note:
n = number of respondents choosing that concern

be concerned about involvement in a program about HIV/AIDS, and 13 (11%) thought that CHAMP seemed boring. Small percentages of respondents considered that CHAMP staff might think that they ($n = 14$; 12%), or their families ($n = 11$; 9%) might be "bad" as concerns about their involvement in CHAMP. Overall, no more than 25% of participants marked any of the concerns presented to them as barriers to involvement.

Table 3 reveals eight major life stressors experienced by the majority of families in the year prior to their involvement in CHAMP.

For each stressor presented, the majority respondents had experienced that stressor in their lives. More than half of the families ($n = 72$; 61%) experienced the death of a family member, and 48 (41%) of these families experienced the death of another relative. Forty (34%) families in the study experienced a family member being seriously ill or injured badly, and 32 (27%) had a family member being beaten or attacked in the past year. A quarter of the sample ($n = 30$; 25%) reported family members having trouble at work, in school, or with authorities, and 24 (20%) had been arrested or gone to jail or court. Twenty-four (20%) respondents reported that someone in their family had a major emotional problem. Moreover, an otherwise positive stressor, "having a new baby come into the family," but which can be a source of stress for many families, was marked by 24 (20%) respondents.

DISCUSSION

The literature on service/program utilization indicates that characteristics of a program may become motivators or barriers to family involvement in behavioral interventions. Several motivators we found reflect what has been found in others studies, such as perceptions of program content and staff, monetary incentives, and logistic conditions (McCormick et al., 2000; Pinto, 2003; Prochaska et al., 1997). However, participants in this study reported specific motivators that have not been cited in the reviewed literature. In relation to the program staff, respon-

TABLE 3. Families Reporting Major Stressors in the Past Year

Stressor (n = 118)	N	Families (%)
Had a family member die	72	61
Had another close relative die	48	41
Had a family member seriously ill or injured badly	40	34
Had someone in family been beaten or attacked	32	27
Had gotten in trouble at work, school, or with authorities	30	25
Had a new baby come into the family	30	25
Had a major emotional problem	24	20
Had been arrested, or gone to court or jail	24	20

dents noted that "nice and friendly" facilitators were an important motivator to their involvement. They also noted that a program that is "fun," that gives food and money, and is scheduled as an after-school activity, all contributed to motivate them to become involved in CHAMP. Since CHAMP may provide fun in many ways, respondents may have perceived communication and socialization as sources of pleasurable feelings called "fun." CHAMP also builds activities around meals and other forms of recreation that may have been perceived as fun, and thus as motivators. Also, as found in other studies, social influence in form of a friend in the program was another motivator to some respondents (Gardner, Hoge, Bennett, Roth, Lidz, Monahan, & Mulvey, 1993).

Some of these motivators, along other conditions known to influence involvement in prevention programs, have been tested elsewhere and found to be significant factors which influence both participation and completion of CHAMP (Pinto, 2003). Therefore, it is recommended that further studies, both to identify other motivators *and* to test them, be carried out as a matter of course in HIV prevention studies. Because involvement of ethnic minority families is usually low, this information will over time help researchers and practitioners better recruit and retain underserved populations.

Participants in this study identified several concerns about their involvement in CHAMP, which have not been reported in other related studies. The related literature shows that most concerns revolve around location, lack of information, and unresponsiveness from providers (Boyd-Franklin, 1993; Leaf et al., 1985; Muecke, 1983). These concerns were not found among CHAMP participants possibly because the program was developed and delivered within the community in which participants reside, and because CHAMP staff strive to help participants understand the content, the goals, and overall objectives of the program (Pinto et al., in press). Nonetheless, participants identify other concerns that need to be accounted for when engaging ethnic minority families.

Adult caregivers indicated that they had concerns about confidentiality, "other people would know my business," and about being judged by program staff. Moreover, they found that not knowing other families in CHAMP, nor the program staff, were also concerns that caused them hesitancy about participation in CHAMP. These concerns were not identified by the majority of respondents. Indeed, no one concern was noted by more than thirty families (25%). These and other, even less frequent concerns are nevertheless important, and must be addressed in HIV prevention programs.

The results also indicate that stressful events in the family were noted as possible barriers to involvement. These stressors reflect many of those already found in the related literature. Note, however, that large numbers of families identified very serious stressors (e.g., death and violence in the family), that may have occurred simultaneously. Single stressors usually do not remain isolated overtime, and a combination of different ones may appear in a family at any point over the course of attempting to involve a family in HIV prevention programming. Socioeconomically disadvantaged families are especially embedded in contexts of multiple stressors, which *together* may have an impact in several areas of family life, including their ability to participate in an HIV prevention program (Dohrenwend, 2000).

One may speculate that families that experience simultaneously more stressors may be less able to get involved and to attend lengthy HIV prevention programs. Therefore, future research needs to continue to identify the impact of stressors and to test how specific stressful events may hinder family participation. Knowing participants' specific sources of stress, researchers and practitioners will be able to provide interventions to help attenuate stress or make referrals to other programs that may be better equipped to help participants. In so doing, health professionals will be better able to recruit and retain families for HIV prevention programs.

It is not possible to discern from the results which sets of motivators and barriers influenced most families in their decisions to become involved in CHAMP. Although limited, these findings are crucial because they reveal various conditions that might facilitate or hinder involvement of ethnic minority families in HIV prevention programs. Nonetheless, other conditions–motivators and barriers–not identified in this study may also influence involvement, and thus should be researched and addressed, in order to improve involvement of families of color in HIV prevention efforts.

REFERENCES

Acosta, F. (1980). Self described reasons for premature termination of psychotherapy by Mexican-American, Black-American Anglo-American patients. *Psychological Reports, 47*, 435-443.

Andersen, R. (1968). *A behavioral model of families' use of health services*. Res. Ser. No. 25, Center for Health Administration Studies, University of Chicago.

Andersen R. M., & Newman, J. (1973). Societal and individual determinants of medical care utilization in the United States. *Milbank Quarterly, 51*, 95-124.

Baekeland, F., & Lundwall, L. (1975). Dropping out of treatment: A critical review. *Psychological Bulletin, 82*, 738-783.

Biglan, A., Matzler, C. W., Wirt, R., Ary, D., Noell, J., Ochs, L., L., French, C., & Hood D. (1990). Social and behavioral factors associated with high-risk sexual behavior among adolescents. *Journal of Behavioral Medicine, 13*, 245-261.

Black, M. M., Ricardo, I. B., & Stanton, B. (1997). Social and psychological factors associated with AIDS risk behaviors among low-income, urban, African American adolescents. *Journal of Research on Adolescent, 7*(2), 173-195.

Boyd-Franklin, N. (1993). Black families. In F. Walsh (Ed.), *Normal family process.* New York: Guilford Press.

Bui, C. T., & Takeuchi, D. T. (1992). Ethnic minority adolescents and the use of community mental health care services. *American Journal of Community Psychology, 20*, 403-417.

Centers for Disease Control and Prevention. (2002a). *AIDS Surveillance Report, 12.* Retrieved April 17, 2002, from http://www.cdc.gov/hiv/stats/hasr1301.pdf

Centers for Disease Control and Prevention. (2002b). *Compendium of HIV Prevention Interventions with Evidence of Effectiveness.* Retrieved April 28, 2002, from *http://www.cdc/hiv/pubs/HIVcompendium/hivcompendium.htm*

Children's Defense Fund. (2000). *The state of America's Children.* Boston: Beacon Press.

Cohen, P, & Hesselbart, C. S. (1993). Demographic factors in the use of children's mental health service. *American Journal of Public Health, 83*, 49-52.

DiLorenzo, T., & Hein, K. (1993). Adolescents: The leading edge of the next wave of the HIV epidemic. In J. L. Wallender, L. J. Siegel (Eds.), *Adolescent Health Problems: Behavioral Perspectives* (pp. 117-140). Advances in Pediatric Psychology. New York: Guilford Press.

Dohrenwend, B. S. (2000). The role of adversity and stress in psychopathology: Some evidence and its implication for theory and research. *Journal of Health and Social behavior, 41*, 1-18.

Flaskerud, J. H. (1986). The effects of culture-compatible intervention on the utilization of mental health services by minority clients. *Community Mental Health Journal, 22*, 127-140.

Gardner, W. P., Hoge, S. K., Bennett, N. S., Roth, L. H., Lidz, C. W., Monahan, J., & Mulvey, E. P. (1993). Two scales for measuring patients' perceptions of coercion during mental hospital admission. *Behavioral Sciences the Law, 11*, 307-322.

Gary, L. E. (1982). Attitudes toward human service organization: Perspectives from an urban Black community. *Journal of Applied Behavioral Sciences, 21*, 445-458.

Greenberg, J., Lifshay, J., Van Devanter, N., Gonzales, V., & Celentano, D. (1998). Preventing HIV infection: The effects of community linkages, time, money on recruiting retaining women in intervention groups. *Journal of Women's Health, 7*, 587-596.

Guerra, N. G., & Tolan, P. H. (1991). Metropolitan Area Child Study. University of Illinois at Chicago.

Jemmott, J. B., & Jemmott, L. S. (1992). Increasing condom-use intentions among sexually active Black adolescent women. *Nursing Research, 41*, 273-279.

Kazdin, A. (1993). Premature termination from treatment among children referred for antisocial behavior. *Journal of Clinical Child Psychology, 31*, 415-425.

Larson, E. G. (1982). Do postcard reminders improve influenza vaccination compliance? *Medical Care, 20*, 639-648.

Leaf, P. J., Livingston, M. M., Tischler, G. L., Weissman, M. M., Holzer II, C. E., & Myers, J. (1985). Contact with health professionals for the treatment of psychological emotional problems. *Medical Care, 23*, 1322-1337.

Lynn, C. J. (2002). *Contextual influences on involvement of urban children families in school-based mental health services.* Unpublished doctoral dissertation, Columbia University School of Social Work, New York.

McCormick, A., McKay, M. M., Wilson, M., McKinney, L., Paikoff, R., Bell, B., Baptiste, D., Coleman, D., Gillming, G., Madison, S., & Scott, R. (2000). Involving families in an urban HIV preventive intervention: How community collaboration addresses barriers to participation. *AIDS Education and Prevention, 12*, 299-307.

McKay, M. M. (1995). Social work engagement: An approach to involving inner-city children their families. Paper presented at the 42nd annual program meeting of the Council of Social Work Education.

McKay, M. M., McCadam, K., & Gonzales, J. (1996). Addressing the barriers to mental health services for inner-city children and their caretakers. *Community Mental Health Journal, 32*, 353-361.

McKay, M. M., Nudelman, & McCadam, K. (1996). Involving inner-city families in mental health services: First interview engagement skills. *Research on Social Work Practice, 6*, 462-472.

McKay, M. M., Stoewe, J., McCadam, K. & Gonzales, J. (1998). Increasing access to child mental health services for urban children their caregivers. *Social Work and Health, 23*, 9-15.

Miller, G. E., & Prinz, R. (1990). Enhancement of social learning family intervention for childhood conduct disorder. *Psychological Bulletin, 108*, 291-307.

Montaño, D. E., Kasprzyk, D., & Taplin, S. H. (1997). The theory of reasoned action the theory of planned behavior. In Glanz, K., Lewis, F. M., and Rimer, B. K. (Eds.) (2nd Ed.). (1997), *Health behavior health education: Theory, research, practice* (pp. 85-112). San Francisco, CA: Jossey-Bass.

Muecke, M. A. (1983). In search of healers. *Western Journal of Medicine, 139*, 835-840.

Pescosolido, B. A. (1992). Beyond rational choice: The social dynamics of how people seek help. *American Journal of Sociology, 97* (New directions in the sociology of medicine), 1096-1138.

Pescosolido, B. A. (1991). Illness careers and network ties: A conceptual model of utilization and compliance. In G. Albrecht, and J. Levy (Eds.), *Advances in Medical Sociology*, Vol. 2, (pp. 164-181). Greenwich, CT: JAI Press.

Pinto, R. M. (2003). *Factors that influence minority women's participation in HIV prevention programs: An ecological perspective.* Unpublished doctoral dissertation, Columbia University School of Social Work, New York.

Pinto, R. M. (2001). HIV prevention for adolescent groups: A six-step approach. *Social Work with Groups, 23*, 81-99.

Pinto, R. M. (2000). Six-step approach to HIV/AIDS prevention in counseling of adolescents. *Journal of HIV/AIDS Prevention & Education for Adolescents & Children, 3,* 49-71.

Prochaska, J. O., Redding, C. A., & Evers, K. E. (1997). The transtheoretical model stages of change. In Glanz, K., Lewis, F. M., and Rimer, B. K. (Eds.) (2nd Ed.), *Health behavior health education: Theory, research, practice* (pp. 60-84). San Francisco, CA: Jossey-Bass.

Romer, D., Black, M., Ricardo, I., Feigelman, S., Kaljee, L., Galbraith, J., Nesbit, R., Homik, R., & Stanton, B. (1994). Social Influences on the Sexual Behavior of Youth at Risk of HIV Exposure. *American Journal of Public Health, 84,* 977-985.

Snow, L. (1983). Traditional health beliefs practices among lower class Black Americans. *Western Journal of Medicine, 129,* 820-828.

Stevenson, H. C. & White, J. J. (1994). AIDS prevention struggles in ethnocultural neighborhoods: Why research partnerships with community based organizations can't wait. *AIDS Education & Prevention, 6,* 126-139.

Tolan, P., Miller, L., & Thomas, P. (1987). *Metropolitan Area Child Study Family Stress Questionnaire.* University of Illinois at Chicago.

Wahler, R. G., & Dumas, J. E. (1989). Attentional problems in dysfunctional mother-child interactions: An interbehavioral model. *Psychological Bulletin, 105,* 116-130.

Webster-Stratton, C. (1985). Predictors of treatment outcome in parent training for conduct disordered children. *Behavioral Therapy, 16,* 223-243.

Windle, C. (1980). Correlates of community mental health center underservice to non-Whites. *Journal of Community Psychology, 8,* 140-146.

Wingood, G. M., & DiClemente, R. J. (2000). The WILLOW program: Mobilizing social networks of women living with HIV to enhance coping and reduce sexual risk behaviors. In W. Pequegnat and J. Szapocznik (eds.), *Working with families in the era of HIV/AIDS,* (pp. 281-298). Thousand Oaks, CA: Sage.

Yen, L., Edington, M. P., McDonald, T., Hischl, D., & Edington, D. W. (2001). Changes in health risks among the participants in the United Auto Workers-General Motors Life Steps health promotion program. *American Journal of Health Promotion, 16,* 7-15.

doi:10.1300/J200v05n01_09

Family-Based HIV Preventive Intervention: Child Level Results from the CHAMP Family Program

Cami K. McBride
Donna Baptiste
Dorian Traube
Roberta L. Paikoff
Sybil Madison-Boyd

Doris Coleman
Carl C. Bell
Ida Coleman
Mary M. McKay

Cami K. McBride, PhD, is affiliated with the Department of Psychology, Rosalind Franklin University of Medicine and Science. Donna Baptiste, PhD, Roberta L. Paikoff, PhD, Sybil Madison-Boyd, PhD, Doris Coleman, LCSW, and Carl C. Bell, MD, are affiliated with the Institute for Juvenile Research, University of Illinois at Chicago. Dorian Traube, CSW, is affiliated with Columbia University. Ida Coleman is affiliated with the CHAMP Collaborative Board-Chicago. Mary M. McKay, PhD, is affiliated with the Mt. Sinai School of Medicine.

Address correspondence to: Donna R. Baptiste, PhD, Institute for Juvenile Research, 1747 West Roosevelt Road, Room 155 (MC747), Chicago, IL 60608 (E-mail: baptiste@uic.edu).

The authors would like to acknowledge the following persons: Emily Folk, Tariq Qureshi and Michelle Ernst for their assistance with the data. The authors are grateful to our community facilitators and mental health interns who tirelessly collected the data and conducted the group sessions. Thanks especially to the CHAMP children and parents who gave their time by participating.

Funding from the National Institute of Mental Health (R01 MH 63662) and the W. T. Grant Foundation is gratefully acknowledged. Dorian Traube is currently a pre-doctoral fellow at the Columbia University School of Social Work supported by a training grant from the National Institutes of Mental Health (5T32MH014623-24).

SUMMARY. Social indicators suggest that African American adolescents are in the highest risk categories of those contracting HIV/AIDS (CDC, 2001). The dramatic impact of HIV/AIDS on urban African American youth have influenced community leaders and policy makers to place high priority on programming that can prevent youth's exposure to the virus (Pequegnat & Szapocznik, 2000). Program developers are encouraged to design programs that reflect the developmental ecology of urban youth (Tolan, Gorman-Smith, & Henry, 2003). This often translates into three concrete programmatic features: (1) *Contextual relevance*; (2) *Developmental-groundedness*; and (3) *Systemic Delivery*. Because families are considered to be urban youth's best hope to grow up and survive multiple dangers in urban neighborhoods (Pequegnat & Szapocznik, 2000), centering prevention within families may ensure that youth receive ongoing support, education, and messages that can increase their capacity to negotiate peer situations involving sex.

This paper will present preliminary data from an HIV/AIDS prevention program that is contextually relevant, developmentally grounded and systematically-delivered. The collaborative HIV/AIDS Adolescent Mental Health Project (CHAMP) is aimed at decreasing HIV/AIDS risk exposure among a sample of African American youth living in a poverty-stricken, inner-city community in Chicago. This study describes results from this family-based HIV preventive intervention and involves 88 African American pre-adolescents and their primary caregivers. We present results for the intervention group at baseline and post intervention. We compare post test results to a community comparison group of youth. Suggestions for future research are provided. doi:10.1300/J200v05n01_10 *[Article copies available for a fee from The Haworth Document Delivery Service: 1-800-HAWORTH. E-mail address: <docdelivery@haworthpress.com> Website: <http://www.HaworthPress.com> © 2007 by The Haworth Press, Inc. All rights reserved.]*

KEYWORDS. Prevent youth exposure to HIV, contextual relevance, developmental groundedness, systemic delivery, Chicago African American youth, developmental ecology of urban youth

INTRODUCTION

Social indicators suggest that African American adolescents are in the highest risk for contracting HIV/AIDS (CDC, 2001). Nationally, African Americans account for over 57% of all new HIV infections

(CDC, 2004). Similarly, AIDS is the fourth leading cause of death among African American young adults–a group likely to have been infected during their adolescent years (CDC, 2001). Notably, a significant majority of reported HIV infection occurs among African American adolescents and young adults living in urban neighborhoods in US cities. For example, in the city of Chicago (where the study discussed in this paper was conducted) over 60% of newly reported HIV-infections occur among African Americans living in the poorest census tracks of the city. Further, inner-city African American youth accounted for more than 50% of all reported adolescent cases of HIV in Chicago (Illinois Department of Public Health, 2001).

The dramatic impact of HIV on urban African American youth has influenced community leaders and policy makers to place high priority on programming that can prevent youth's exposure to the virus (Pequegnat & Szapocznik, 2000). Program developers are encouraged to design programs that reflect the developmental ecology of urban youth (Tolan, Gorman-Smith, & Henry, 2003). This often translates into three concrete programmatic features: (1) *Contextual relevance* embedding messages and strategies specifically tailored for youth living in an urban context, many of whom are growing up in poverty-stricken communities with high levels of social toxicity. The multiple and co-occurring risks for these youth underscore the need to address risks holistically (Bell, Flay, & Paikoff, 2002). (2) *Developmental-groundedness*–recognizing that urban youth face significant different risks and challenges as they move from younger to more mature phases of adolescence. Many preadolescents are not *actually* engaged in sexual behavior (Paikoff, 1996), but are indirectly exposed to the same risk factors that are stronger lures for older youth. Older youth are often in more potent risk situations and hence decision-making about sexual choices become more complex. Correspondingly, prevention programs must prepare youth to recognize risk situations, as well as to negotiate situations once they are unfolding (Hains & Herrman, 1989). (3) *Systemic Delivery*–working in proximal systems in which youth decision making unfold. For most youth, these systems include family and peer contexts. Families are often considered to be urban youth's best hope to grow up and survive multiple dangers in urban neighborhoods (Pequegnat & Szapocznik, 2000). Hence, centering prevention within families may ensure that youth receive ongoing support, education, and value messages that can increase their capacity to negotiate peer situations involving sex.

Utilizing this framework, this article will present preliminary data from an HIV/AIDS prevention program that is contextually relevant, developmentally grounded and systemically-delivered. The Collaborative HIV/AIDS Adolescent Mental Health Project (CHAMP) is aimed at decreasing HIV/AIDS risk exposure among a sample of African American youth living in a poverty-stricken, inner-city community in Chicago. The CHAMP Program is distinctive because of a high intensity researcher-community collaboration that became the vehicle for designing the developmentally timed, family-based HIV/AIDS prevention program customized for urban youth. CHAMP taps into the construct of contextual relevance by teaming with community members to design an intervention that is laden with symbols, vocabulary, and topics indigenous to the neighborhood where the intervention is being implemented. All CHAMP curriculum is delivered by age group with material specifically targeted to the developmental tasks of pre adolescence and early-adolescence respectively. This ensures developmental appropriateness of each group. Finally, CHAMP is systematically delivered in neighborhood schools with facilitators from the community. Additionally, families are recruited by their fellow community members. This strategy eases the possibility of distrust of university based researchers and ensures the longevity of the intervention as the community has a sense of ownership. In prior publications, Madison and colleagues (2000) describe the collaborative partnership framework that under girds the CHAMP approach to prevention. In addition, Baptiste et al. (2004) describe how researcher and community members collaborated to design and deliver programs targeting youth at two developmental nodes, pre and early adolescence.

THE CHAMP PRE-ADOLESCENT PROGRAM

The CHAMP preadolescent program was designed for urban African American youth ages 9-11, and is based on the idea that prevention should begin early, to equip youth to resist pressure to engage in unprotected sexual activity, and by extension prevent HIV risk exposure. The program involves having youth participate with parents and/or other adult caregivers who can steer them through pubertal changes, increases in romantic thoughts and feelings, and social pressure to engage in risky behavior, which may involve sexual activity. In a prior paper, we noted that while less than 3% of urban pre-adolescents report actually engaging in sex, many have thought about it and are in *sexual possibility situations*–where youth are alone with other youth in private settings without adult supervision. (Paikoff, 1996). Therefore, our preadolescent program focuses on: (a) increasing parent/caregivers' and youth comfort in discussing puberty and the development of romantic or sexual feelings; (b) reducing time spent in *sexual possibility situations*; (c) increasing parental effectiveness around supervision and monitoring of youth in general, and of sexual possibility situations, in particular; (d) clarifying family values about sexual choices; and (e) increasing parent and youth's knowledge about risks related to HIV/AIDS.

The preadolescent program is structured as a Multiple Family Group (MFG) intervention in which 6-8 families participate together. MFGs are designed to increase inter and intra family support and mutual aid, to decrease stigma parents and youth may experience about being involved in a group discussing sensitive family issues, and to create supportive, parent and youth peer-groups to problem solve about prevention strategies. The twelve MFG sessions in the preadolescent program are structured comparably. Families first meet together for about twenty minutes to focus on the topic of the meeting. This is followed by simultaneous parent and youth break out sessions which last for approximately 45 minutes. Youth sessions are aimed at creating a peer microcosm to practice negotiation and refusal skills in peer pressure situations. Youth role play scenarios that typically occur in urban settings. Further, they practice strategies for handling these situations also for talking with their parents about them (see Madison et al., 2000; McKay et al., 2000 for a more complete description).

Simultaneously, parents are also holding related discussions. Parents discuss monitoring strategies to reduce *sexual possibility situations* and problem solve about strategies to help youth deal with social pressure in an urban context. Parents are encouraged to support each other within groups, and outside of groups around the idea that mutual-aid and encouragement can enhance parenting overall. Further, parents also prepare to discuss sensitive topics with their youth by talking with other group members and the CHAMP facilitators. Following parent and youth break out groups, each family holds a discussion to allow parents and youth to exchange ideas on the day's topic and to make an action plan that would be implemented out-of-group. A detailed summary of the goals, topics and activities of each session in the preadolescent curriculum is included in Table 1.

FAMILY INFLUENCES ON HIV/AIDS RISK BEHAVIOR

In this paper we focus on components of this conceptual model that relate to family influence on preadolescent HIV/AIDS risk exposure. Next, Figure 1 presents our conceptual model of family influences on HIV/AIDS risk behavior. Sexual possibility situations (hereafter abbreviated as SPSs), defined as private, mixed sex, unsupervised situations, represent one possible gateway to early sexual activity and HIV/AIDS risk exposure (Paikoff, 1996). As children mature into older adolescents, SPSs become more normative and developmentally appropriate as youth become interested in dating and romantic relationships. However, participation in SPSs at an *early* age represents a risk for younger children who are not cognitively or developmentally prepared for early sexual activity. Hence, the CHAMP intervention program encourages parents to improve their monitoring skills with the goal of reducing the number of opportunities that youth have to participate in SPSs. While the theoretical value of SPSs is clear, empirical support for the links between SPSs and actual sexual activity exists as well. DiLorio and colleagues (2004) found that SPS were associated with actual sexual behavior in a sample of 11 to 14 year old African American adolescents.

Sexual Possibility Situations and Peer Pressure

We used Situations of Sexual Possibility as our key intervention outcome and explored several key theoretical mediators addressed as targets of the intervention. At the level of the child, we investigated the role of peer pressure. As part of the intervention, the CHAMP program develops peer resistance skills in the youth. Numerous studies have demonstrated that youth who can refuse the unwanted pressure of peers are less likely to engage in risky behaviors (Billy & Udry, 1985; Keefe, 1992; Romer et al., 1993; Dahlberg, 1998; Kung & Farrell, 2000; Walker-Barnes & Mason 2001; Fuemmeler et al., 2002). We assessed how likely youth are to break off a friendship when faced with unwanted peer pressure. Since sexual risk often occurs in peer contexts, the child's ability to refuse unwanted pressure and discontinue these friendships with pressuring peers is an important marker of the child's assertiveness skills.

TABLE 1. The Champ Pre-Adolescent Program

Session Topic	Session Objectives	Parent Group Activities	Child Group Activities	Family Interaction Tasks
Session 1: *Working Together to Keep Our Kids Safe!*	• To introduce the CHAMP Program • To help families feel comfortable with facilitators and with each other • To discuss dangers and threats to kids in the community • To identify ways in which families can help youth	• Parents lists: dangers in the community • Threat of HIV/AIDS in the community • How families can help kids to withstand risks • Guidelines for being in the CHAMP program • How being in CHAMP can help	• Kids list: What they believe parents worry about • Dangers for kids in the neighborhood • Danger of HIV/AIDS in the community • How being in CHAMP can help	Each family sits together • Parents and kids compare list of dangers in the community • Parents and kids make a list of how families can protect kids • Families share ideas with each other
Session 2: *Where Are We Going?* *Paperwork!*	• To explain the purposes of research and assessment measures • To explain confidentiality • To complete pre-test family and risk measures	• Complete Pre Assessments	• Complete Pre Assessments	• None
Session 3: *Talking and Listening To Each Other*	• To introduce "sexual possibility situations" • To identify how good parent/child communication deter sexual possibility situations • To discuss children's peer pressure experiences	• Parents discuss: what a sexual possibility situation is • Sexual possibility situations at home, and outside the house • How sexual possibility situations are linked to HIV risk • Strategies to decrease sexual possibility situations at home and away from home	• Kids discuss what peer pressure is • List peer pressure situations • Share stories of peer pressure situations	Each family sits together • Kids share list of peer pressure situations • Talk about the *Johnson Family*. Tanya faces a peer pressure situation • Discuss how talking and listening to each other is connected to HIV
Session 4: *Keeping Track of Kids–Part 1*	• To discuss importance of parental supervision and monitoring • To have parents and children exchange information using the CHAMP Family Game • To complete process measures	• Parents discuss: benefits of close monitoring • Monitoring strategies for home, school, neighborhood • Monitoring sexual possibility situations • Prepare for family game	• Kids discuss benefits to tell parents about themselves • Easy and hard things to tell • Role play telling parents hard things • Prepare for the family game	Each family sits together • Kids share their list of things that are "hard to tell" • Families play the family game • Families discuss how keeping track of kids is connected to preventing HIV • Complete process measures
Session 5: *Keeping Track of Kids–Part 2*	• To help parents identify safe and unsafe neighborhood areas • To help parents identify their children's positive and negative peer relationships • To discuss positive and negative neighborhood and peer environments	• Parents draw a community map and identify places to avoid • Parents list friends and associates of their children and indicate people to avoid	• Kids list qualities of a good friend and not so good friend • Share stories about ending friendships	Each family sits together • Parents share maps and explain about places/people to avoid • Talk about the *Johnson Family*. Tarik is faced with breaking off an undesirable friendship

209

TABLE 1 (continued)

Session Topic	Session Objectives	Parent Group Activities	Child Group Activities	Family Interaction Tasks
Session 6: *Who Can Help Us Raise Our Children?*	• To identify current supports and resources for parenting • To identify ways to get additional parenting support • To discuss how support in CHAMP can help families protect kids against HIV	• Parents identify supportive people in their lives • Think of additional support they need • Discuss ways to find additional support • Talk about how support can assist in preventing HIV	• Kids identify people who support their families • Identify people they talk to about different scenarios • Identify way in which people support them personally • List ways having supporters can prevent HIV	Each family sits together • Families talk about the *Johnson Family Cartoon*: The family talks about finding more support • Each family prepare to make a videotape to thank support people • Families make and then view videos
Session 7: *Rules Keep Kids Safe*	• To make connections between rules and children's safety • To help families evaluate current rules • To strengthen rule-making in families • To encourage families to acknowledge when rules are kept • To complete process measures	• Parents list rules in the home, for school and community • Evaluate whether rules are working • Strategize about ways to reward kids who keep rules • Analyze why rules may not be kept • Review principles of a good rule	• Kids discuss why rules are helpful • List rules for home, school and in the community • Identify easy and hard rules to follow • Role play talking with parents about hard to follow rules	Each family sits together • Kids share list of rules that are easy and hard to follow • Families discuss *The Johnson Family Cartoon*: Tarik struggles to keep a rule. Mom compliments him for trying • Complete process measures
Session 8: *Growing Up: Talking About Puberty*	• To review puberty information • To prepare parents to talk about puberty with their children • To prepare children to talk with their parents about puberty	• Parents discuss puberty changes • Role play answering kids questions about changes • Give each other feedback	• Kids discuss puberty changes • Make a list of questions they want answers to • List people they can talk to about puberty	Each family sits together • Kids hare their list of puberty questions/Parents answer • Families talk about *Johnson Family Cartoon*: Tanya and Tarik tease each other about puberty changes
Session 9: *What We Need to Know About HIV/AIDS*	• To present facts about HIV risks • To present information about transmission and prevention • To help parents answer children's questions accurately	• Parents identify HIV risks in the community • List myths and facts about HIV • List safe and unsafe behaviors	• Kids identify HIV risks in the community • List myths and facts • List safe, unsafe behaviors	Each family sits together • Families discuss the *Johnson Family Cartoon*: Tanya and Tarik's aunt dies of AIDS
Session 10: *Growing Up: Preparing Kids for Adolescence*	• To help parents identify children's transitions to adolescence • To clarify values and how they impact children • To help families prepare for about transitions to adolescence	• Parents draw kids lifelines through adolescence • Identify timing of events (e.g., sleeping over, going out alone, dating, having a boyfriend, etc.) • Parents discuss reasons for timing	• Kids draw their lifelines through adolescence • Identify timing of events (e.g., sleeping over, going out alone, dating, having a boyfriend • Discuss reasons for timing	Each family sits together • Parents and kids exchange ideas on lifelines • Families discuss the *Johnson Family Cartoon*: The older brother of Tany's friend sends Tanya a romantic letter
Session 11: *Paperwork and More Paperwork!*	• To remind families why data is collected • To help families understand the value of research • To complete post test measures	• Complete Post-Assessments	• Complete Post-Assessments	• None
Session 12: *A Celebration!*	• To celebrate the completion of families' time in CHAMP • To help families plan ways to keep in touch with each other	• Parents: review lessons learned in CHAMP • Discuss how information will be used to help kids avoid HIV	• Kids review lessons learned in CHAMP	• Ending celebration • CHAMP thanks and compliments families • Certificates of participation

FIGURE 1. A Conceptual Model of Family Influences on HIV/AIDS Risk Exposure

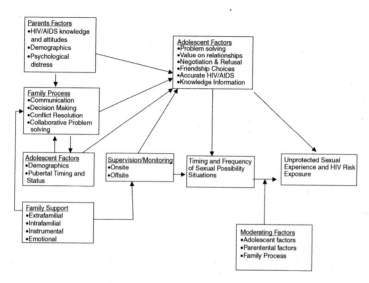

Sexual Possibility Situations and Family Processes

We also explored two elements of family process, as reported by the youth, who participated: parental control and family conflict. Parental control addresses who makes decisions in the family regarding key family issues. Paikoff et al. (1997) did not find an association between parental control and situations of sexual possibility. However, Kapungu et al. (in preparation), in a longitudinal study, found that boys of families with greater parental control were less likely to reach sexual debut in early adolescence. In terms of family conflict, McBride et al. (2003) found that both self-reported and observed family conflict at pre-adolescence, with some results moderated by pubertal development, predicted sexual debut at early adolescence. Early sexual debut has been linked to greater sexual risk because younger adolescents who are also less likely to use condoms and have greater numbers of lifetime partners (Rodrigue, Tercyak, & Lescano, 1997).

The constructs discussed here are only a portion of the key variables in the theoretical model. Each of the constructs is a component of the intervention and is hypothesized to change as a result of participation in the intervention. McKay and colleagues (2004) discuss findings related to key outcomes based on the report of parents in the same sample.

Findings reveal that parents who participated in the intervention reported that they were more likely to make decisions in the family, had improvements in parental monitoring, as well as in family communication and comfort related to family communication. Hence these findings indicates the importance of increasing parents' capacity for control and decision-making, as well as reducing family conflict so that parents may protect their developing teens. This paper builds on findings of McKay and colleagues (2004) by examining key outcomes based on the child's report

METHODS

Participants

The CHAMP Family Program sample of youth and their families (n = 324) were identified to participate in the CHAMP Family Program at the end of the 1995/1996 school year. Youth attended one of four elementary schools, located adjacent to large, high rise subsidized housing projects and within 11 blocks of each other. All of these schools are 99% African American and over 90% poverty (as indicated by children's qualification for free lunches). Approximately 75% of families in the community are female-headed households, and 63% of adult caregivers have not worked in the last year.

Of the 324 eligible 4th and 5th graders (92% of youth on class rosters at 4 elementary schools, all with active parent consent), 274 (85%) of their families could be located and invited to participate. We did not continue to track the remaining 15% of youth since they represented moves to other communities or whose address we were never able to determine. Approximately 73% of families located completed the entire CHAMP Family Program (n = 201). An additional 26 families completed pre/posttest assessments and some portion of the intervention (for a total of 86% of families located). Only the first three cohorts of youth and their families are included in the current study (n = 100).

Approximately 60% of the sample is female and 40% is male. Almost 76% of parents reported a family income of less than $14,000. Three quarters of adult caregivers completed high school and 8% of parent figures had attended some college. Approximately 17% of the adult caregivers are between the ages of 25 and 29 years, indicating that they were teenagers at the time of the target child's birth.

Youth involved in the comparison group in the current study, consists of 315 non-overlapping 4th and 5th graders drawn from the same community during the 1993/1994 school year. This sample of youth and their families were involved in the CHAMP Family Study, a longitudinal examination of family and mental health factors related to HIV risk exposure during the transition to adolescence (and did not receive the preventative intervention). The longitudinal examination consisted of yearly interviews only. Of the 315 eligible youth, all parents were invited to learn more about the longitudinal study. Approximately 92% ($n = 290$) of parents responded to project outreach efforts. Two hundred sixty-four families (91% of contacted families) participated fully in a three-hour interview. From this sample of 4th and 5th grade children who completed questionnaires, we selected a random sample of 104 children to serve as a comparison sample. This comparison sample, which consisted of 60% girls and 40% boys, completed questionnaires with their female caregiver.

These caregivers were also primarily biological mothers as well as grandmothers, aunts and older siblings. Approximately 57% of the youth comparison sample is female and 43% is male. Approximately 60% of the families are headed by unmarried mothers. Approximately 90% of families reside in federally subsidized housing apartments and have incomes less than $14,000. Approximately 46% of adult caregivers reported completing high school or GED. Fifty-four percent of adult caregivers were employed in the last year. A comparison between the experimental and comparison samples is provided in Table 2.

Measures

Frequency in Situations of Sexual Possibility. This measure is derived from a gated behavioral interview developed by Paikoff (1995) that inquires about the amount of time the pre-adolescent spends in unsupervised, mixed sex, private situations–sexual possibility situations. This scale taps how often during the week that youth find themselves in these situations of sexual possibility. An index score is created by summing across three items answered by the child: how often, how long, and how many times the child is in unsupervised situations with children of opposite sex. DiIorio et al. (in press) using an index of SPS found an alpha reliability of .66. Higher scores indicate that a child is in a situation of sexual possibility more often.

Relationship Maintenance. This scale is completed by the pre-adolescent about whether they would keep or break off a friendship under 7

TABLE 2. Comparison of Samples

	CHAMP Family Program ($n = 201$)	Comparison ($n = 264$)
Gender		
Males	40%	43%
Females	60%	57%
Percent Female Headed Household	73%	60%
Family Income < $14,000	76%	90%
Adult Caregiver Employed	70%	54%

situations of pressure from a friend. Pressure situations include making fun of another friend, skipping school, smoking cigarettes, drinking alcohol, etc. Each item is answered using a 4 point Likert type scale that includes (1) Definitely would break off the friendship, (2) Probably would keep the friendship, (3) Probably would break off the friendship, and (4) Definitely would break off the friendship.

Parental Control. This questionnaire, completed by the pre-adolescent, asked questions related to 17 parenting issues (e.g., chores, bedtime, friends); responses were made on a 4-point Likert scale. For each parenting issue, youth were asked whether their parents (a) tell their child exactly what to do (restrictive control), (b) discuss the issue and then have the final say (firm control), (c) discuss the issue and then the child has the final say (responsive control), or (d) leave it up to the child to decide (low control). Scores can range from 17 to 68, higher scores indicating low control. Paikoff et al. (1997) found inter-item reliability was high (alpha = .76). The scale has been used previously with diverse adolescents (Holmbeck & O'Donnell, 1991).

Average Intensity of Discussion (Family Conflict): Average intensity of discussion between parent and child was assessed using the Issues Checklist, brief version (Holmbeck & O'Donnell, 1991; Robin & Foster, 1989). Children indicated if they had discussed 17 possible issues (i.e., curfew, homework, choice of friends) with their caregivers during the past two weeks. For each issue discussed, participants indicated how many times the issue had been discussed in the past two weeks, and how "hot" (intensity) the discussions were using a five point Likert scale, which ranged from 1 (calm) to 5 (angry). Average intensity of discussions was calculated by computing the mean of the intensity ratings for the 17 issues discussed. Total scores ranged from 17-16, with higher scores indicating greater conflict. Inter-item reliability was .77 for the child report.

RESULTS

For each variable measured, we conducted paired t-tests of the pre and post data from the intervention group. Table 3 presents the results of these analyses ($n = 88$). On the Parental Control scale, there was a significant change in who makes the decisions in the family, $t = 2.70, p <$ .01, such that on average, after receiving the intervention, parents were making more decisions in their families, as opposed to the children. On the Relationship Maintenance scale, which measured the child's response to peer pressure, there was a significant change, $t = -2.53, p <$ .01, such that children reported after receiving the intervention, they were more likely to break off a friendship in response to peer pressure. There were no significant pre-post changes in the Family Conflict measure or in the frequency of situations of sexual possibility for the intervention group.

We next compared the post-test scores from the intervention group to scores from the comparison group. These results are summarized in Table 4. The children in the intervention group reported significantly lower scores on the Parental Control scale, $t = 5.60, p < .001$, suggesting that the parents in the intervention group are making more decisions in their families than the parents in the comparison group. The children in the intervention group reported that they were in situations of sexual possibility significantly less often, $t = 3.22, p < .01$, n = 88, than children in the comparison sample ($n = 315$). Interestingly, children in the intervention group reported a significantly higher level of Family Conflict, $t = -2.97, p < .01$, than the comparison group. There was no signif-

TABLE 3. Pre vs. Post Comparison of Intervention Group Only

Variable	Pre M (S.D.)	Post M (S.D.)	t (df)	p
Family Conflict	1.95 (0.68)	1.98 (0.77)	−0.34 (87)	ns
Decision Making	1.92 (0.47)	1.77 (0.52)	2.70 (86)	.01
Relationship Maintenance	3.68 (0.32)	3.77 (0.26)	−2.53 (85)	.01
Frequency in SSP	0.89 (2.98)	0.35 (1.69)	1.51 (84)	.14

SSP = Situations of Sexual Possibility

TABLE 4. Post Intervention vs. Comparison Group

Variable	Intervention M (S.D.)	Comparison M (S.D.)	t (df)	p
Family Conflict	2.03 (0.81)	1.71 (0.79)	−2.97 (219)	.01
Decision Making	1.79 (0.53)	2.17 (0.47)	5.60 (219)	.001
Relationship Maintenance	3.77 (0.26)	3.84 (0.27)	1.77 (188)	.08
Frequency in SSP	0.35 (1.69)	1.67 (3.74)	3.22 (187)	.01

icant difference between the intervention and comparison groups on the Relationship Maintenance scale.

DISCUSSION

Social indicators suggest that African American adolescents are in the highest risk categories of those contracting HIV/AIDS (CDC, 2001). One potential method of curtailing HIV transmission is via strategic community prevention programs. However, for these programs to be successful they must contain three concrete programmatic features: (1) *Contextual relevance*; (2) *Developmental-groundedness*; and (3) *Systemic Delivery*. Because families are considered be urban youth's best hope to grow up and survive multiple dangers in urban neighborhoods (Pequegnat & Szapocznik, 2000), centering prevention within families may ensure that youth receive ongoing support, education, and value messages that can increase their capacity to negotiate peer situations involving sex. The CHAMP Family Program not only centers its prevention efforts at the family level in order to prevent early adolescent sexual debut, it is also designed and administered within the community to ensure cultural relevance and develop unique systems of care. Moreover, CHAMP is designed to meet the needs of children at various developmental levels to ensure that they acquire appropriate and viable strategies for social problem solving and family communication.

Results from this study suggest that participation in the CHAMP Family Program was positively associated with parental decision making within the family, thereby potentially improving the influence that parents have in their children's lives. Results also revealed that youth reported an improvement in their abilities to resist peer pressure. Both of these findings suggest that changes in two key mechanisms related to risk taking were associated with participation in the intervention. We also found that relative to a comparison group, the children in the intervention group were in sexual possibility situations less often and had parents with higher levels of parental control in their families.

LIMITATIONS

As with any quasi-experimental design, our findings may be criticized for threats to internal validity. Specifically the intervention sample may have improved over time, regardless of the intervention. To address this threat we compared the intervention sample to a comparison group of similar adolescents from the same community. We were able to avoid a lack of comparability between the samples by comparing the samples across a number of dimensions to demonstrate their multiple similarities; the children from the two groups did not differ in terms of age or gender and attended the same schools. Their parents had similar levels of education, had similar levels of income and they lived in the same neighborhoods.

IMPLICATIONS FOR HIV PREVENTION RESEARCH

These results are promising given that multiple studies have shown that adolescents who are involved with their parents and interact about high-risk behavior have been found to more successfully negotiate peer pressure social situations and resist engaging in high-risk behavior than adolescents who do not communicate with their parents (Holtzman & Rubinson, 1995; Farrell & White, 1998; Romer et al., 1994; Pick & Palos, 1995; Hutchinson & Cooney, 1998; Somers & Paulson, 2000). Communicating with their adolescents may be one of the most effective ways caregivers can protect their adolescents from making poor decisions that may impact their lives (Mueller & Powers, 1990; Holtzman & Rubinson, 1995).

By discussing possible high-risk situations and appropriate negotiation skills, parents may be able to increase the likelihood that their adolescent will implement these skills outside of the family unit. Ideally these discussions will lead to increased confidence for the adolescent and subsequent perceived self efficacy in social situations.

The multiple and co-occurring risks for urban youth underscore the need to address HIV risk holistically (Bell, Flay, & Paikoff, 2001) Future studies in the area of HIV prevention could benefit from implementing programs that embed messages and strategies specifically tailored for youth living in an urban context, many of whom are growing up in poverty-stricken communities with high levels of social toxicity, thus providing and element of contextual relevance to the inter- vention. Moreover, recognizing that urban youth face significantly different risks and challenges as they move from younger to more mature phases of adolescence requires researchers to cultivate developmentally grounded interventions that prepare youth to recognize risk situations, as well as to negotiate situations according to their current level of skills (Hains & Herrman, 1989). Finally, researchers should design interventions that will be delivered in the proximal systems in which youth decisions unfold. For most youth these include family and peer systems. More specifically, interventions that actively involve family members and strategies that enhance protective family processes are needed.

It is important to note that results indicating greater levels of family conflict in this study's intervention group relative to the comparison group were unexpected. We speculate that a finer analysis of this finding might indicate that the overall level of conflict among the intervention families may have been raised because they were addressing difficult issues more frequently than the comparison sample.

REFERENCES

Baptiste, D., Paikoff, P., McKay, M., Madison-Boyd, S., Bell., C., Coleman, D. & The CHAMP Board. (2004) Collaborating with an urban community to develop an HIV/AIDS prevention program for Black youth and families. (*Behavior Modification, 29*(2): 370-416. Sage. CA.

Bell, C.C., Flay, B., & Paikoff, R. (2002) Strategies for Health Behavioral Change. In J. Chunn (Ed.) *The Health Behavioral Change Imperative: Theory, Education, and Practice in Diverse Populations*. New York: Kluwer Academic/Plenum Publishers, p. 17-40.

Billy, J.O.G., & Udry, J.R. (1985). The influence of male and female best friends on adolescent sexual behavior. *Adolescence, XX* (77), 21-32.

Centers for Disease Control. (2001). *HIV/AIDS surveillance report*. Atlanta: Center for Infectious Disease Control.

Dahlberg, L.L. (1998). Youth violence in the United States: Major trends, risk factors, and approaches. *American Journal of Prevention Medicine, 14* (4), 259-272.

DiLorio, C., Dudley, W.N., Soet, J.E., & McCarty, F. (2004). Sexual possibility situations and sexual behaviors among young adolescents: The moderating role of protective factors. *Journal of Adolescent Health, 35*(6), 11-20.

Fuemmeler, B.F., Taylor, L.A., Metz, A.E.J., & Brown, R.T. (2002). Risk-taking and smoking tendency among primarily African American school children: Moderating influences of peer susceptibility. *Journal of Clinical Psychology and Medical Settings, 9* (4), 323-330.

Hains A.A., & Herrman L.P. (1989) Social cognitive skills and behavioral adjustment of delinquent adolescents in treatment. *Journal of Adolescence, 12* (3), 323-328.

Hutchinson, M.K., & Cooney, T.M. (1998). Patterns of parent-teen sexual risk communication: Implications for intervention. *Family Relations, 47* (2), 185-194.

Holmbeck, G.N., & O'Donnell, K. (1991). Discrepancies between perceptions of decision making and behavioral autonomy. *New Directions for Child Development, 51,* 51-69.

Holtzman, D., & Rubinson, R. (1995). Parent and peer communication effects on AIDS-related behavior among U.S. high school students. *Family Planning Perspectives, 27* (6), 235-247.

Illinois Department of Health (2001). *http://www.idph.state.il.us/.* Retrieved 8/12/04.

Kapungu, C.K., Holmbeck, G.N., & Paikoff, R.L. (in preparation). Longitudinal association between parenting practices and early sexual risk behaviors among urban African American adolescents: The moderating role of gender.

Keefe, K. (1992). Perceptions of normative social pressure and attitudes toward alcohol use: changes during adolescence. *Journal of Studies on Alcohol,* January, 46-54.

Kung, E.M., & Farrell, A.D. (2000). The role of parents and peers in early adolescent substance use: an examination of mediating and moderating effects. *Journal of Child and Family Studies, 9* (4), 509-528.

Madison, S. M., McKay, M. M., Paikoff, R. L., & Bell, C.C. (2000). Basic research and community collaboration: Necessary ingredients for the development of a family-based HIV prevention program. *AIDS Education and Prevention, 12,* 281-298.

McBride, C. K., Paikoff R. L., & Holmbeck G. N. (2003). Individual and familial influences on the onset of sexual intercourse among urban African American adolescents. *Journal of Consulting and Clinical Psychology, 71* (1), 159-167.

McKay, M., Paikoff, R., Baptiste, D., Bell, C., Coleman, D., Madison,S., McKinney, L. & CHAMP Collaborative Board (2004). "Family-level impact of the CHAMP Family Program: A community collaborative effort to support urban families and reduce youth HIV risk exposure." *Family Process, 43*(1), 79-93.

McKay, M., Baptiste, D., Coleman, D., Madison, S., Paikoff, R. & Scott, R. (2000). Preventing HIV risk exposure in urban communities: The CHAMP Family Program in W. Pequegnat & Jose Szapocznik (Eds). In *Working with families in the era of HIV/AIDS.* California: Sage Publications.

Mueller, K.E., & Powers, W.G. (1990). Parent-child sexual discussion: perceived communicator style and subsequent behavior. *Adolescence, XXV* (98), 469-482.

Paikoff, R. L., McKay, M. (1995). *The Chicago HIV Prevention adolescent mental health project (CHAMP) family-based intervention.* National Institute of Mental Health, Office on AIDS and William. T. Grant Foundation.

Paikoff, R. L., Parfenoff, S.H., Greenwood, G. L., & McCormick, A. (1997). Parenting, parent-child relationships, and sexual possibility situations among urban

African American preadolescents: Preliminary findings and implications for HIV prevention. *Journal of Family Psychology, 11,* 11-22.

Paikoff, R. L. (1996). Early heterosexual debut: Situations of sexual possibility during the transition to adolescence. *American Journal of Orthopsychiatry, 65,* 389-401.

Pequegnat. W. & Szapocznik, J. (Eds.). (2000). *Working with Families in the Era of HIV/AIDS.* CA: Sage publications.

Pick, S., & Palos, P.A. (1995). Impact of the family on the sex lives of adolescents. *Adolescence, 30* (119), 667-675.

Robin, A. L., & Foster, S. L. (1989). Self-report measures. *Negotiating parent-adolescent conflict* (pp. 295-328). New York: Guilford Press.

Rodrigue, J. R., Tercyak, K. P., & Lescano, C. M. (1997). Health promotion in minority adolescents: emphasis on sexually transmitted diseases and the human immunodeficiency virus. In D. K. Wilson, J. R. Rodrigue & W. C. Taylor (Eds.), *Health-promoting and health-compromising behaviors among minority adolescents* (pp. 87-105). Washington, DC: American Psychological Association.

Romer, D., Black, M., Ricardo, I., Feigelman, S., Kalijee, L., Galbraith, J. et al. (1993). Social influences on the sexual behavior of youth at risk for HIV exposure. *American Journal of Public Health, 84* (6), 977-985.

Tolan, P.H., Gorman-Smith, D., & Henry, D.B. (2003). The developmental ecology of urban males' youth violence. *Developmental Psychology, 39*(2), 274-291.

Walker-Barnes, C.J., & Mason, C.A. (2001). Perceptions of risk factors for female gang involvement among African American and Hispanic women. *Youth and Society, 32* (3), 303-326.

doi:10.1300/J200v05n01_10

Addressing Urban African American Youth Externalizing and Social Problem Behavioral Difficulties in a Family Oriented Prevention Project

William M. Bannon, Jr.
Mary M. McKay

SUMMARY. The current article examines the secondary effects of an inner-city Community-University Collaborative HIV-Prevention and Adolescent Mental Health Family Program (CHAMP) in reducing externalizing (i.e., aggressive and rule-breaking behavior) and social problem behaviors for children with significant levels of externalizing behavior.

William M. Bannon, Jr., MSW, is affiliated with the Columbia University School of Social Work. Mary M. McKay, PhD, is affiliated with Mount Sinai School of Medicine, Departments of Psychiatry & Community Medicine, CHAMP Collaborative Board.

Address correspondence to: Mary M. McKay, PhD, Mount Sinai School of Medicine, Department of Psychiatry & Community Medicine, 1425 Madison Avenue, NY, NY 10029 (E-mail: mary.mckay@mssm.edu).

Without the contributions of CHAMP Collaborative Board members and participants, this work would not have been possible.

Funding from the National Institute of Mental Health (R01 MH 63662) and the W.T. Grant Foundation is gratefully acknowledged. William Bannon is currently a pre-doctoral fellow at the Columbia University School of Social Work supported by a training grant from the National Institutes of Mental Health (5T32MH014623-24).

[Haworth co-indexing entry note]: "Addressing Urban African American Youth Externalizing and Social Problem Behavioral Difficulties in a Family Oriented Prevention Project." Bannon, William M. Jr., and Mary M. McKay. Co-published simultaneously in *Social Work in Mental Health* (The Haworth Press, Inc.) Vol. 5, No. 1/2, 2007, pp. 221-240; and: *Community Collaborative Partnerships: The Foundation for HIV Prevention Research Efforts* (ed: Mary M. McKay, and Roberta L. Paikoff) The Haworth Press, Inc., 2007, pp. 221-240. Single or multiple copies of this article are available for a fee from The Haworth Document Delivery Service [1-800-HAWORTH, 9:00 a.m. - 5:00 p.m. (EST). E-mail address: docdelivery@haworthpress.com].

Data were provided by parents for a sample of 50 youth assigned to the CHAMP Family Program and 299 comparison children. Among the CHAMP Family Program participants at pretest, 40% ($n = 20$) of parents reported their children exhibited significant levels of externalizing behavior. Among the comparison group, 38% ($n = 113$) of parents reported their children exhibited significant levels of externalizing behavior. There was a significant reduction in child externalizing scores for children in the CHAMP Family Program from pretest to posttest, bringing their mean scores of externalizing behavior from clinical to sub-clinical levels. Posttest only comparisons revealed that children in the CHAMP Family Program had significantly lower externalizing behavior scores than children in the comparison group. Analyses of child social problems indicated mixed results. Implications for urban mental health and prevention programs are discussed. *doi:10.1300/J200v05n01_11 [Article copies available for a fee from The Haworth Document Delivery Service: 1-800-HAWORTH. E-mail address: <docdelivery@haworthpress.com> Website: <http:// www.Haworth Press.com>* © *2007 by The Haworth Press, Inc. All rights reserved.]*

KEYWORDS. Secondary effects of CHAMP, reducing externalizing and social problem behavior, implications for urban mental health and prevention programs, pretest to posttest reduction of externalizing behavior

National data indicate that while there has been an overall reduction in the level of violence in recent years, there has not been a comparable reduction in delinquent and violent behavior involving adolescent youth (Guerra, Huesmann, Tolan, Van Acker, & Eron, 1995; Hennes, 1998; Rachuba, Stanton, & Howard, 1995). For example, surveillance data indicate a steady decline in rates of arrest for violent crimes among young adults, while there has been a comparable increase in rates of arrest for disruptive acts among young adolescents (Hennes, 1998). Adolescent disruptive behavior is especially problematic for minority inner-city youth (Tolan, Guerra, & Kendall, 1995). For example, among a sample of elementary age predominantly African American students living in an urban area, over one-third had been involved in a physical fight at school (Cotton et al., 1994). In another study involving over 1,000 inner-city youth, rates of disruptive, aggressive, and delinquent behavior were found to be approximately 40% (Tolan & Henry, 2000).

Significant levels of the delinquent and aggressive behavior evidenced by urban children, can often be connected with exposure to the stressors associated with the inner-city environment, most notably poverty, community violence, inadequate child serving resources, under supported schools, substance abuse and multiple health epidemics (Attar, Guerra, & Tolan, 1994; Gorman-Smith, Tolan, & Henry, 1999; Hess & Atkins, 1998; Weist, Acosta, & Youngstrom, 2001). Thus, it seems for many urban and minority adolescents, especially those living in poverty, externalizing behaviors have become symptomatic of coping with the daily pressures associated with living in the inner-city (Prothrow-Stith, 1995). Additionally, there is reason to believe that high levels of externalizing behavior coupled with exposure to urban stressors are associated with the development of significant other social problem behaviors (Cohen, 2002), that may further compromise children's well-being (Best, 1994).

Child developmental research has identified a clear link between a range of externalizing behaviors in adolescence, such as violence, delinquency, truancy, stealing, and later deviant behaviors in adulthood, notably drug abuse and criminal activity (Elliot et al., 1996). Additionally, the presence of social and peer relational difficulties have been linked with serious ongoing difficulties, particularly as youth enter adolescence. For example, a higher frequency of social problems in grade-school has been associated with the onset of academic failure and eventual school dropout (Alexander, Entwisle, & Dauber, 1993; Alexander, Entwisle, & Kabbani, 2001) in mid to late adolescence. Thus, a central focus for urban mental health providers and child mental health researchers has become the design, delivery, and testing of interventions that can effectively reduce externalizing behaviors that emerge at pre and early adolescence (Dishion & Kavanagh, 2002; Dishion, Nelson, & Kavanagh, 2003), as well as other related problematic behaviors (Bradock & McPartland, 1992; O'Brien, 1991), in order to enhance urban youth mental health outcomes.

Past research has identified a number of family processes that appear protective in relation to development for inner-city African American youth. For example, parental monitoring has emerged in the literature as one of the most consistently cited correlates of lower levels of child behavioral problems, including delinquency and aggression (Barnes & Farrel, 1992; Palmer & Hollin, 2001). Research suggests that parents of disruptive youth are often not aware of their children's activities, companions, or physical location (Patterson & Stouthamer-Loeber, 1984), which often leaves children "free" to become involved with deviant

peers (Dishion, Capaldi, Spracklen, & Li, 1995). Other familial characteristics have been associated with lower levels of behavioral difficulties for urban youth of color including parent-child interaction (Hanlon
et al., 2004) and family connectedness (Kerr et al., 2003). Thus, a number of recent interventions have focused on strengthening these family
processes as a means of reducing problematic behavior in high-risk
youth (Dishion & Kavanagh, 2002; Dishion et al., 2003),

The current study considers the secondary effect of The Collaborative HIV-prevention and Adolescent Mental health Project (CHAMP)
Family Program in reducing problem behaviors among a sample of
low-income urban African American youth. The CHAMP Family Program is a family-based HIV preventive and mental health promoting intervention meant to reduce risk taking activity by urban youth in the 4th
and 5th grades (9 to 11 years of age) living in inner-city neighborhoods
(Madison, McKay, Paikoff, & Bell, 2000; McKay, Baptiste, Coleman,
Madison, Paikoff, & Scott, 2000). The youth oriented prevention literature indicates that risk taking among youth, particularly related to risky
sexual activity, is inversely related to the presence of many of the same
family processes that are associated with other problematic behaviors in
youth (e.g., externalizing and social problem behaviors). For example,
past research has revealed that urban youth sexual risk taking behavior
of urban youth is associated with levels of family monitoring (Romer et
al., 1994; Stanton et al., 2000), parent-child interaction (e.g., communication concerning sexual risk topics; Jaccard & Dittus, 1991), and inversely related to levels of family conflict (Black, Ricardo, & Stanton,
1997). A key component of the CHAMP Family Program is the strengthening of a range of family processes in order to reduce sexual risk taking
behavior among youth (Madison et al., 2000; McKay et al., 2000).

Over the last decade, a number of prevention programs similar to
CHAMP that seek to impact youth HIV exposure, have demonstrated
efficacy in enhancing youth outcomes for urban adolescents and their
families (Centers for Disease Control, 2001). However, the consideration of how these interventions simultaneously impact youth problem
behaviors, is largely unstudied. This is unfortunate, since HIV preventive interventions may hold promise for impacting youth problem behaviors due to the fact that these programs attempt to strengthen the
same family processes associated with pro-social adolescent behavior.
Therefore, to explore this potential, the purpose of the current study is to
determine what impact, if any, the CHAMP Family Program interven-

tion has on problematic behaviors evidenced by African American youth that reside in low-income urban environments.

METHODS

Research Design

The current research study involves a posttest-only comparison of two samples of African American youth, 4th and 5th graders, drawn from the same inner-city community. Posttest comparisons were conducted between the sample of youth that received the CHAMP Family Program and a cohort of youth living in the inner-city community that participated in a NIMH longitudinal study, but were not involved in the intervention. The posttest data for the comparison group was collected the year prior to the data collection related to CHAMP. Thus, a quasi-experimental research design is employed.

Setting and Sample

The CHAMP sample of youth and their families ($n = 324$) were identified to participate in the CHAMP Family Program at the end of the 1995/1996 school year. Of the 324 eligible 4th and 5th graders (92% of youth on class roster at 4 elementary schools, all with active parent consent), 274 (85%) of their families could be located and invited to participate. We did not continue to track the remaining 15% of youth since they represented moves to other communities or an address we were never able to determine. Approximately 73% of families located completed the entire CHAMP Family Program ($n = 201$). Of these, 53% ($n = 107$) of youth and families participated in the research associated with CHAMP. Ultimately, 53% ($n = 50$) of completed all assessments and their data was available for analysis.

Table 1 summarizes CHAMP Family Program participant characteristics. Approximately 60% of children in the sample of children are female. Seventy-three percent of families are headed by unmarried mothers. Almost 76% of parents reported family income less than $14,000. Three-quarters of adult caregivers completed high school and 8% of parent figures had attended some college. Approximately 17%of the adult caregivers are between the ages of 25 and 29 years, indicating that they were teenagers at the time of the target child's birth.

TABLE 1. Comparison of Samples

	CHAMP Family Program (n = 201)	Comparison (n = 308)
Child gender		
Male	40%	43%
Female	60%	57%
Percent of female headed households	73%	60%
Family income < $14,000	76%	90%
Adult caregiver employed	70%	54%

The second sample, serving as the comparison group in the current study, consists of 315 non-overlapping 4th and 5th graders drawn from the same community during the 1993/1994 school year. This sample of youth and their families were involved in an earlier survey of family and mental health factors related to HIV risk exposure during the transition to adolescence among urban, minority youth (Paikoff, 1995). Of the 315 youth and families eligible to participate in this study, approximately 98% ($n = 308$) participated in the comparison group study interview. Of those, 97% ($n = 299$) of cases were available for analysis.

Of the comparison group, 57% of children of the sample are female. Approximately, 60% of families are headed by unmarried mothers. Approximately 90% of families reside in federally subsidized housing apartments and have annual incomes less than $14,000. Approximately 46% of adult caregivers reported completing high school or a GED. Fifty-four percent of adult caregivers were employed in the last year. A comparison between the two samples is provided in Table 1. Youth from both samples attend one of four elementary schools, located adjacent to large high-rise subsidized housing projects within 11 blocks of each other. Ninety-nine percent of the children who attend these schools are African American and over 90% of these children live in poverty (as indicated by children's qualification for free lunches).

Description of the CHAMP Family Program Intervention

The CHAMP Family Program family-based intervention was created to reduce the spread of HIV among low-income African American youth by strengthening family relationship processes, such as family communication, social support, and parental monitoring skills (see McKay et al., 2000, for a complete description), which have been linked to a reduction of youth sexual risk taking behavior (Black et al., 1997; Jaccard & Dittus, 1991; Romer et al., 1994; Stanton et al., 2000). The program was developed in collaboration with parents and elementary school representatives from the target community. The intervention is developmentally timed (9 to 11 years of age) for children just prior to the onset of puberty, when an increase in sexual possibility situations is likely. The program incorporates a 12-week sequence of meetings in which families meet once per week to engage in discussions related to: (a) sexual possibility situations; (b) information relevant to puberty and HIV/AIDS; and (c) family communication (see Table 2 for specific content focused on in each of the 12 sessions).

Each program meeting lasts approximately 90 minutes and consists of three blocks of discussions. In the first thirty minutes, the specific meeting topic is introduced and discussed among children and families together. During the second thirty-minute interval, separate parent and child only groups are convened that focus on in-depth exploration of the topic and skills building. The final thirty-minute block consists of a family practice activity delivered in a multiple-family group format. Throughout the program, discussions and structured activities/games are used to enhance participant interest and engagement (Madison et al., 2000; McKay et al., 2000).

Delivery of the CHAMP Family Program Intervention

Each CHAMP family group, consisting of approximately 10 families each, is facilitated by program leaders. The program leaders are comprised of one or two mental health interns (BA or MA level) and one or two community consultants/parent co-facilitators. Criteria for selection of parent co-facilitators include: (a) parent/teacher's aid of children at one of the targeted schools, or referral by a collaborative board member; (b) NOT parenting or teaching children eligible for program participation; and (c) commitment made by the community consultant to devote at least one calendar year to co-facilitating groups with mental health interns in this project, as well as to continue contact with the targeted community even if the consultant should relocate or change jobs. Criteria for mental health interns include: (a) enrollment in or completion of a program aimed at mental health services provision; (b) commitment to devote a calendar year of internship to program delivery; and (c) commitment to co-delivering groups with community facilitators in a community setting.

TABLE 2. Outline of the CHAMP Family Program

Session 1	Getting to know the CHAMP Family Program: Working together to keep our kids safe
Session 2	Where are we going? Paperwork?
Session 3	Talking and listening to each other
Session 4	Keeping track of kids–Part I
Session 5	Keeping track of kids–Part II
Session 6	Who can help us raise our children?
Session 7	Rules keep kids safe
Session 8	Growing up: Talking about puberty
Session 9	What we need to know about HIV/AIDS
Session 10	Growing up: Preparing our kids for adolescence
Session 11	Where are we ending up? Paperwork and more paperwork!!
Session 12	A celebration!! Where we have been and where we go from here

Program leaders are trained extensively (e.g., approximately 40 hours) in group facilitation and process, as well as context and sequencing of program delivery, in human subjects' issues and rights (e.g., confidentially), and in basic rationale for consistency of implementation and evaluation. In addition, program leaders receive weekly, ongoing training, supervision, and on-site weekly monitoring to ensure adherence to intervention protocol.

Procedures

Participants in the CHAMP Family Program were assessed following an introduction to the program (week 2, pretest) and at the completion of the program (week 11, posttest). Data gathered at pretest and posttest data collection points are presented here for CHAMP family program participants. All information was obtained from parents and youth separately. Each child or adult participant completed paper-pencil instruments in small groups of six to eight program participants, with research staff reading each item aloud.

For those included in the comparison sample, youth and their adult caregivers were interviewed during the 4th or 5th grade school year, approximately twelve months earlier. Youth and their adult caregiver were interviewed separately with a one to one ratio of participant to research staff. All survey items were read aloud to the participant. In both the CHAMP Family Program and comparison samples, participants were compensated monetarily for their time and transportation costs.

Measurements

The *Child Behavior Checklist* (CBC-L/6-18; Achenbach & Edelbrock, 1983) is a widely used parent report form that measures problem behavior in children. The CBCL/6-18 uses a hierarchical factor structure in which eight first-order factors (i.e., Anxious/Depressed, Withdrawn/Depressed, Somatic Complaints, Social Problems, Thought Problems, Attention Problems, Rule-Breaking Behavior, and Aggressive Behavior) load on two higher order factors (i.e., Internalizing Behavior and Externalizing Behavior). Only the higher order factor for Child Externalizing behavior (possible range = 0-52) and the first order factor for child Social Problems (possible range = 0-14) are used in these analyses. The instrument also contains cutoff values representing levels of significance for child externalizing behavior that place children in one of three categories: (1) non-clinically significant (< 12); (2) sub-clinically significant (12-15); and (3) clinically significant (> 16) levels of externalizing behavior. Cronbach Alpha levels were high for pretest (alpha = .90) and posttest (alpha = .87) CHAMP Family Program participants in regard to child externalizing behavior. However, ratings of internal consistency for the social problem first-order factor completed by CHAMP Family Program participants at pretest (alpha = .69) and posttest (alpha = .57) tended to be lower. Cronbach Alpha ratings for the comparison group were acceptable in regard to both child externalizing (alpha = .91) and social problem scores (alpha = .70).

Statistical Analysis

Data were only analyzed for children with significant levels of mental health need. A significant level of child mental health need was defined as a child receiving a score on the CBC-L indicating a sub-clinical or clinical level of externalizing behavior for (CHAMP Family Program participants considered at pretest). Once these children were identified, changes between mean ratings for the CHAMP Family Program participants from pretest to posttest for externalizing CBC-L scale scores were examined using paired sample t-tests. Likewise, changes in pretest and posttest mean social problem scores for the CHAMP Family Program participants were examined using paired sample t-tests. Next, t-tests were used to examine the differences in child externalizing behavior and social problem mean scores between the CHAMP Family Program participants at posttest and the comparison group.

RESULTS

Of the fifty families that participated in the CHAMP Family Program, 40% ($n = 20$) of youth were rated by parents as exhibiting levels of externalizing behavior above the cutoff point for a subclinical level of mental health need. Thus, their data was analyzed for the current study. Bivariate analyses were conducted to determine if children above and below the clinical cutoff point for mental health need differed by important demographic characteristics for CHAMP Family Program participants. Children having a clinically significant amount of child externalizing behavior (yes/no) did not differ significantly by child gender (χ^2 (1) = 1.61, p = .20), single-parent status (χ^2 (1) = .28, p = .60), parent education (< high school, high school, > high school; χ^2 (2) = .09, p = 98), parent employment status (employed/unemployed; χ^2 (1) = .52, p = .47), or if the family received public assistance (χ^2 (1) = .98, p = .32). Of the 299 parents who provided data concerning their child's externalizing behavior in the comparison group, 38% (n = 113) reported CBC-L externalizing scores that were above the cutoff point for mental health need and had their data analyzed.

Table 3 displays summaries of statistical tests examining mean changes in child behavioral difficulties for children in the CHAMP Family Program from pretest to posttest. Mean child externalizing behavior scores of children with mental health need in the CHAMP Family Program were well-above the sub-clinical level (M = 17.7, SD = 5.0). However, post-test scores indicated that this same group of children had significantly lower mean scores (M = 14.6, SD = 5.9) at post-test (t (19) = 2.34, p < .05). In fact, mean scores reflected that the average child in the experimental group exited the clinically significant classification of externalizing behavior and entered the sub-clinical range of child externalizing behavior. Statistical analysis of the first order factor scale examining social problems also represented a significant reduction in pretest (M = 6.4, SD = 2.1) to posttest (M = 5.1, SD = 2.4) mean scores values (t (19) = 2.61, p < .05).

Table 2 presents post-test only score comparisons examining mean differences in child behavioral difficulties for children in the CHAMP Family Program group and comparison group. Mean values for the

TABLE 3. Means, Standard Deviations, and t-test Values for CHAMP Family Group Pretest and Posttest Scores

Variable	Pretest ($n = 20$)	Posttest ($n = 20$)	t	Possible Range
Externalizing Scores	17.7	14.6	2.34*	0-52
	(5.0)	(5.9)		
Social Problem Scores	6.4	5.1	2.61*	0-14
	(2.1)	(2.4)		

Note. Standard deviations are in parentheses.
*$p < .05$.

comparison group indicate a clinically significant amount of child externalizing behavior ($M = 19.7$, $SD = 6.5$). Bivariate analyses revealed that the comparison group had significantly higher amount of child externalizing behavior, ($t (131) = 3.29, p < .001$), when compared to the mean ratings of the CHAMP Family Program group ($M = 14.6$, $SD = 5.9$). However, analysis revealed that no significant differences existed between mean values for the CHAMP Family Program group ($M = 5.1$, $SD = 2.4$) and comparison group ($M = 5.4$, $SD = 2.6$) in relation to mean ratings of child social problems.

DISCUSSION

The objective of the current study was to examine the potential impact of participation in the CHAMP Family Program on the problematic behavior evidenced by urban minority youth. Bivariate tests of means revealed that children in the CHAMP Family Program had a significant reduction in their mean levels of externalizing behavior from pre to post with their mean scores lowering from a clinical to subclinical level of mental health need. Additionally, at posttest the children in the CHAMP Family Program had significantly lower externalizing score means relative to youth in the comparison group. The data indicated that among children in the community with significant mental health need, those who had been in the CHAMP Family program evidenced significantly better mental health in comparison to those who had not. Considering the significant levels of externalizing behavior regularly identified among these youth (Barone, Weissberg, Kasprow, & Voyce, 1995;

TABLE 4. Means, Standard Deviations, and t-test Values for Posttest Only Score Comparisons for the CHAMP Family Program Group and Comparison Group

Variable	CHAMP Family Program Group ($n = 20$)	Comparison Group ($n = 113$)	t	Possible Range
Externalizing Scores	14.6 (5.9)	19.7 (6.5)	3.29***	0-52
Social Problem Scores	5.1 (2.4)	5.4 (2.6)	.49	0-14

Note. Standard deviations are in parentheses.
***$p < .001$.

Tolan & Henry, 1996), programs such as the CHAMP Family program may be of great benefit to urban low-income communities.

Bivariate tests of means also revealed that youth in the CHAMP Family program experienced a significant reduction in mean social problem scores. However, at posttest the children in the CHAMP Family program did not evidence significantly lower social problem mean scores in comparison to children in the comparison group. Therefore, the potential for CHAMP to reduce child social problems is inconclusive and requires further examination.

The association of participation in the CHAMP Family Program with reduced levels child externalizing behavior suggests that this program is a potentially useful tool in enhancing urban adolescent mental health. Several aspects of the program may have contributed to its association with reduced problematic youth behavior. At a basic level, the CHAMP Family Program targeted specific family processes (i.e., parental monitoring, parent-child interaction, family support, family connectedness, family communication) that have been previously associated with a lower levels of youth problematic behaviors (Dishion & Kavanagh, 2002; Dishion, Nelson, & Kavanagh, 2003). However, a number of other features of the CHAMP program may have also contributed to child behavioral outcomes and warrant mention.

First, the ability of the CHAMP Family Program to broach, address, and attempt to enhance the targeted family processes among families was been largely contingent on the strong community collaborative effort that was the foundation for the design of the program. The discussion of topics related to familial processes among urban minority families can be challenging. This may be especially true in reference to the discussion of explicit sexual behaviors, which is among the topics addressed in the CHAMP family program. Many families may have never openly discussed several of these topics, consider them too personal to discuss, and/or considered their discussion inappropriate (Kleinman, 1988; Marin, 1993). Additionally, youth likely recognize that drug and alcohol use are behaviors that are considered shameful and punishable for people in their age group and may be even more determined not to refrain from broaching these subjects. The community collaborative-based research design used in the CHAMP Family Program linked researchers (e.g., university based personnel) with agencies and other community members (e.g., parents, teachers) that had trusting relationships with urban African American youth and their families. Subsequently, these institutions and persons were essential in building rapport, enhancing engagement, and facilitating the discussion of private and sexually intimate behaviors between urban families and those involved in the collaborative research. This community-researcher association created ways of identifying sexual and drug risk behaviors (Madison et al., 2000; McKay, in press; McKay et al., 2000) among urban youth that were key in crucial in addressing the family processes that are associated with a reduction in youth problematic behavior.

Second, the community collaborative design also contributed to the CHAMP Family Program by informing the project of specific community needs. There is accumulating evidence that projects must consider the stressors, scarce contextual resources, and core values of the participants in the targeted community if programs are to engage and enhance outcomes for the families within that area (Aponte, Zarskl, Bixenstene, & Cibik, 1991; Fullilove & Fullilove, 1993; Fullilove, Green, & Fulliove, 2000; McLoyd, 1990; Schensul, 1999; Secrest et al., 2004). Research projects may be best informed of these elements by the community members themselves. Thus, through including community members in the design, implementation, and key decisions being made in the CHAMP Family Program, the project was likely better received by the community (McKay, in press; McKay et al., 2000), more effective in engaging families in the intervention, and may have enhanced project outcomes. More specifically, child behavioral outcomes may have been enhanced as community members were available to inform CHAMP Family Program activities (e.g., topical discussions), so that the program may have been better geared to the specific behavioral needs of the children in the targeted community.

Third, the CHAMP Family Program had an enhanced ability to engage and provide services to youth in the community that may have been in need of services for some time. Thus, the initial provision of behavioral treatment through the CHAMP Family Program may have satisfied a long-standing need for services and had a more dramatic role in reducing child problem behavior. Studies have indicated that in spite of their elevated level of mental health need, low-income inner-city African American youth are actually less likely to receive mental health services in comparison to White children or youth in more economically stable areas due to a number of financial, perceived, logistic, and concrete barriers (Chow, Jaffee, & Snowden, 2003; Griffin, Cicchetti, & Leaf, 1993; Kazdin, 1993; Kataoka, Zhang, & Wells, 2002; McKay, & Bannon, 2004; National Institute of Mental Health, 2001; Regier et al., 1993). For example, African American families have often been faced with problems in mental health service availability in their community. Many families may not use child mental health services because the treatment they need is simply not available in their community (US Public Health Service, 1999; 2000; 2001). Thus, because the CHAMP Family Program was readily available to these families, this issue was circumvented.

Additionally, a short supply of African American mental health service providers also limits the availability of services African Americans families (US public health service, 1999; 2000; 2001). Research has indicated that many African Americans prefer African American providers (Cooper-Patrick et al., 1999; Komaromy, Grumbach, Drake, Vrazizan, & Lurie, 1996; Moy & Bartman, 1995). However, it is estimated that among the general population of clinically trained mental health professionals only 2% of psychiatrists, 2% of psychologists, and 4% of social workers are African American (Holzer, Goldsmith, & Ciarlo, 1998). Thus, African American parents may be unlikely to be successful locate needed or preferred child mental health providers considering this small pool of available professionals. However, the CHAMP Family Program effectively addresses these issues as the program is provided directly in the community and is delivered by fellow community residents all of whom are also African American.

Another frequent problem in encouraging minority families to utilize child mental health services is a distrust of majority cultural institutions (Gamble, 1993; Klonoff & Landrine, 1997), such as those who attempt to provide mental health services in low-income urban communities.

These misgivings are based upon a history of abuse minority communities have suffered through programs aimed at improving health implemented by larger mainstream institutions (Dalton, 1989; Friemuth, Quinn, Thomas, Cole, Zook, & Duncan, 2001; Stevenson & White, 1995; Stevenson et al., 1995; Thomas & Quinn, 1991). The community collaborative approach within the CHAMP Family may better garner the trust of a targeted community over traditional mainstream services as community members are involved in program design, delivery, and supervision. Additionally, research has indicated that children of color often received misdiagnoses (Garretson, 1993) for mental health problems due to the lack of availability of culturally competent services, which may understandably dissuade families from using services (US Public Health Service, 1999; 2000; 2001). The CHAMP collaboration may also help providers understand the needs of the community better to help create more culturally competent services, which may enhance service use among families. Thus, the CHAMP Family Program may not only be associated with better child mental health outcomes (i.e., less externalizing and social problem behavior), but the design of the program may also support service provision among this vulnerable population of youth.

LIMITATIONS

A number of limitations hampered the current study, primarily due to problems related to missing data. The use of pencil and paper self-administered questionnaires among participants in CHAMP Family program resulted in a high proportion of families being eliminated from analyses because subjects did not provide complete data. A larger sample of comparable youth in both the CHAMP Family Program would have given the current study greater statistical power to detect trends within this population. Additionally, a larger sample of subjects in the CHAMP Family Program would also allow a more in-depth examination of how behavioral outcomes differed by other study variables (e.g., family race, child age, child sex, parent mental health outcomes).

CONCLUSION

In spite of these limitations, the current study does contribute to the existing urban child mental health literature examining child problematic behaviors. Data revealed that the CHAMP Family Program was associated with reductions in levels of externalizing behavior among inner-city low-income African American youth with significant mental health need. The program effects on reducing social problem behavior are somewhat inconclusive and require further examination. Future research needs to be conducted with larger and more representative samples so that trends and outcomes (e.g., child mental health) within urban communities of color can be better observed. The design and delivery of the CHAMP Family Program, particularly in regard to community collaboration aspect, may have contributed to reducing obstacles to urban child mental health services and enhanced child outcomes. Urban child mental service practitioners and researchers should consider the potential of the tools (e.g., community collaborative design) used in CHAMP when attempting to create conditions to foster community use of effective child mental health services.

REFERENCES

Achenbach, T. M.,& Edelbrock, C. (1983). *Manual for the Child Behavior Checklist and Revised Child Behavior Profile.* Burlington: University of Vermont.

Alexander, K. L., Entwisle, D. R., & Dauber, S. L. (1993). First-grade classroom behavior: Its short- and long-term consequences for school performance. *Child Development, 64*, 801-814.

Alexander, K. L., Entwisle, D. R., & Kabbani, N. S. (2001). The dropout process in life course perspective: Early risk factors at home and school. *Teachers College Record, 103*, 760-822.

Aponte, H.J., Zarskl, J., Bixenstene, C., & Cibik, P. (1991). Home/community based services: A two-trier approach. *American Journal of Orthopsychiatry, 61*, 403-408. 224.

Attar, B. K., Guerra, N. G., & Tolan, P. H. (1994). Neighborhood disadvantage, stressful life events, and adjustment in urban elementary-school children. *Journal of Clinical Child Psychology, 23*, 391-400.

Barnes, G. M. & Farrell, M. P. (1992). Parental support and control as predictors of adolescent drinking, delinquency, and related problem behaviors. *Journal of Marriage & the Family, 54*, 763-776.

Barone, C., Weissberg, R. P., Kasprow, W., & Voyce, C. K. (1995). Involvement in multiple problem behaviors of young urban adolescents. *Journal of Primary Prevention, 15*, 261-283.

Best, J. (1994). *Troubling children: Studies of children and social problems.* New York: Aldine de Gruyter.

Black, M., Ricardo, I., & Stanton, B. (1997). Social-psychological factors associated with AIDS risk behaviors among low income, urban, African American adolescents: Implication for intervention. *Journal of Research of Adolescence, 7,* 173-195.

Braddock, J. H. & McPartland, J. (1992). *Educating at risk youth: Recent trends, current status, and future needs.* Washington, DC: Panel on high-risk youth, Commission on Behavioral and Social Science, and Education, National Research Council.

Centers for Disease Control and Prevention (2001). *Compendium of HIV Prevention Interventions with Evidence of Effectiveness.* Atlanta, GA: Author.

Chow, J. C., Jaffee, K., & Snowden, L. (2003). Racial/Ethnic Disparities in the Use of Mental Health Services in Poverty Areas. *American Journal of Public Health, 93,* 792-797.

Cohen, C. I. (2002). Poverty, social problems, and serious mental illness. *Psychiatric Services, 53,* 899-900.

Cooper-Patrick, L., Gallo, J. J., Powe, N. R., Steinwachs, D. M., Eaton, W. W., & Ford, D. E. (1999). Mental health service utilization by African Americans and whites: The Baltimore Epidemiologic Catchment Area follow-up. *Medical Care, 37,* 1034-1045.

Cotton, N.U. Resnick, J., Browne D.C. et al. (1994). Aggression and fighting behavior among African American adolescents: Individual and family factors. *America Journal of Public Health, 84,* 618-622.

Dalton, H. L. (1989). AIDS in blackface. *Daedalus, 118,* 205-227.

Dishion, T. J., Capaldi, D., Spracklen, K. M., & Li, F. (1995). Peer ecology of male adolescent drug use. *Development & Psychopathology, 7,* 803-824.

Dishion, T. J. & Kavanaugh, K. (2002). The Adolescent Transitions Program: A family-centered prevention strategy for schools. In J. B. Reid, G. R. Patterson (eds.) et al. *Antisocial behavior in children and adolescents: A developmental analysis and model for intervention* (pp. 257-272). Washington, DC, US: American Psychological Association.

Dishion, T. J., Nelson, S. E., & Kavanagh, K. (2003). The Family Check-Up With High-Risk Young Adolescents: Preventing Early-Onset Substance Use by Parent Monitoring. *Behavior Therapy, 34,* 553-571.

Elliot, D. S., Wilson, W. J., Huizinga, D., Sampson, R. J. et al. (1996). The effects of neighborhood disadvantage on adolescent development. *Journal of Research in Crime & Delinquency, 33,* 389-426.

Freimuth, V. S., Quinn, S. C., Thomas, S. B., Cole, G., Zook, E., & Duncan, T. (2001). African American's views on research and the Tuskegee syphilis study. *Social Science & Medicine, 52,* 797-808.

Fullilove, M. T. & Fullilove, R. E., III. (1993). Understanding sexual behaviors and drug use among African Americans: A case study of issues for survey research. In D. G. Ostrow & R. C. Kessler (Eds.), *Methodological Issues in AIDS Behavioral Research* (pp. 117-132). New York: Plenum Press.

Fullilove, R. E, Green, L., & Fullilove, M. T. (2000). The Family to Family program: A structural intervention with implications for the prevention of HIV/AIDS and other community epidemics. *AIDS, 14* (Suppl 1), S63-S67.

Gamble, V. N. (1993). A legacy of distrust: African Americans and medical research. *American Journal of Preventive Medicine, 9* (6, Suppl), 35-38.

Garretson, D. J. (1993). Psychological misdiagnosis of African Americans. *Journal of Multicultural Counseling & Development, 21,* 119-126.

Gorman-Smith, D., Tolan, P. H., & Henry, D. (1999). The relation of community and family to risk among urban-poor adolescents. In P. Cohen, C. Slomkowski (Eds.) et al. *Historical and geographical influences on psychopathology* (pp. 349-367).

Griffin, J. A., Cicchetti, D., & Leaf, P. J. (1993). Characteristics of youth identified from a psychiatric case register as first-time users of services. *Hospital and Community Psychiatry, 44,* 62-65.

Guerra, N. G, Huesmann, L. R., Tolan, P. H., Van Acker, R., & Eron, L. (1995). Stressful events and individual beliefs as correlates of economic disadvantage and aggression among urban children. *Journal of Consulting & Clinical Psychology, 63,* 518-528.

Hanlon, T. E., Bateman, R. W., Simon, B. D., O'Grady, K. E., & Carswell, S. B. (2004). Antecedents and Correlates of Deviant Activity in Urban Youth Manifesting Behavioral Problems. *Journal of Primary Prevention, 24,* 285-309.

Hennes, H. (1998). A review of violence statistics among children and adolescents in the United States. *Pediatric Clinical Northern America, 45,* 269-280.

Hess, L. E. & Atkins, M. S. (1998). Victims and aggressors at school: Teacher, self, and peer perceptions of psychosocial functioning. *Applied Developmental Science, 2,* 75-89.

Holzer, C. E., Goldsmith, H. F., & Ciarlo, J. A. (1998). Effects of rural-urban county type on the availability of health and mental health care providers. In R. W. Manderscheid & M. J. Henderson (Eds.), *Mental health, United States,* Rockville, MD: Center for Mental Health Services.

Jaccard J. & Dittus, P. (1991). *Parent-teen communication: Toward the prevention of unintended pregnancies.* New York: Springer Verlag.

Kataoka, S. H., Zhang, L., & Wells, K. B. (2002). Unmet need for mental health care among US children: Variation by ethnicity and insurance status. *American Journal Psychiatry, 159,* 1548-1555.

Kazdin, A. (1993). Premature termination from treatment among children referred for antisocial behavior. *Journal of Clinical Child Psychology, 31,* 415-425.

Kerr, M. H., Beck, K., Shattuck, T. D., Kattar, C., & Uriburu, D. (2003). Family involvement, problem and prosocial behavior outcomes of Latino Youth. *American Journal of Health Behavior, 27,* S55-S65.

Kleinman, A. (1988). *Rethinking psychiatry: From cultural category to personal experience.* New York: Free Press.

Klonoff, E. A. & Landrine, H. (1997). Distrust of Whites, acculturation, and AIDS knowledge among African Americans. *Journal of Black Psychology, 23,* 50-57.

Komaromy, M., Grumbach, K., Drake, M., Vrazizan, K., & Lurie, N. (1996). The role of black and Hispanic physicians in providing health care for underserved populations. *New England Journal of Medicine, 334,* 305-310.

Madison, S., McKay, M., Paikoff, R.L. & Bell, C. (2000). Community collaboration and basic research: Necessary ingredients for the development of a family-based HIV prevention program. *AIDS Education and Prevention, 12,* 281-298.

Marin, G. (1993). Defining culturally appropriate community interventions: Hispanics as a case study. *Journal of Community Psychology, 21,* 149-161.

McKay, M. (in press). "Collaborative child mental health services research: Theoretical perspectives and practical guidelines." In K. Hoagwood (Ed.). *Collaborative research to improve child mental health services.*

McKay, M. M. & Bannon, W. M., Jr. (2004). Evidence Update: Engaging Families in Child Mental Health Services. *Child and Adolescent Psychiatry Clinics of North America, 164.*

McKay, M., Baptiste, D., Coleman, D., Madison, S., Paikoff, R. & Scott, R. (2000). Preventing HIV risk exposure in urban communities: The CHAMP Family Program in W. Pequegnat & Jose Szapocznik (Eds). *Working with families in the era of HIV/AIDS.* California: Sage Publications.

McLoyd, V. C. (1990). The impact of economic hardship on Black families and children: Psychological distress, parenting, and socioemotional development. *Child Development, 61,* 311-346.

Moy, E., & Bartman, B. A. (1995). Physician race and care of minority and medically indigent patients. *Journal of the American Medical Association, 273,* 1515-1520.

National Institute of Mental Health (2001). *Blueprint for Change: Research on Child and Adolescent Mental Health.* Rockville, MD: U.S. Department of Health and Human Services Administration, Center for Mental Health Services, National Institutes of health, National Institute of Mental Health.

O'Brien, M. (1991). *Promoting successful transition in school: A review of current intervention practices.* Lawrence, KS: Kansas University Early Childhood Research Institute.

Paikoff, R. L. (1995). Early heterosexual debut: Situations of sexual possibility during the transition to adolescence. *American Journal of Orthopsychiatry, 65(3),* 389-401.

Palmer, E. J. & Hollin, C. R. (2001). Sociomoral reasoning, perceptions of parenting and self-reported delinquency in adolescents. *Applied Cognitive Psychology, 15,* 85-100.

Patterson, G. R. & Stouthamer-Loeber, M. (1984). The correlation of family management practices and delinquency. *Child Development, 55,* 1299-1307.

Prothrow-Stith, D.B. (1995). The epidemic of youth violence in America: Using public health prevention strategies to prevent violence. *Journal of Health Care of the Poor and Underserved, 6,* 95-101.

Rachuba, L., Stanton, B., & Howard D. (1995). Violent crime in the United States: An epidemiologic profile. *Archives of Pediatric Adolescence Med 149,* 953-960.

Regier, D. A., Narrow, W. E., Rae, D. S., Manderscheid, R. W., Locke, B., & Goodwin, F. K. (1993). The de facto US mental and addictive disorders service system: Epidemiologic Catchment Area prospective 1-year prevalence rates of disorders and services. *Archives of General Psychiatry, 50,* 85-94.

Romer, D., Black, M., Ricardo, I., Feigelman, S. et al. (1994). Social influences on the sexual behavior of youth at risk for HIV exposure. *American Journal of Public Health, 84,* 977-985.

Schensul, J. J. (1999). Organizing community research partnerships in the struggle against AIDS. *Health Education & Behavior, 26,* 266-83.

Secrest, L. A., Lassiter, S. L., Armistead, L. P., Wyckoff, S. C., Johnson, J., Williams, W. B. et al. (2004). The Parents Matter! Program: Building a successful investigator-community partnership. *Journal of Child & Family Studies, 13,* 35-45.

Stanton, B. F., Li, X., Galbraith, J., Cornick, G., Feigelman, S., Kaljee, L., & Zhou, Y. (2000). Parental underestimates of adolescent risk behavior: A randomized, controlled trial of a parental monitoring intervention. *Journal of Adolescent Health, 26,* 18-26.

Stevenson, H. C., Davis, G., Weber, E., Weiman, D. et al. (1995). HIV prevention beliefs among urban African American youth. *Journal of Adolescent Health, 16,* 316-323.

Stevenson, H. C. & White, J. J. (1994). AIDS prevention struggles in ethnocultural neighborhoods: Why research partnerships with community based organizations can't wait. *AIDS Education & Prevention, 6,* 126-139.

Thomas, S. B. & Quinn, S. C. (1991). The Tuskegee Syphilis Study, 1932 to 1972: Implications for HIV education and AIDS risk education programs in the Black community. *American Journal of Public Health, 81,* 1498-1505.

Tolan, P. H. & Henry, D. (1996). Patterns of psychopathology among urban poor children: Co-morbidity and aggression effects. *Journal of Consulting and Clinical Psychology, 64,* 1094-1099.

Tolan, P. H. & Henry, D. (2000). *Patterns of psychopathology among urban poor children: Community, age, ethnicity and gender effects.* Manuscript submitted for publication. University of Illinois at Chicago.

Tolan, P. H., Guerra, N. G., & Kendall, P. C. (1995). Introduction to Special Section: Prediction and prevention of antisocial behavior in children and adolescents. *Journal of Consulting & Clinical Psychology, 63,* 515-517.

U.S. Public Health Service (1999). *Mental Health: A Report of the Surgeon General.* Rockville, MD: U.S. Department of Health and Human Services Administration, Center for Mental Health Services, National Institutes of health, National Institute of Mental Health.

U.S. Public Health Service (2000). *Report of the Surgeon General's Conference on Children's Mental Health: A National Action Agenda.* Washington, DC: Department of Health and Human Services.

U.S. Public Health Service (2001). *Mental Health: Culture, Race, and Ethnicity A Supplement to Mental Health: A Report of the Surgeon General.* Rockville, MD: U.S. Department of Health and Human Services Administration, Center for Mental Health Services, National Institutes of health, National Institute of Mental Health.

Weist, M. D., Acosta O. M., & Youngstrom, E. A. (2001). Predictors of violence exposure among inner-city youth. *Journal of Clinical Child Psychology, 30,* 187-198.

doi:10.1300/J200v05n01_11

PART II

A Commentary on the Triadic Theory of Influence as a Guide for Adapting HIV Prevention Programs for New Contexts and Populations: The CHAMP-South Africa Story

Carl C. Bell
Arvin Bhana
Mary McKernan McKay
Inge Petersen

Carl C. Bell, MD, is affiliated with the Department of Psychiatry, School of Medicine and School of Public Health, University of Illinois at Chicago. Arvin Bhana, PhD, is affiliated with the Human Sciences Research Council, South Africa. Mary McKernan McKay, PhD, is Professor of Social Work in Psychiatry & Community Medicine, Mt. Sinai School of Medicine. Inge Petersen, PhD, is affiliated with the University of Durban-Westville, South Africa.

Address correspondence to: Mary M. McKay, PhD, Professor of Social Work in Psychiatry & Community Medicine, Mount Sinai School of Medicine, One Gustave L. Levy Lane, New York, NY 10029 (E-mail: mary.mckay@mssm.edu).

The authors thank the staff of the Collaborative HIV/AIDS Prevention and Adolescent Mental Health Project (CHAMP), and members of the CHAMP Collaborative Board for their extraordinary efforts. The authors are also indebted to the many families who have participated in their research.

This work is supported by the National Institutes of Mental Health (R01 MH64872).

[Haworth co-indexing entry note]: "A Commentary on the Triadic Theory of Influence as a Guide for Adapting HIV Prevention Programs for New Contexts and Populations: The CHAMP-South Africa Story." Bell et al. Co-published simultaneously in *Social Work in Mental Health* (The Haworth Press, Inc.) Vol. 5, No. 3/4, 2007, pp. 243-267; and: *Community Collaborative Partnerships: The Foundation for HIV Prevention Research Efforts* (ed: Mary M. McKay, and Roberta L. Paikoff) The Haworth Press, Inc., 2007, pp. 243-267. Single or multiple copies of this article are available for a fee from The Haworth Document Delivery Service [1-800-HAWORTH, 9:00 a.m. - 5:00 p.m. (EST). E-mail address: docdelivery@haworthpress.com].

SUMMARY. The purpose of this paper is to illustrate how the Collaborative HIV Prevention and Adolescent Mental Health Project-South Africa (CHAMPSA) began and to present some of the results from this South African version of CHAMP. This paper informs readers of a number of lessons about international program translation. The first important lesson is that there are universal principles of health behavior change that seem to be useful across cultures. The implementation of these principles, however, needs to be informed by an in-depth understanding of local cultural contexts. The second important lesson is that it is possible to undertake large-scale, scientifically sophisticated community-based prevention research in developing countries through international collaborative research projects. It is the authors' hope that this mixture of science, service, and business will inspire other public health, community mental health, research, and business professionals to develop international prevention interventions that can be shown to be effective, and disseminated on a wide scale. doi:10.1300/J200v05n03_01 *[Article copies available for a fee from The Haworth Document Delivery Service: 1-800-HAWORTH. E-mail address: <docdelivery@haworthpress.com> Website: <http://www.HaworthPress.com> © 2007 by The Haworth Press, Inc. All rights reserved.]*

KEYWORDS. CHAMPSA beginnings, international program translation, universal principles of health behavior change, effective development of international prevention interventions, large-scale community-based prevention research

The purpose of this paper will is to illustrate how the Collaborative HIV Prevention and Adolescent Mental Health Project-South Africa (CHAMPSA) began and to present some of the results from this South African version of CHAMP. It is the authors' hope that this mixture of science, service, and business will inspire other public health, community mental health, research, and business professionals to develop international prevention interventions that can be shown to be effective, and disseminated on a wide scale. This work is being achieved via a team of community stakeholders, academicians, business people, and community mental health service providers on a mission to "save lives, make a difference, make some money, and have some fun" (Bell, 2004).

This work has its origins in the professional socialization (Griffith and Delgado, 1979) of its authors as we were trained to believe the best way to "Save Lives" was to combine clinical service with the basic tenants of public health supported by community-based research. Thus, CHAMPSA's ultimate goal is to foster the development of a service model to disseminate culturally sensitive evidence-based prevention services to underserved communities as shown in Figure 1.

For several decades the lead author has been involved in providing improved services to underserved populations and providing relevant research on African American mental health issues (U.S. Public Health Service, 2001; Bell & Williamson, 2002). The results of these efforts are evident in the completed research conducted on various topics. For example, the misdiagnosis of African Americans with manic depressive illness (Bell and Mehta, 1980; 1981), children exposed to violence (Bell & Jenkins, 1991; Jenkins and Bell, 1994), the prevalence of isolated sleep paralysis in African Americans (Bell et al., 1984; Bell et al., 1986; Bell et al., 1988), and the management of violence in psychiatric emergency services (Bell & Palmer, 1982; Bell, 2000) have all been areas of study. In South Africa, our colleagues are involved in similar efforts in mental health policy development to promote access to mental health care for underserved populations, as well as initiatives to stem the tide of HIV within largely Black community college settings (e.g., Bhana et al., 1998; Bhana et al., 2002; Parry et al., 2004; Petersen, 2004; Petersen et al., 2002a, Petersen et al., 2002b, Petersen et al., 2004).

Lessons learned from these collective experiences indicated a need for theoretical and methodological sophistication to capture the multiple levels of influence and interest in community-based research. The lead author's

FIGURE 1. Service Model

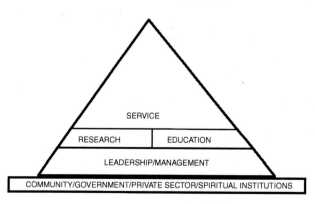

involvement as Co-Investigator of the Chicago African American Youth Health Behavior Project at the University of Illinois at Chicago also known as ABAN AYA (NICHHD HD30078) made it apparent that in order to produce community-based research that is scientifically acceptable, an organization must have a methodological, statistical. research grant, and administrative infrastructure to support it (Flay et al., 2004),

It also became clear that establishing the efficacy of an intervention did not equate with the intervention being disseminated as a service. Therefore, our task was to develop a research program that overcame these obstacles by developing a dissemination plan along with completing the research. These early lessons informed the original Collaborative HIV Adolescent Mental Health Program (CHAMP) in Chicago as well as the CHAMP replication in New York (see McKay et al., 2000; Madison et al., 2000 for a complete discussion of CHAMP).

CHAMP-USA

As one of the basic tenets of community psychiatry consisted of making partnerships with community stakeholders, it was extremely important not to do research that exploited the community, thus the concept of the Collaborative Board was developed within CHAMP. It was also important that, if the developed prevention intervention proved efficacious and effective, it would be disseminated to the community. Accordingly, the CHAMP Principle Investigator (Dr. Paikoff) and Co-Investigators (Drs. McKay and Bell) decided that the best way to accomplish these goals was to develop a team of research and mental health professionals and community partners. This group would form a Collaborative Board and the process would be facilitated by a community-based service businessman and service provider (the lead author). As a result, Drs. Paikoff, McKay, and Bell along with a group of talented project directors and community partners began to develop CHAMP on the Southside of Chicago. When one of the Co-Investigators (Dr. McKay) moved to New York, CHAMP migrated East and to Chicago's Westside while still being driven by the basic principles developed by the original CHAMP from Chicago's Southside.

Theoretical Model Underpinning CHAMP

As Aban Aya and CHAMP Southside continued to progress, and CHAMP New York and CHAMP Westside began developing, the Theory of Triadic Influence (TTI) (Bell, Flay, & Paikoff, 2002) was used to guide the expansion. CHAMP increasingly adopted this ecological approach by understanding risk behavior as being a product of multiple streams of influence–an intra-personal stream linked to biology/personality, a social normative stream linked to the social/inter-personal situation, and a cultural attitudinal stream linked to the socio-cultural environment (Flay and Petraitis, 1994). TTI provides an integration of multiple well-accepted sociological and psychological theories of behavior and behavior change. TTI incorporates sociological theories of social control and social bonding (Akers, Lanza-Kaduce, & Rado- sevich, 1979; Elliott et al., 1985), peer clustering (Oetting & Beauvais, 1986), cultural identity (Oetting & Beauvais, 1990-91), psychological theories of attitude change and behavioral prediction (Fishbein & Ajzen, 1975; Ajzen, 1985), personality development (Digman, 1990), social learning (Akers, Lanza-Kaduce, & Radosevich, 1979; Bandura, 1977; 1986), and other integrative theories (see Petraitis, Flay and Miller (1995) for a review of many such theories).

TTI includes five "tiers" of "causes" of behavior that range from very proximal to distal to ultimate, including: (1) cultural-environmental influences on knowledge and values; (2) social situation contextual influences on social bonding and social learning; and (3) interpersonal influences on self determination/control and social skills (see Figure 2).

In addition to the direct influences of these streams, there are important inter-stream effects and influences that flow between tiers. The theory is intended to account for factors that have direct and indirect effects on behavior, both new behaviors and standard behavior. Experiences with related behaviors and early experiences with a new behavior lead to feedback loops through all three streams, adding to the prior influences of these streams. This integration of existing theories leads to a meta-theoretical view that suggests higher order descriptions and explanations of health behavior, that in turn suggest new approaches for health promotion and disease prevention.

While being theoretically sound, the Triadic Theory of Influence was too complicated to be used for guidance in the field. Being pragmatic, the lead author used the TTI to develop seven field principles that are necessary for any successful universal health behavior intervention (Bell, Flay, & Paikoff, 2002). The seven fields *(in italics)* include: (1) *re-building the village*–consisting of developing and expanding community partnerships and coalitions through a level of community organization around health behavior issues (derived from the "cultural/attitudinal stream" and "social/normative stream" of TTI), (2) *providing access to health care*–ad-

FIGURE 2. Theory of Triadic Influence

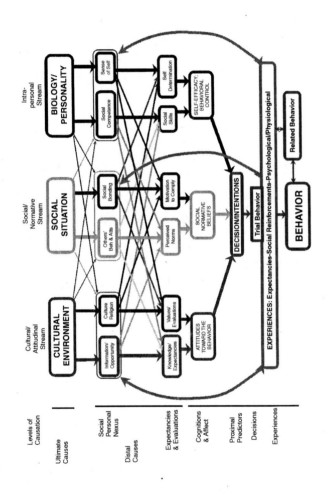

dresses highly influential, individual-level risk factors that require a community-level service (derived form the "biology" in the Intra-personal stream of TTI), (3) *improving bonding, attachment, and connectedness dynamics*–within the community and between stakeholders (derived from the "social bonding" in the social/normative stream of TTI), (4) *improving self-esteem and self-respect* ("sense of self" in the intrapersonal stream of TTI), (5) *increasing social skills of target recipients* ("social skills" in the intra-personal stream of TTI), (6) *reestablishing the adult protective shield and monitoring problem behaviors* ("others' behavior and attitudes" in the social/normative stream of TTI), and (7) *minimizing the residual effects of trauma* ("behavioral control-self-management skills and affect regulation" in the intra-personal stream of TTI).

These seven field principles can guide academic/community partnerships to actualize the Theory of Triadic Influence and to base their intervention on sound scientific theory. Bell et al. (2002) suggest these seven universal field principles of behavior change have been found to be effective in promoting resiliency & behavior change in youth in a number of community-based projects. These include *the Chicago Public School Violence Prevention Program (Bell et al., 2001), the DCFS McLean County, IL Project (Bell & McKay, 2004),* and *Project Liberty in New York City (http://www.mhanc.org/ProjectLiberty/projectliberty.htm).*

CHAMP SOUTH AFRICA

History of Collaboration

In 1999, when Dr. David Satcher was the Surgeon General of the United States, he made it clear that to be effective public health needed to be practiced on an international scale. As Dr. Satcher put it "Germs don't need passports," and such leadership helped federal research institutions such as the National Institute of Mental Health to recognize their responsibility to help developing countries grow research infrastructures (e.g., methodological, statistical and grant administration competencies). As a result of leadership coming from Drs. Satcher and, then NIMH Director, Steve Hyman, Drs. Willo Pequegnat and Ellen Stover convened a South African-United States Workshop entitled, "Setting an agenda and creating partnerships for behavioral research on HIV prevention in the South African Medical Research Council: Exploring collaboration with the National Institute of Mental Health."

This event, sponsored by the South African Medical Research Council and the Center for Mental Health Research on AIDS, National Institute of Mental Health, National Institutes of Health, U.S. Public Health Service was held November 1, 2000 in Durban, South Africa.

It became clear that while our South African colleagues were very good at "hitting the ground running," i.e., doing the same type of useful, pragmatic, community-based research the senior author had done for years, they were similarly looking for ways to address complex levels of risk influences, as well as to have access to large grants necessary to undertake scientifically sophisticated community-based research.

It was at that meeting that the senior author met the future Co-Investigators of "Using CHAMP to Prevent Youth HIV Risk in a South African Township (NIMH 5 RO1 MH64872-02)" for the first time. At the meeting, Dr. Pequegnat encouraged the U.S. investigators to collaborate with South African research colleagues in developing an R-O1 grant application to conduct HIV prevention research in South Africa. An outcome of the meeting was a partnership between the US investigators, Drs. Bell and McKay and the South African investigators, Drs. Bhana and Petersen in the writing of an NIMH R-O1 grant to determine if CHAMP could be adapted to South Africa.

We had a comprehensive, theoretically driven and scientifically tested community-based primary prevention intervention for the prevention of HIV risky behaviors in adolescents which took into account multiple levels of risk and protective influences for youth in South Africa. We recognized that while South African theory and models of health behavior change were adequate, they were not as recognizable by U.S. grant reviewers as were the theories underpinning the Theory of Triadic Influence. TTI was suggested to be the best theoretical basis for the grant submission. Although, legitimately skeptical that a U.S. theoretical model would have currency in South African culture, after many discussions regarding the model and, more importantly, illustrating how the field principles were potentially universal, the South African Co-Investigators agreed to use the TTI as the basis for adapting CHAMP to South Africa.

Adaptation of CHAMP for South African Context– Establishing a Theoretical Context

First Field Principle

Our South African colleagues endorsed the importance of social capital in facilitating health and enhancing behavior change within the social normative stream of TTI (McKnight, 1997; Campbell, 2002). Thus, we incorporated the concept of social capital (which broadly refers to the investment one makes in membership of a social group, which secures relational & material benefits) into the social normative stream of TTI. Improving the "community protective shield" through *re-building the village* is the first field principle emphasized in the CHAMPSA program. This essentially refers to building social capital within communities. In CHAMPSA's case this involved using the CHAMPSA Collaborative Board to assist persons in making an investment in membership of a social group to secure relational and material benefits (Hawe & Sheill, 2000). Communities with high levels of social capital have also been found to have fewer incidents of risky health behaviors (Bell, 2001, Flay et al., 2004). Furthermore, communities with high levels of social capital are more likely to provide a 'health-enabling community' which supports the renegotiation of health enhancing peer and social norms through facilitating the development of a collective critical consciousness (Campbell, 2002).

Second Field Principle

The second field principle is *improving bonding, attachment and connectedness dynamics*. Sexual behavior and gender identities are socially constructed and strongly influenced by group based social identities and peer influences. Renegotiation of such identities can not occur at an individual level, and needs to occur collectively by people in peer group settings (Campbell & McPhail, 2002). "It is through the development of bonding social capital that a group of people takes the first step towards developing a critical consciousness of the material and symbolic obstacles to their health and well-being, and begin to develop both insight and the confidence to address these obstacles" (Campbell, 2002, p. 57). In this respect CHAMPSA attempts to build health enhancing peer social networks amongst child participants.

Third Field Principle

Also within this stream of influence is the third field principle of the need to *re-establish the adult protective shield* through strengthening parental supervision and monitoring skills. Low levels of parental warmth, acceptance and affection have been found to be associated with high levels of conflict, hostility and risky behaviors later in life (Bell, 2001). In relation to this aspect, a major effort of the CHAMPSA program is to improve the connectedness between South African parents and their children so that family communication, family problem solving, skills building, parental monitoring, and other important protective factors can be easily taught through the process of cooperative or team learning within the family.

Field principles guiding behavior change within the intra-personal stream include *minimizing the residual effects of trauma. Minimizing trauma* requires access to *health and social services.* The early identification of children who have been exposed to trauma and providing them with assistance to cope with the stressor, is likely to reduce risky behavior later in life (Bell, 2001). The association between childhood trauma and its impact on adult health outcomes is well established by the Adverse Childhood Experience (ACE) Study (Felitti et al., 1998). This pivotal study noted that adults who had experienced four or more of the seven categories of adverse experiences of childhood (e.g., physical abuse, psychological abuse, sexual abuse, violence against the respondent's mother, living with household members who were substance abusers, mentally ill or suicidal, and reported ever being imprisoned) had a 3.2-fold increased risk for fifty or more sexual intercourse partners, and a 2.5-fold increased risk for having a STD history compared with persons who experienced none of the adverse childhood experiences. Thus, the CHAMPSA program seeks to provide social support for traumatized children and their families and assist youth and families with addressing their grief from loss through ensuring access to a psychological referral service.

Furthermore, *improving self esteem/self-respect* by increasing self-efficacy and *increasing social skills* are also important interventions within the intra-personal stream. Self-efficacy is important to promote as a protective factor against engaging in risky sexual behavior situations, thus we placed an emphasis on recognizing dangerous situations and refusal skills within the CHAMPSA program. Finally, the impact of cultural/societal stream influences informs attitudes toward behavior. CHAMPSA addresses attitudes which promote high risk behavior and employs community facilitators who are the bearers of their culture, values, and standards that have protected the indigenous people over the years.

Based on the Theory of Triadic Influence and given these multiple risk influences for engaging in risky sexual behavior, similar to ABAN AYA (Flay et al., 2004; Ngwe et al., 2004), CHAMPSA was designed to be multi-layered, including individually based interventions, peer and family group interventions, as well as community-based interventions.

Stages of Adapting CHAMP

Three distinct stages characterized the adaptation of CHAMP for the South African context. Stage one involved doing a rapid focused ethnographic study of the dynamics underpinning the spread of HIV/AIDS within the Valley of a Thousand Hills, a semi-rural area in KwaZulu-Natal (Paruk et al., 2002). Findings from this study suggested the theoretical principles underpinning the original CHAMP program had relevance for the South African context. Within the intra-personal stream and the social/normative stream of TTI, the following thematic issues emerged: disempowerment of parents; poor communication between parents and children and punitive parenting styles; poor knowledge of HIV/AIDS and its transmission; loss of family members and significant distrust of others within the community (i.e., no *connectedness*). Within the cultural/attitudinal stream of TTI, major themes that emerged included poor information and knowledge about HIV/AIDS associated with attitudes which promote high risk behaviour as stigmatic attitudes towards people with AIDS and "scape goating" females and people living outside of the immediate neighbourhood for spreading the virus. The perception was that community leadership (*adult protective shield*) and social networks (the need to *rebuild the village*) were weak and unable to contain anxieties about HIV/AIDS. This resulted in fear of the many risks and vulnerabilities within the home and community, with sexual abuse highlighted as a prominent threat. Multiple deaths of friends and neighbors caused by the HIV virus exacerbated this sense of vulnerability in the community (Paruk et al., 2002). These characteristics are represented in the person/situation-centered matrix in Figure 3 based on the TTI.

As indicated in Figure 3, the findings of the focused ethnographic study suggest that at the level of intra-personal influences, low levels of *self-esteem* and self-respect as well as low levels of self-efficacy plus the unresolved grief also contributed to high-risk behavior.

Establishing Protective Shields

In relation to social situation contextual influences, the findings suggest a weak *"adult protective shield"* as there was significant parental disempowerment, poor parent-child communication, punitive parenting styles, poor parental monitoring, and inadequate adult role models. Be-

FIGURE 3. Person/Situation Centered Matrix of Findings of the Focused Ethnographic Study

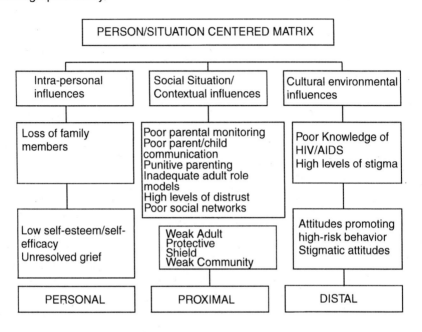

cause the shredded nature of the community's social fabric, apparent from the low levels of trust and social networks within the community, the concept of a weak *"adult protective shield"* was broadened to include the concept of a weak *"community protective shield"* in an effort to highlight the low levels of social cohesion and associated low levels of social control in existence within the community. The high levels of stigma associated with the HIV/AIDS epidemic in South Africa also weakened the community's formal and informal social cohesion and control.

Using the findings of the focused ethnographic study, CHAMPSA attempted to address the three levels of risk influence highlighted in the person/situation centered matrix derived from TTI. The adaptation and implementation of the CHAMPSA manual and multiple family group intervention addresses individual and family/interpersonal influences. At the level of intra-personal influences, the CHAMPSA manual focuses on strengthening the resistance of pre-adolescents so they may resist negative peer influences through improving self-esteem and self-efficacy particularly with respect to assertive and refusal skills in adolescence. Also at this level, owing to the high level of stress and distress from the high AIDS mortality rates in South African, the CHAMPSA team thought it was important to add a grief component to the manual and to provide *access to health services*, particularly psychological counseling through the implementation of a referral psychological service.

In relation to social situation contextual influences, the CHAMPSA intervention seeks to improve family processes such as strengthening communication between youth and their parents (particularly around sensitive topics such as puberty, sexuality and HIV) as well as facilitating health-enhancing peer social networks amongst the child participants. The manual also includes exercises to improve parental monitoring and supervision of peer relations in addition to keeping track of youth whereabouts and activities. Thus, the program facilitates the establishment of protective peer networks as well as a strong *"adult protective shield."* Strengthening these family and peer processes are understood to also offer youth protection from negative peer influences during adolescence, with early sexual experiences being found to be significantly contextually influenced (Paikoff, 1995). Thus, the focused ethnographic study's qualitative findings significantly informed the development of the first adapted version of the CHAMPSA manual.

We also sought to facilitate a more health enabling community context through strengthening social cohesion. Sampson, Raudenbush and Earls (1997) refer to social cohesion as collective efficacy, which is essentially a willingness among neighbors to act on behalf of the common good of the neighborhood. This can strengthen the "community protective shield" and create a more health enabling community, which in turn enables or supports health-enhancing behavior (Campbell, 2000).

CHAMPSA seeks to foster social cohesion through engaging community leaders on the Board, as well as involve family participants delivering the manualized program in social action events and activities related to strengthening families and collective efficacy. While such activities help to build social competence amongst the participants, they also facilitate transference of newly learned skills, behaviors and attitudes beyond the program walls.

At the level of cultural environmental influences, there are likely to be attitudes that tend to promote high-risk behavior given the poor knowledge of HIV transmission. The CHAMPSA program is used to improve HIV/AIDS knowledge and reduce stigmatizing attitudes by raising participants' awareness of the reasons underpinning the development of such attitudes as well as their consequences.

Developing the CHAMP-SA Manual

Using key informants (i.e., community leaders, community health workers, social workers, teachers, and parents) from the target community, the appropriateness of the content and exercises of the first CHAMPSA manual was evaluated and from this process the second version of the CHAMPSA manual was developed. The second version was piloted on 94 families in both an urban and semi-rural site, and the focus group information from this pilot informed the third and final CHAMPSA manual which is being used in the main study.

Most of the topics covered in the original CHAMP manual were incorporated in the adaptation. These included: parenting styles; monitoring of children; improving communication between parents and children (particularly on sensitive topics such as puberty); identifying and developing strategies to keep children safe in high risk situations; ensuring appropriate knowledge and understanding of HIV transmission and biological progression to AIDS; and building social networks. Based on the focused ethnographic findings of disempowerment of parents in relationship to parenting their children as well as high levels of stigma and loss within the community, CHAMPSA investigators felt it was important to include sessions on parental and children's rights and responsibilities and how to deal with stigma and bereavement.

The implementation of the CHAMPSA manual utilizes Freireian principles of participatory adult education where behavior change is understood to emerge from a process of critical reflection on one's own lived experience leading to the development of critical consciousness (Freire, 1970). Small group participatory experiential learning facilitates this process through an iterative process of discussion and discovery and has been successfully used by Campbell and MacPhail (2002) in behavior change programs with youth. The delivery of the program in which several families participate in a group setting has been found to be effective with urban populations participating in both prevention and treatment interventions (McKay et al., 1998; Tolan & McKay, 1996).

Exercises to facilitate this process are presented through the CHAMPSA manual that is an open-ended participatory cartoon narrative. A cartoon-based story line runs throughout the program, with participating families closing the narrative in each session through engaging in exercises using the characters in the narrative. The narrative method consisted of first establishing an authentic setting, creating a set of credible, 'typical' (as opposed to stereotypical) characters and then introducing topics found from the findings of the focused ethnographic study. The use of simplified iconic cartoon characters facilitates identification with the characters in the cartoon family, allowing for sensitive topics, which would otherwise be difficult to engage with, to be discussed through the characters. This process provides some 'distance' from the issue. (Bhana et al., 2004). For example, in session 2, the son in the AmaQuawe family (S'bu) is goaded to sniff some glue by some of his "friends." He tells his aunt about his issues as she is someone he feels he can talk to. This facilitates a family discussion that supports S'bu's self-respect earned from his self-efficacy at using his "refusal skills" to avoid this risky health behavior (see Illustration 1).

Each session is accompanied by a workbook, which families take home. Home assignments assist in facilitating consolidation of the material learned in each session as well as facilitating involvement of non-participating family members (typically fathers or adult males).

The Pilot Study

Families were recruited by inviting them to an information meeting at schools, via notices sent home with the children. Families were assigned to an intervention or comparison group based on their availability over a 10-week period. Our procedures emphasized an informed consent process. We drew samples from three areas, Cato Manor, an urban shack settlement ($n = 30$), Embo ($n = 41$) and Molweni ($n = 53$), both semi-rural areas in the Valley of a Thousand Hills. A total of 124 families participated in the pilot phase of the study. The measures consisted of AIDS Transmission Knowledge, AIDS Myth Knowledge, Parental Communication Styles, Hard-To-Talk About, Social Networks, and Stigma scales (Bhana et al., 2004). All the measures were adapted to take account of language and cultural idiosyncrasies. The Social Networks measure was not applied to children. Table 1 shows the reliability estimates for the various child scales (The reliability estimates for the adult scales are reported in Bhana et al., 2004).

Pilot Results

Multivariate repeated measures Analysis of Variance was used to assess for significant differences between the intervention and comparison groups across the pre- and post-test assessments using the measures above. In line with the theoretical framework adopted by CHAMPSA, the findings reflect both proximal and distal effects where significant

Illustration 1

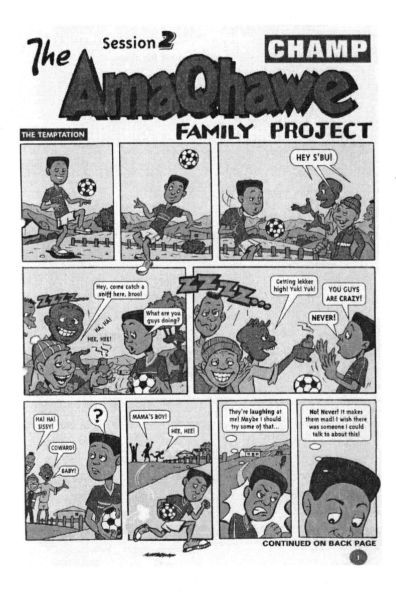

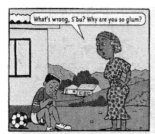
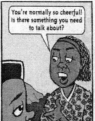
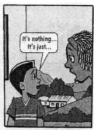
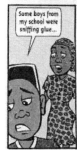
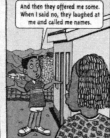
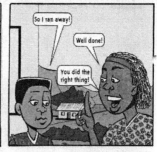
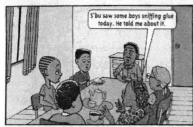
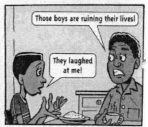
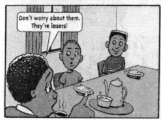
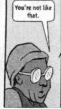
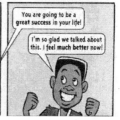

TABLE 1. Reliability Estimates

Child Scales	Alpha
Stigma (5 items)	.81
AIDS Myth Knowledge (7 items)	.53
AIDS Transmission Knowledge (5 items)	.70
Parental Communication (11 items)	.74
Hard to Talk About (Frequency) (7 items)	.88

differences were found between the intervention and comparison group (see Tables 2 and 3).

In general, the findings from the pilot study indicate that the measures were successfully translated given the obtained reliability estimates. Among adults, except for stigmatic attitudes, AIDS transmission knowledge, AIDS myth knowledge, parental communication, frequency of hard- to-talk about issues, and social networks improved significantly compared to the control group. Similarly, for children AIDS transmission knowledge, stigmatic attitudes, and frequency of hard-to-talk about issues showed significant gains over the control group. The differences in findings on AIDS myth between adults and children attests to parents being generally uninformed about the AIDS virus. Children also did not think that their parents' communication with them had changed over the 10 week period between test and retest. Theoretically, the CHAMPSA adaptation impacted positively on cultural environmental influences as well as on contextual influences. These results are encouraging as they intimate a successful translation of the CHAMP program to local contexts. It is expected that similar findings will emerge out of the main study.

Desired Outcomes

However, the challenge of moving science to service still remains in the South African context, even though it has become clearer in the USA that from the outset, partnerships with community stakeholders and/or not-for-profit agencies can facilitate dissemination efforts. For example, using the CHAMPSA principles in McClean County, the Community Mental Health Council was able to significantly change the removal of 24.1/1,000 African American children from their homes by child protective services in McLean County, Illinois (the statewide average was 4.3/1,000). This goal was achieved by first doing a careful assessment of the service environment and contextual factors in McLean County. Next, using the seven field principles used to actualize CHAMPSA (derived

TABLE 2. Summary Table of Intervention Effect Scores for Adults

Variable#	Intervention Change	Control Change	Intervention Effect
AIDS Transmission Know	0.93	0.13	.80 **
AIDS Myth Knowledge	1.6	1.43	.17 ***
Stigma	1.02	0.63	.39 §
Parental Communication	0.68	0.36	.32 **
Hard to Talk About	−1.38	−0.76	−.62 *
Social Network Support	−1.5	−2.08	−.58 **

TABLE 3. Summary Table of Intervention Effect Scores for Children

Variable	Intervention Change	Control Change	Intervention Effect
AIDS Transmission Know	0.39	0.33	.06 **
AIDS Myth Knowledge	0.06	−0.42	−0.36 §
Stigma	2.69	−0.39	2.30 *
Parental Communication	0.35	0.18	.17 §
Hard to Talk About	−2.89	−0.66	

\# The change score represents the mean for the variable at Time 2 minus the mean for the variable at Time 1. The Intervention Effect is the change score for the intervention group minus the change score for the comparison group.
Key: § - Not significant;
*$p < 0.05$
**$p < 0.01$
***$p < 0.001$

from the Theory of Triadic Influence) for guidance, CMHC's business professionals developed a business plan to change the excessive removal of African American children from their homes. We actualized the business plan by using existing service systems via improving their quality and introducing new services per the direction of the theory/model. Finally, using new statistical methodology, examine the outcome after the business intervention. Two years after the intervention began, the results revealed a decrease in the number of children being removed (11.1/1,000) (Redd et al., in press).

Based on our prior research and programmatic experience, it is our belief that we are able to move scientific findings into the field by having business professionals create a business plan to move the "science into service." Professionals should develop a business executive summary consisting of who the company is and who are the leaderships and managers and their strengths; what the objectives are and how they will be accomplished successfully; and if you need financing how much you need and how the loan will be repaid. There should be a summary of the nature of the organization's core business and administrative infrastructure of the business. A description of the mission along with long-term and short-term goals; the company's model for doing business which should contain the reason the company is unique and on the cutting edge; the strategy of the short-term and long-term objectives of the business plan; the strategic relationships that will make the plan go forward, and the internal and external risks to the plan. The services should be described along with the service growth plan.

Once it is determined that the intervention is efficacious and the method of delivering "multiple family groups" by using community facilitators are deemed to be effective, a major objective of CHAMPSA is to disseminate its work. A business plan for this work is in development. This is envisaged to be achieved through existing health and social welfare resource infrastructures within South Africa. Community facilitators will be trained to deliver the program using the manual with the support of community service psychologists employed within the public/private sectors.

CONCLUSIONS

CHAMPSA has taught us a number of lessons. The first important lesson is that there are universal principles of health behavior change that seem to be useful across cultures. The implementation of these principles, however, needs to be informed by an in-depth understanding of local cultural contexts. The initial focused ethnographic study proved to be invaluable in preparing for the adaptation of CHAMP-USA for the South African context. An understanding of cultural contexts goes beyond merely changing language to firstly ensuring that content-specific issues appropriate to the cultural context are covered, and secondly, that the method of delivery is acceptable and facilitative of behavior change within the target population. Given the low literacy levels as well as sensitivity related to discussion of issues of a sexual nature, a cartoon storyline incorporating Freirian principles of adult education was used to deliver the CHAMPSA program.

The second important lesson is that it is possible to undertake large-scale, scientifically sophisticated community-based prevention research in developing countries through international collaborative projects. This collaboration is vital for harnessing financial resources as well as building research infrastructure through developing statistical, methodological, grant, and administrative core capacities within the developing context.

Former Surgeon General (1977-1981), Dr. Julius Richmond has noted that in order to institutionalize interventions, three forces need to be present (Figure 4). We have already addressed the need of having a knowledge base or good science behind the intervention being institutionalized. The issue of having an "implementation limb" or an "effector limb" has also been addressed in our discussion of the need to develop a sound business plan. Finally, using a metaphor, we want to briefly discuss the role of developing a "public will" by using marketing principles.

Congress invited the senior author, who at the time was Chairman of the National Commission on Correctional Health, to give testimony to the as a national expert on correctional health care (April 28, 1992). Going with a serious public health mission of trying to get the House of Representatives Subcommittee on Labor, Health & Human Services Education and Related Agencies of the Appropriations to understand that they needed to have federal funding follow a delinquent child into the detention center, the senior author set off for Washington, D.C. (1992). The idea was to provide federal funding for evidence-based psychiatric or medical services for incarcerated children who had a mental illness or physical illness. The Chair of the committee, after fifteen minutes of allotted speaking time, bangs his gavel and says Congress appreciates your testimony, next please. The next national expert gave a rousing testimony about work accidents and why more money was needed to make employment safer. He got the same treatment–fifteen minutes, bang goes the gavel, and 'Congress appreciates your testimony, next please.' Finally, Mary Tyler Moore comes in to get some

FIGURE 4. Developing Public Will

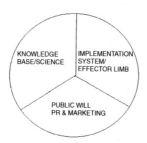

money for juvenile diabetes (she has diabetes). Six additional Congressmen come out of the back room. She gets an hour and fifteen minutes. The Chair adjourned the meeting so the Congressmen could take individual and group shots with Ms. Moore. Everybody had a question for Mary. Everybody loved Mary's show. Because of the public will Mary's marketing created, juvenile diabetes got increased funding from Congress. We are not marketing what works. We expect people to read our scientific publications and say–'Oh this intervention is so wonderful. I am going to have my staff try it.' It is not going to happen that way. We have to create science-based interventions, have support for delivery, develop a business and dissemination plan and create public will if we are going to prevent the spread of HIV.

REFERENCES

Akers Krohn, MD, Lanza-Kaduce, L & Radosevich, M (1979). Social learning and deviant behavior: A specific test of a general theory. *American Sociological Review*, 44, 636-655.

Ajzen, I (1985). From decisions to actions: A theory of planned behavior. In Kuhl J & Beckmann J (Eds.), *Action-control: From cognition to behavior*, pp. 11-39. Heidelberg: Springer.

Bandura, A (1986). *Social Foundations of Thought and Action*. Englewood Cliffs, NJ: Prentice Hall.

Bandura, A (1977). *Social Learning Theory*. Englewood Cliffs, NJ: Prentice Hall.

Bell, CC (2001). Cultivating Resiliency in Youth. *Journal of Adolescent Health*, Vol. 29: 375-381.

Bell, CC (ed.). (2000). *Psychiatric Aspects on Violence: Understanding Causes and Issues in Prevention and Treatment*. San Francisco: Jossey-Bass.

Bell, CC, Dixie-Bell, DD & Thompson, B (1986). Further studies on the prevalence of isolated sleep paralysis in Black subjects. *Journal of the National Medical Association*, Vol. 78, No. 7: pp. 649-659.

Bell, CC, Flay, B, & Paikoff, R (2002). Strategies for health behavioral change. In J. Chunn (Ed.) *The Health Behavioral Change Imperative: Theory, Education, and Practice in Diverse Populations*. New York: Kluwer Academic/Plenum Publishers, pp. 17-40.

Bell, CC, Hildreth, C, Jenkins, EJ, & Carter, C (1988). The relationship between isolated sleep paralysis, panic disorder, and hypertension. *Journal of the National Medical Association*, Vol. 80, No. 3: pp. 289-294.

Bell, CC & Jenkins, EJ (1991). Traumatic stress and children. *Journal of Health Care for the Poor and Underserved*, Vol. 2, No. 1: pp. 175-188.

Bell, CC, & Mehta, H. (1980). The misdiagnosis of black patients with manic depressive illness. *J Natl. Med Assoc.* ; 72: 141-145.

Bell, CC, & Mehta, H (1981). Misdiagnosis of black patients with manic depressive illness. *J Natl. Med Assoc.* ; 73: 101-107.

Bell, CC, Shakoor, B, Thompson, B, Dew, D, Hughley E, Mays, R, & Shorter-Gooden, K (1984). The prevalence of isolated sleep paralysis in Blacks. *Journal of the National Medical Association*, Vol. 76, No. 5: pp. 501-508.

Bell, CC, & Williamson, J (2002). Psychiatric services across the millennium: A celebration of 50 Years of *Psychiatric Services Journal*-Special Populations. *Psychiatric Services*, Vol. 53, No. 4: 419-424.

Bhana, A, Flisher, AJ, & Parry, CDH (1998). School survey of substance use among students in Grades 8 and 11 in the Durban metro region. *Southern African Journal of Child and Adolescent Mental Health*, 11, 131.

Bhana, A, Parry, CDH, Myers, B, Plüddeman, A, Morojele, NK, & Flisher, AJ (2002). The South African Community Epidemiology Network on Drug Use (SACENDU) project, phases 1-8-cannabis and mandrax. *South African Medical Journal*, 92 (7), 542-547.

Bhana, A, Petersen, I, Mason, A, Mahintsho, Z, Bell, C, & McKay, M (2004). Children and youth at risk: Adaptation and pilot study of the CHAMP (*Amaqhawe*) programme in South Africa, *African Journal of AIDS Research (AJAR)*, 3(1): 33-41.

Campbell, C (2002). *Letting them die. How HIV/AIDS prevention programmes often fail.* Cape Town: Double Storey.

Campbell, C & MacPhail, C (2002). Peer education, gender and the development of critical consciousness: participatory HIV prevention by South African youth. *Social Science & Medicine*, 55, 331-345.

Digman, JM (1990). Personality structure: Emergence of the five-factor model. *Ann Rev of Psychology*, 41:417-440.

Elliott, DS, Huizinga, D, & Ageton, SS (1985). *Explaining Deliquency and Drug Use.* Beverly Hills: Sage.

Felitti, VJ, Anda, RF, Nordenberg D, Williamson, DF, Spitz, AM, Edwards, V, Koss, MP, & Marks, JS (1998). Relationship of child abuse and household dysfunction to many of the leading causes of death in adults. The Adverse Childhood Experiences (ACE) Study. *American Journal of Preventative Medicine* 14: 245.

Fishbein, M & Ajzen, I (1975). *Belief, Attitude, Intention and Behavior: An Introduction to Theory and Research.* Reading, MA: Addison-Wesley.

Flay, BR, Graumlich, S, Segawa, E, Burns, J, Amuwo, S, Bell, CC, Campbell, R, Cowell, J, Cooksey, J, Dancy, B, Hedeker, D, Jagers, R, Levy, SR, Paikoff, R, Punwani, I, & Weisberg, R (2004). The ABAN AYA Youth Project: Effects of comprehensive prevention programs on high risk behaviors among inner city African American youth: A randomized trial. *Archives of Pediatrics and Adolescent Medicine*, Vol. 158, No. 4: pp. 377-384.

Flay, BR & Petraitis, J (1994). The theory of triadic influence: A new theory of health behavior with implications for preventive interventions. In Albrecht GS (Ed.) *Advances in Medical Sociology, Vol IV: A Reconsideration of models of health behavior change.* Greenwich, CN: JAI Press, pp. 19-44.

Freire, P (1970). *Pedagogy of the Oppressed.* New York: Seabury Press.

Griffith, E, Delgado, A (1979). On the professional socialization of black psychiatric residents in psychiatry. *J Med Educ*; 54: 471-476.

Hawe, P & Sheill, A (2000). Social capital and health promotion: a review. *Social Science and Medicine, 51*: 871-885, .

Human Rights Watch. (2001). *Scared at school: Sexual violence against girls in South African schools*. New York: Human Rights Watch.

Jenkins EJ, Bell CC (1994). Violence exposure, psychological distress and high risk behaviors among inner-city high school students. In: Friedman S, ed. *Anxiety Disorders in African Americans*. New York, NY. Springer Publishing, 76-88.

Madison, S, McKay, M, Paikoff, RL & Bell, C (2000). Community collaboration and basic research: Necessary ingredients for the development of a family-based HIV prevention program. *AIDS Education and Prevention, 12*, 281-298.

McKay, M, Baptiste, D, Coleman, D, Madison, S, Paikoff, R & Scott, R (2000). Preventing HIV risk exposure in urban communities: The CHAMP Family Program in W. Pequegnat & Jose Szapocznik (Eds). In *Working with families in the era of HIV/AIDS*. California: Sage Publications.

McKay MM, Stoewe, J, McCadam, K & Gonzales, J. (1998). Increasing access to child mental health services for urban children and their caregivers. *Health and Social Work*, 23 (1): 9-15.

McKnight, J (1997). A twenty-first century map for healthy communities and families. *Families in Society: The Journal of Contemporary Human Services, 78* (2): 1-27.

Ngwe, JE, Liu, LC, Flay, BR, Segawa, E, Amuwo, S, Bell, CC, Campbell, R, Cowell, J, Cooksey, J, Dancy, B, Hedeker, D, Jagers, R, Levy, SR, Paikoff, R, Punwani, I, & Weisberg, R. (2004). Violence Prevention among African American adolescent males. *American Journal of Health Behavior*, Vol. 28 (Supple 1): pp. S24-S37.

Oetting, ER & Beauvais, F (1990-91). Orthogonal cultural identification theory: The cultural identification of minority adolescents. International Journal of the Addictions, 25 (5A & 6A), 655-685.

Oetting, ER & Beauvais, R. (1986). Peer cluster theory: Drugs and the adolescent. J of Counseling and Dev, 65,.17-22.

Paikoff, RL (1995). Early heterosexual debut: Situations of sexual possibility during transition to adolescence. *Am J Orthopsychiatry*, 65(3), 369-393.

Parry, CDH, Myers, B, Morojele, NK, Flisher, AJ, Bhana, A, Donson, H, Plüddemann, A (2004). Trends in adolescent alcohol and other drug use: findings from three sentinel sites in South Africa (1997-2001). *Journal of Adolescence*, 27, 429-440.

Paruk, Z, Peterson, I, Bhana, A, Bell, C, & McKay, M (2002). A Focused Ethnographic Study to Inform the Adaptation of the NIMH Funded CHAMP Project in South Africa. In Manfredi R (Ed). XIV International AIDS Conference. Bologna, Italy: Monduzzi Editore S.p.A. (ISBN 88-323-2709-0), p. 295-298.

Petersen, I (2004). Primary level psychological services in South Africa: Can a new psychological professional fill the gap? Health Policy and Planning, 19(1), 33-40.

Petersen, I, Bhagwanjee, A, Bhana, A, & Mahintsho, Z (2004). The Development and Evaluation of a Manualised participatory HIV/AIDS risk reduction programme (Sex and Risk) for Tertiary Level Students: A pilot study. *African Journal of AIDS Research*, in press.

Petersen, I, Bhagwanjee, A, Roche, S, Bhana A, & Joseph S (2002a). *Sex & Risk: Facilitator's Manual: An HIV/AIDS risk reduction programme for tertiary level students*. Community Mental Health Programme, School of Psychology, University of Durban-Westville, Durban.

Petersen, I, Bhagwanjee, A, Roche, S, Bhana, A, & Joseph, S (2002b). *Sex & Risk: Student Workbook: An HIV/AIDS risk reduction programme for tertiary level students.* Community Mental Health Programme, School of Psychology, University of Durban-Westville, Durban.

Petraitis, J, Flay, BR & Miller, TQ (1995). Reviewing theories of adolescent substance abuse: Organizing pieces of the puzzle. *Psychological Bulletin,* 117(1), 67-86.

Redd, J, Suggs, H, Gibbons, R, Muhammad, L, McDonald, J, & Bell, CC (in press). *The Bloomington Model: A Plan to Strengthen Families and Decrease the Need for Protective Custody.*

South African Institute of Race Relations. (1997). *The 1996/7 Survey of South Africa.* Johannesburg: S.A. Institute of Race Relations.

Sampson, RJ, Raudenbush, SW, & Earls, F (1997). Neighborhoods and violent crime: A multilevel study of collective efficacy. *Science* 277: 918-924.

Tolan, PH & McKay, MM (1996). Preventing aggression in urban children: An empirically based family prevention program. *Family Relations,* 45, 148-155.

U.S. Public Health Service (2001). *Mental Health: Culture, Race, and Ethnicity: A Supplement to Mental Health: A Report of the Surgeon General.* Rockville, MD: U.S. Public Health Service.

doi:10.1300/J200v05n03_01

Transferring a University-Led HIV/AIDS Prevention Initiative to a Community Agency

Donna Baptiste
Dara Blachman
Elise Cappella
Donald Dew
Karen Dixon
Carl C. Bell
Doris Coleman

Ida Coleman
Bridgette Leachman
LaDora McKinney
Roberta L. Paikoff
Lindyann Wright
Sybil Madison-Boyd
Mary M. McKay

Donna Baptiste, PhD, Dara Blachman, PhD, Elise Cappella, PhD, Carl C. Bell, MD, Doris Coleman, MSM, Ida Coleman, Bridgette Leachman, LaDora McKinney, Roberta L. Paikoff, PhD, and Lindyann Wright, MA, are affiliated with the Institute for Juvenile Research, University of Illinois at Chicago. Donald Dew, MSW, and Karen Dixon, EdD, are affiliated with Habilitative Systems Incorporated (HSI). Sybil Madison-Boyd, PhD, is affiliated with the University of Chicago. Mary M. McKay, PhD, is affiliated with Columbia University.

Address correspondence to: Donna R. Baptiste, PhD, Institute for Juvenile Research, 1747 West Roosevelt Road, Room 155 (MC747), Chicago, IL 60608 (E-mail: baptiste@uic.edu).

The authors thank the staff of the Collaborative HIV/AIDS Prevention and Adolescent Mental Health Project (CHAMP); members of the CHAMP Collaborative Board; and the staff of Habilitative Systems Incorporated (HSI) for their extraordinary efforts. The authors are also indebted to the many families who have participated in their research.

This work is supported by the National Institute of Mental Health (5R01-MH50423; 5R01-MH55701) and the William T. Grant Foundation.

[Haworth co-indexing entry note]: "Transferring a University-Led HIV/AIDS Prevention Initiative to a Community Agency." Baptiste, Donna et al. Co-published simultaneously in *Social Work in Mental Health* (The Haworth Press, Inc.) Vol. 5, No. 3/4, 2007, pp. 269-293; and: *Community Collaborative Partnerships: The Foundation for HIV Prevention Research Efforts* (ed: Mary M. McKay, and Roberta L. Paikoff) The Haworth Press, Inc., 2007, pp. 269-293. Single or multiple copies of this article are available for a fee from The Haworth Document Delivery Service [1-800-HAWORTH, 9:00 a.m. - 5:00 p.m. (EST). E-mail address: docdelivery@haworthpress.com].

SUMMARY. Given the urgent need for HIV/AIDS interventions that will reverse current infection trends among urban minority youth, identifying effective and socially relevant approaches is of primary concern. HIV/AIDS prevention initiatives that are housed in, and led by, communities may address the limits of laboratory-based inquiry for this complex and socially-situated health issue. In this article, we describe the process of moving a researcher-led, HIV/AIDS prevention research program–the Collaborative HIV/AIDS Adolescent Mental Health Project (CHAMP)–from a university laboratory to a community mental health agency with the goal of strengthening program access, effectiveness, and sustainability over time. We outline the framework, timeline, and responsibilities involved in moving the program, research, and technology from its original university base to a local community agency. From the challenges faced and lessons learned during this complex transfer process, we hope to enhance understanding of ways in which we can narrow the gap between academic and community leadership of HIV/AIDS prevention research. doi:10.1300/J200v05n03_02 *[Article copies available for a fee from The Haworth Document Delivery Service: 1-800-HAWORTH. E-mail address: <docdelivery@haworthpress.com> Website: <http://www.HaworthPress.com> © 2007 by The Haworth Press, Inc. All rights reserved.]*

KEYWORDS. HIV/AIDS prevention, technology transfer, community based prevention, translational research

The unabated spread of HIV/AIDS among urban minority youth has influenced academic and community level initiatives aimed at decreasing youths' vulnerability to the virus. Community groups and agencies are implementing outreach efforts such as HIV/AIDS information and awareness campaigns (CDC, 2000). Likewise, prevention scientists are conducting research studies to delineate factors linked to youths' HIV/AIDS risk reduction (Pequegnat & Szapocznik, 2000). But despite academic and community responses to youth's HIV/AIDS prevention needs, there is a surprising lack of integration between the two. Prevention strategies detailed in scientific studies rarely find their way to community agencies and groups, and interventions shown to be efficacious under laboratory-style conditions in academic settings yield disappointing results in community-based trials (Jensen, Hoagwood & Trickett, 1999). On the other side, agencies and groups in communities hardest hit by HIV/AIDS target youth with innovative programs, but scant data are collected to document program efficacy; therefore, little is known about why these programs work or whether they will work in other contexts (Kellam & Langevin, 2003).

Given the urgent need for HIV/AIDS interventions that will reverse current infection trends among urban minority youth, identifying those that demonstrate efficacy *and* real world relevance is of primary concern (Schensul, 1999; Stevenson & White, 1996). Further, the complexities surrounding HIV/AIDS prevention and the limits of laboratory-style inquiry for a health issue that is socially situated, have highlighted the need to develop prevention approaches that are based in, and led by, communities (Mutchler, 2000; Schensul, 1999).

Clearly, community-agency driven HIV/AIDS prevention programs may lead to wider dissemination of prevention messages and strategies (Galbraith, Ricardo, & Stanton et al., 1996; Schenshul, 1999; Stevenson & White, 1994). Agencies can troubleshoot aspects of a program's design and delivery that affect its viability in a setting, thus leading to more effective outreach among targeted groups. Further, agencies may be more apt than academic research teams to retain proven programs within their infrastructure, enhancing the likelihood that a specific program will be sustained over time (Galbraith et al., 1996; Goark & Mccall, 1996). But many community-based agencies interested in leading HIV/AIDS prevention question whether empirically-validated information and ideas can be infused into their initiatives and how agency perspectives and control over research can be merged with a scientific approach. Academic researchers who value community input also wonder how information generated within the academy can be disseminated to agencies and groups leading HIV/AIDS prevention efforts and how a scientific approach will unfold within an agency's climate and culture (Goark & Mccall, 1996; Neumann & Sogolow, 2000; Schensul, 1999).

In this paper, we describe a program of HIV/AIDS research, the Collaborative HIV/AIDS Adolescent Mental Health Project (CHAMP) that is designed to address questions such as those listed above and to narrow the gap between academic and community leadership of HIV/ AIDS prevention. One view guiding our work is that academic and community HIV/AIDS initiatives are not inherently incompatible nor are they necessarily synergistic. We believe that a scientific focus can be integrated into community-driven programs and that the merger is a valuable goal for the field of HIV/AIDS prevention research.

More recently, there has been increasing interest in fostering community leadership of prevention research, and some researchers have provided theoretical overviews and important themes and recommendations for facilitating this goal (e.g., Altman, 1995; Everhart & Wandersman, 2000). Still, there is a dearth of information about community leadership of research programs specifically focused on preventing HIV/AIDS. In prior publications we have described our efforts to work along these lines. Madison, McKay, Paikoff and Bell (2000) and McKay et al. (2000) discuss the framework for the academic-community collaborative approach in HIV/AIDS risk reduction with urban adolescents. This was the starting point for infusing community leadership at the "ground floor" in the CHAMP initiative. Further, Baptiste et al. (2005) describe how researcher and community ideas and values have been blended to create and implement the CHAMP interventions in urban neighborhoods in Chicago.

As necessary as these steps have been, they have been insufficient in facilitating full community leadership of this HIV/AIDS prevention program. Whereas community members have been involved in a high-intensity collaboration with researchers, the work has been centered within a university's walls and shaped by its culture. Specifically, in many university settings, individual initiative and work flexibility are likely to be valued, rules and procedures are often more implicit than explicit, the power structure is not strictly hierarchical, and the bottom line is often knowledge rather than sustainability or effectiveness. CHAMP has not been led by or adapted to fit the format, pattern, and cadence of a community agency, which is likely to have different structures, values, and expectations (Swisher, 2000). In this article, we discuss our attempts to take this additional step–moving CHAMP from a university to a community setting–a phase critical to the evolution of our ideas about HIV/AIDS prevention initiative.

In sum, this article describes our efforts to transfer CHAMP from its base at the University of Illinois at Chicago to Habilitative Systems Incorporated (HSI), a community mental health center in urban Chicago. We begin by providing brief overviews of both CHAMP and HSI. Then, we discuss our framework for transfer, along with the timeline, constituents, roles, and responsibilities in the planning process. Finally, we summarize the challenges we experienced in this undertaking and offer recommendations that, we hope, will help to guide others.

OVERVIEW OF CHAMP

CHAMP is a research program designed to identify factors related to HIV/AIDS risk exposure among youth living in high sero-prevalent urban communities, with the aim of implementing preventive interventions that can increase youths' protection against the virus. The CHAMP research program involves three studies: (a) a longitudinal survey of family and contextual factors related to youths' HIV/AIDS risk in a low-income community in Southside Chicago (Paikoff et al., 1993; 1998); (b) a longitudinal evaluation of a family-based intervention involving 4th-7th graders and their families in the same community (Paikoff et al., 1995); and, (c) a replication/transfer study involving two new communities, one in the Bronx, New York, and the other on Chicago's Westside (McKay et al., 2000). Two international research studies have been derived from CHAMP, an efficacy trial of a CHAMP-style intervention in Trinidad and Tobago in the Caribbean (Baptiste et al., 2006; Voisin et al., 2006) and a similar research project in urban and rural communities in South Africa (Bhana et al., 2004; Paruk et al., 2002). In this article, we focus on our Chicago work–more specifically the study designed to transfer leadership of CHAMP Family Program to a community agency.

A core element underlying all CHAMP studies is *academic-community collaboration*. In keeping with this principle, we have followed a series of steps to ensure intensive community involvement. First, we established a Community Collaborative Board comprised of members of the academic research team, as well as community constituents. Community members on the board include such individuals as staff and parents within selected schools, staff of mental health and other youth- serving agencies in the community, residents-at large, and clergy (Madison, McKay, Paikoff & Bell, 2000). Second, we designed an intervention using both basic research and a synergy of academic and community ideas. A temporary board subcommittee comprising researchers and community members distilled and refined the core ideas to be packaged into a manualized curriculum (Baptiste et al., 2006). Third, facilitator teams involving both university and community members delivered the program and collected intervention and process data from youth and parents. Prior to implementation and while the program was underway, facilitators were jointly trained to negotiate the complexities of this collaborative relationship. Fourth, the Community Collaborative Board oversees ongoing dissemination activities. Notably, board members are involved with researchers in drafting and/or reviewing papers, such as this one, and presenting at professional meetings. Our Collaborative Board and/or specific members are named as co-authors on most of our publications (e.g., McKay et al., 2004).

TRANSFERRING CHAMP

We identified the goal of transferring CHAMP to a community agency early in the development of the first study on Chicago's Southside. The first CHAMP Collaborative Board recognized this goal in its mission statement: "If a community likes the program, the research staff will help the community find ways to continue the program on its own" (CHAMP mission statement, May 1996). Thus, in the early stages of this study, we began to pave the way for the transfer. For example, we received grant funding to enhance leadership development among community board members (Madison, McKay & the CHAMP Board, 1998). Academic leaders of the project identified a list of "tangible and intangible skills" required for key roles and responsibilities, and community members shadowed these leaders to learn these skills. Selected board members were trained as supervisors or team coordinators in anticipation of future leadership roles in CHAMP. Finally, early in the fourth year of the study, we submitted a grant proposal to secure funding for replication/transfer in two new communities. The grant proposal included a plan to mentor and train community members to assume full responsibility for delivering the intervention as it was being replicated in the new setting. We expected community leaders to be responsible for the day-to-day research operation (with consultation from university researchers) and envisioned that the last year of the study would involve preparations to move the entire initiative to a community agency–in particular, Habilitative Systems Incorporated (HSI).

OVERVIEW OF HSI

Habilitative Systems, Incorporated (HSI) is a human service agency on the West Side of Chicago involved in the development and implementation of a range of programs serving African American adults and children. HSI was founded in 1978 by several church members and has grown to incorporate over 50 programs serving more than 7,000 people in 14 sites across Chicago. The mission of HSI is to be the "premier behavioral health and human service organization, providing an array of responsive services that promote consumer self-sufficiency" (HSI Annual Report, 2002, p. 1). The overarching purpose is to work toward the alleviation of human suffering through the development and delivery of resources that foster "dignity, self-sufficiency, and empowerment."

HSI seeks to promote such independence and responsibility among mentally, physically, socially, and emotionally disabled persons in order that they may become fully contributing members of society. HSI also endeavors to provide a continuum of care that appears seamless, as clients are moved through a comprehensive and broad range of services across four divisions. Table 1 describes HSI's divisions and programs and notes the division in which CHAMP will be situated.

OUR FRAMEWORK FOR TRANSFER

Models for integrating academically-driven prevention programs into community agencies are discussed within a range of fields and/or movements (e.g., prevention science, translation research, technology transfer) with the goal to broaden the impact of efficacious prevention programs through large-scale dissemination and implementation of such programs. A review of these approaches is beyond the scope of this paper. However, we highlight common themes (irrespective of the differences in terminology, framework, and content area) and indicate how these themes have played out in our work.

Ensuring a good academic-agency fit. Common across many frameworks is the notion that effective transfer of programs involves ensuring a good fit between the academic program and the mission, goals, and needs of the community agency. For example, Swisher (2000) argues that successful adoption of an academic program by an agency involves considering how the program can be integrated into the agency's central mission and adapted to the "usual pattern and cadence of the activities" rather than included as a separate project (p. 971). Similarly, Olds (2002) suggests that the program must fit the community's needs as well as the agency's mission and goals, and that the community and agency must be "fully knowledgeable and supportive of the program" (p. 169). This issue, the goodness-of-fit between CHAMP and HSI, also has been important in our work. CHAMP researchers approached HSI–an agency located in the targeted community–in part because it articulated HIV/AIDS prevention as an aspect of its core mission (HSI Annual Report, 2003). In addition, HSI recently had altered its service philosophy to include evidence-based treatments designed to maximize accountability and improve client outcomes. In a related vein, the organization already was involved in partnerships with academic researchers. Finally, the Chief Executive Director (CEO) of HSI has focused attention on the health risks for urban children and has strengthened the

TABLE 1. Habiliatative Systems Incorporated (HSI) Programs and Services

Children and Family Services Care Center **	Behavioral Health Care Center	Residential Services Care Center	Disabilities Management Care Center
Teen Parenting	Case Management	Community Individual Living Arrangements	SBC Bill Payment Center
Youth Enhancement Services? • Delinquency Prevention? • Safe Nights/Finish Lines? • Target Ready	Child and Adolescent Mental Health Services	Assertive Community Treatment Programs	Developmental Training Work Services
Day Care Program	HIV Education/Prevention	Emergency Housing	Supported Employment
Extended Family Services	Residential and Outpatient	Transitional Homeless Shelter	Employment Training
Housing Advocacy	Substance Abuse	MISA Services	Vocational Evaluation
Child Protective Services	Client/Family Support Services	Extended Treatment Residential Program	Earnfare Placement Services
**CHAMP	Case Coordination		Sheltered Employment

**Division where CHAMP is located

organization's commitment to providing quality services to urban children and their families through a variety of school- and community-based programs. Thus, HSI welcomed CHAMP's family-based approach to prevention, one emphasizing ongoing collection of evaluation data to assess the program's efficacy/effectiveness. The agency expressed a view that, with a few changes, CHAMP would fit comfortably within the agency's Children and Family Services Care Division whose mission is "to help urban children, youth, and families stay together, become independent, and develop to their full potential" (HSI annual report, 2002, p. 1).

Early planning for sustainability within the agency. Researchers (e.g., Neumann & Sogolow, 2000) have noted that successful transfer requires investments in people, relationships, and time, as well as coordination around such critical issues as staffing and funding. These issues are viewed as affecting an agency's ability to sustain a transferred program within its infrastructure. But agencies often lack the technical assistance, staff support, and implementation resources that are available in well-funded prevention trials (Spoth, Kavanagh, & Dishion, 2002). They also may grapple with issues such as high staff turnover and lack of adequate space, facilities, and equipment, which can undermine a program's long-term viability (Kellam & Langevin, 2003; Swisher, 2000).

These issues were relevant to our process. It was clear to us that, apart from outside consultation, a well-trained, supervised, and supported staff was a necessary prerequisite to maintaining a program within an agency's service delivery model (Olds, 2002; Swisher, 2000). Accordingly, over a three-year period, researchers and academic staff mentored and trained three community members to assume leadership roles at the agency. Our training and mentorship was via a hands-on method. Community leaders ran a small replication study and performed all leadership tasks. Although HSI's staff will decide the scope of training and support offered community members as they lead CHAMP at the agency, researchers will continue to provide both support and some training, especially during the transition period, as community leaders acclimate to the agency culture.

Heller (1990) and Swisher (2000) also advise that funding options should be sorted out early to prevent interruptions once transfer occurs. Along these lines, Kellam and Langevin (2003) recommend conducting long-term cost-benefit analyses of transferred programs to match resource allocation to service delivery needs. Although this latter aspect–long-term budgeting for CHAMP–is still unresolved, we have made financial and budgetary arrangements for the short-term. Undoubtedly, HSI needs time to establish a secure financial base for the CHAMP program. Therefore, we moved the program to the agency approximately 18 months before the end of grant funding. All grant monies to fund salary, wages, benefits, program delivery, and data collection then move from the university to the agency to underwrite agency expenses for those 18 months. Although HSI will direct some of its own resources to sustain the program, we fully expect the agency to seek external support to keep it going. In fact, HSI's leaders already have begun to do this.

Build in continuous quality improvement. Elias (1997) notes that an ongoing and iterative cycle of implementation, monitoring, evaluation, feedback, and adaptation of an intervention can help to assure its sustainability in a transfer process. Thus, a preventive intervention is transferred with a specific set of principles and practices related to continuous evaluation and modification of the program, with the ultimate goal of improving impact on health and social behavior. Olds (2002) recommends collecting "real-time information" on implementation of the intervention and its achievement of benchmarks to guide continuous quality improvement (p. 169). Schoenwald and Hoagwood (2001) provide a useful framework for moving evidence-based practices into real world use at a community site. They suggest researchers investigate how aspects of the intervention, those delivering it, those participating in it, the delivery mode, and the organization itself must be modified for effective implementation in a community setting.

We also believe that continuous quality improvement is key to CHAMP's sustainability within HSI; thus, we are transferring the technology to make programming improvements over time. For example, community leaders recently have adapted our 12-session intervention, usually delivered mid-week, into four Saturday sessions of longer duration. This adaptation was in response to the reality that parents in our population have returned to the workforce and are not available for mid-week sessions. We also felt a shortened program would better fit the agency's infrastructure. The capacity that community leaders have demonstrated to distill and condense core program components into a format that better fits population and agency demands is an example of a "quality control" approach. Community leaders piloted the adapted version of the CHAMP intervention and made refinements to the program manual and assessments. The knowledge gained from these experiences will move with them to the agency.

Balancing program adaptation with fidelity. Researchers (e.g., Kelly et al., 2000) suggest that the "core elements" driving a program's effectiveness should be identified prior to transferring it to another setting. Core elements are best identified empirically but, at the least, should be readily apparent from the theoretical model that guides the research. In a similar vein, others have offered guidelines for balancing program fidelity with program adaptation or program tailoring for another setting. For example, Domitrovich and Greenberg (2000) suggest that researchers specify active ingredients and change mechanisms. Once these mechanisms have been identified, other aspects of the intervention may be more flexible and adaptable based on the needs of the setting and population in which the intervention is being delivered. A related recommendation is that intervention adaptations and revisions should be carefully documented in order to determine their impact on the design and effectiveness of programs (Domitrovich & Greenberg, 2000).

We have attempted to identify both core and flexible aspects of our program while training and mentoring community leaders to grasp CHAMP's theoretical model of change. Within the four-session adaptation of the program developed to match parents' schedules and agency resources, community leaders evaluated ways to retain the core elements while adapting the program structure. Core elements of our intervention include: (a) a structure involving multiple family groups and breakout components for parents and youth, (b) content involving attention to family supports and parental monitoring, HIV/AIDS information, a discussion of family rules, attention to increasing parent/child comfort in discussions of sensitive issues, and (c) research involving careful data collection (Baptiste et al., in press).

A common theme in all of the above areas is the necessity for academic researchers to pursue true collaboration with community partners–ideally from the beginning of the process to the end. Indeed, we agree that insufficient community ownership leads to a model of *doing for* instead of *doing with* the community (Everhart & Wandersman, 2000; Kellam & Langevin, 2003). As suggested by others, the interpersonal relationships behind our partnership have been key to facilitating honest discussion and reconciliation of differences with respect to timelines, priorities, and logistics (Rotheram-Borus, Rebchook, & Kelly et al., 2000). We have held extensive discussions to plan for the transfer of CHAMP. These meetings have helped to ensure that all constituents are active participants in decision-making. In the pages that follow we provide a detailed summary of our planning process.

PLANNING TO TRANSFER CHAMP

Timeline

Our efforts to transfer CHAMP from the university to a community agency began five years after we first launched the program. We spent an additional six years in planning CHAMP's move from the University to the agency. Notwithstanding the challenges we encountered over the six years, as evident from the timeline below, we achieved significant milestones that brought us closer to this end goal.

Year 1: The Southside Community Collaborative Board identifies transfer of the CHAMP research initiative from the University of Illinois at Chicago to a community agency as a concrete goal, and a decision is made to apply for grant funding to pursue it. The Board discusses and ratifies the idea, and over a 12-month period the grant application is developed. This includes finding a suitable host agency for CHAMP (HSI); reviewing literature about transfer of programs, and preparation of a RO1 application that includes parallel goals of (a) replicating the CHAMP program in the Bronx, New York, and (b) transferring CHAMP out of the university to the agency in Chicago. The proposal is written and submitted to the National Institute of Mental Health (NIMH) Office on AIDS, and it identifies a primary strategy to effect program transfer, that is, mentorship and training of community members who can join agency as leaders of the initiative.

Year 2: Funding is successful and administrative and budgetary structure is developed to achieve specific aims of the research. One aim is to replicate the CHAMP in New York and that operation is launched as a parallel but separate initiative. In relation to the second aim, program transfer in Chicago, researchers submit the Institutional Review Board (IRB) application. This IRB requests that researchers submit three distinct applications to oversee human subject protections for the multi-layered research activities. These applications spell out procedures collection of both qualitative and quantitative research aspects, an appropriate and ethical structure for mentorship of community leaders, and methods and measures related to conducting the small replication study. The IRB applications require multiple revisions that delay the start of program activities. However, recruitment and selection of potential community leaders begins. The Southside Community Collaborative Board determines the appropriate entry-level education and experience for Project Director (PD) and Co-community leader positions. The PD is expected to train and mentor four community members slated to become the future leaders of CHAMP at the agency. The training arena will be implementation of a small replication of the CHAMP program on Chicago's West Side in close proximity to the agency. A personnel sub-committee of the board prepares job descriptions, advertises the PD community leader positions, and recruits and selects applicants. At the end of the recruitment process, IRB approvals are secured.

Year 3: The replication study that is the training ground for community leaders is scheduled to begin, but multiple obstacles are encountered that further delays plans for transfer. These include: (a) competing researcher priorities including critical carry-over tasks from the initial CHAMP research;[1] (b) researchers' inexperience in developing an adequate framework for the training/mentorship of community members; (c) a lack of clarity on roles and responsibilities in the initiative, especially those related to mentorship; (d) illness of the Project Director; (e) interpersonal conflicts; and (f) personnel turnover. In a series of conflict resolution sessions, we contemplate an early transfer of the project to the agency. However, this is not feasible because community leaders are inadequately trained to assume leadership of CHAMP; the agency is not yet ready to incorporate CHAMP within its infrastructure; and the fiscal and budgetary resources for transfer are not in place. Instead, researchers and community leaders develop an alternative training/ mentoring plan involving various individuals and including researchers in mentorship/roles.

A framework begins for mentorship of community leaders via hands-on involvement in the intervention replication. The replication includes most aspects related to adapting and delivering the CHAMP pre-adolescent family intervention. These include (a) development of a Westside Community Board, (b) recruitment of schools and participants (4th/5th grade students and their parents), (c) a pilot to refine the intervention for the Chicago Westside community, (d) revisions to the program manual, and (e) preparation for data collection.

The Chief Executive Director (CEO) of HSI is selected to chair the CHAMP Westside Board and this marks the first concrete step towards transfer. In the role of chairperson, the agency's director is orientated to all aspects of the CHAMP initiative, including to the community leaders who will eventually join the agency.

Year 4: Community leaders continue their involvement in every aspect of program replication. Each Co Project Director (CPD) has increasing responsibility for leading one primary and one secondary aspect of managing CHAMP (e.g., coordinating the Community Collaborative Board; subject recruitment). Under the oversight of the PD and/or researchers' CPDs are immersed in setting up overall and specific project goals and activities; establishing timelines; developing contingency plans; and evaluating progress. This process involves iterative action-reflection cycles. The impending goal of moving the program to the agency is an underlying theme that causes some tensions; as yet, no formal meetings are planned to discuss it.

Year 5: The goal of transfer is now a regular part of discussions among researchers and academic staff. There is a fair amount of consensus among this group that transfer will occur, but disagreement as to the timing and pacing of it. There are even some concerns about whether it should occur at all.

The CPDs are not active participants in the discussion about transfer and continue to receive mentorship and training via the replication. Their knowledge and skills related to managing the program is increasing. For example, community leaders display sound knowledge and skills in developing relationships with selected schools; recruiting early adolescents and parents for the study; and recruiting, selecting and training facilitators. However, they seem less prepared to lead other key aspects of CHAMP, for example, training facilitators in data collection; archiving collected data; supervising facilitators to competently deliver the intervention; and independently handling unordinary interpersonal situations that occur during the conduct of the research. There is a recognition of a need for more intensive training and mentorship of community leaders around "less concrete" tasks related to leading CHAMP and discussions are held to determine the best methods to achieve this. However, the resignations of two key mentors within CHAMP affect morale of all and threatens the project's stability. The feeling that the project should move to the agency resurfaces but there are still tensions and conflicts about the timing and pacing of transfer.

An external event–a confirmed date for the move of faculty, clinical and research staff, and university research labs, including CHAMP, to a newly-acquired building–becomes the catalyst that propels the board, researchers, agency staff, and CPDs to enter the active phase of transfer planning. Whereas many issues are as yet unresolved, there is consensus among all that CHAMP's move to HSI is close.

Year 6: The first of several project-wide meetings are held to begin formal discussions related to transferring CHAMP to HSI. Although there are still disagreements as to exactly when staff and infrastructure will move out of the university, there is consensus that formal planning should begin and involve all stakeholders–agency staff, board members, community leaders, and research staff. Community leaders remain involved in the program's replication and have acquired advanced skills related to its operation; however, they face recruitment challenges that illuminate questions about the program's viability, especially in light of its prospective transfer to the agency. A decision is made to revise the program to better fit agency resources and community needs. A curriculum sub-committee, led by a community member, adapts and pilots a shortened version of the CHAMP intervention.

The Westside Community Collaborative Board ratifies transfer to HSI and the agency's Executive Board of Directors discusses how CHAMP can be incorporated into its programs. Monthly transfer planning meetings involving the primary constituents (agency staff, researchers, community leaders, and board members) begin at the agency. Early meetings focus on broad issues such as overall mission and philosophy, level of board involvement in the process, processes of decision-making, and the fit between agency and program goals. Later meetings focus on the logistical issues of transfer such as moving staff, fiscal restructuring, and IRB revisions, along with a specific action plan and timeline for the move. Approximately eight months after formal planning sessions begin, community leaders, equipment, supplies, and other CHAMP resources are relocated to the agency and post-transfer planning begins.

Constituents, Roles, and Responsibilities

The timeline above indicates that transferring CHAMP to HSI has been both *time* and *labor* intensive, involving more than 70 individuals over a sustained period in discussions and negotiations on a variety of levels. There were clear constituents that have been critical to the process, and multiple roles and responsibilities have emerged throughout.

We needed an effective chairperson of our transfer planning group and HSI's CEO assumed this role. Key agency officials served as an integral supporting cast. These officials included the following: (a) HSI's Chief Operating Officer, responsible for hammering out the details related to moving personnel and resources, and securing the agency's IRB approval; (b) HSI's Director of Budgets, who worked with CHAMP's Budget Administrator to effect a transfer of fiscal resources; (c) HSI's Clinical Director of the Child and Family Services Care Center, slated to become the direct supervisor of the community leaders; and (d) HSI's human resources manager, who oriented community leaders to the agency's employee policies, salary and benefits, and requisite employment paperwork.

CHAMP researchers and academic staff, usually only indirectly responsible for human resource and fiscal aspects of grants/contracts, took on matching roles to those at the agency. There were three broad roles with concomitant responsibilities. First, researchers provided general oversight over the transfer process on the University's side. This involved securing IRB approvals related to moving the project, transferring existing data, and communicating with the funding source (National Institute of Mental Health) and University officials about the impending change in the project's status. Second, researchers helped to prepare community leaders for the psychological and pragmatic issues related to leaving the university culture and forming new attachments with agency personnel (Glisson, 2002). These discussions focused on areas such as community leaders' readiness to assume leadership of the project, to work with increased autonomy, and to move the resources needed to run the program at the agency. Third, CHAMP's budget administrator arranged for the transfer of fiscal and budgetary aspects of the project, moving CHAMP's assets and resources (money, equipment, etc.) out of the university and into the agency.

Finally, the community leaders themselves were critical players in planning for their move to HSI. Their perspectives illuminated the personal impact of moving from one organizational culture to another. Early in the planning process, community leaders developed a list of questions that helped to organize transfer planning discussions. We include a sample of unedited questions here as an example of latent issues that were a significant part of our discussions:

1. What will the CHAMP model look like at HSI?
2. What elements will be kept and what will be given up?
3. Does HSI have another plan for CHAMP (e.g., will it be combined with some of their other programs?)
4. How will HSI ensure that CHAMP is recognizable when at the agency? (suggested name CHAMP HSI)
5. What will be staff's pay rate, will it be higher, the same or lower as at the University?
6. What type of benefit plan would be at HSI? Specifically, how would benefits like medical insurance, retirement, dental, vacation, and sick, rate of employee's contribution compare to the University's?
7. What type of training/mentoring would staff get at HSI? Who will do the training/mentoring?
8. Which IRB will be in charge of CHAMP if it moves?
9. How would university staff be involved when the project moves?
10. What role will the CHAMP board playing in transfer? How will Board members continue to be involved after transfer?

Members of the Westside Community Collaborative Board also attended planning meetings and helped to reconcile the various interests and agendas of other constituents. Board members' observations led to refinement of our ideas. Although some of these issues are not fully resolved, our initial contemplation of them has enhanced the philosophical and logistical perspectives related to transferring CHAMP. For example, Board members who were not involved at the time HSI was selected as the permanent home for the project pressed for additional details about why the agency was selected. This had been a "taken-for-granted" decision, but the inquiry facilitated new discussions about the compatibility between CHAMP and HSI, bringing even greater insight into the goodness-of-fit.

Similarly, board members asked about the role of a Community Collaborative Board under HSI's leadership. Because the Community Board has been a highly celebrated aspect of CHAMP's work, this question facilitated discussion on the potential involvement of community members at the agency. HSI's administrators agreed to establish a research committee as part of its Quality Assurance Coordinating Committee (QACC), an internal, employee-based committee that oversees organizational functioning and reports to the governing board of directors. (Figure 1 details QACC's structure and potential placement of

CHAMP staff. Figure 2 describes HSI's Board of Directors and where CHAMP Board members may be incorporated.) Notably, as part of both of these boards, CHAMP staff and community board members have the opportunity to oversee other agency initiatives in addition to continuing their involvement with CHAMP.

In sum, planning to transfer CHAMP to HSI has, by no means, been a linear process unfolding smoothly over time. On the contrary, we have experienced major interpersonal conflicts, terminations and resignations, and multiple and ongoing disagreements related to transplanting community leaders to a new setting. Our planning process has been fraught with inconsistencies and ambiguities, many of which are yet to be resolved. Despite challenges, we have been united by a commitment to finding a permanent home for CHAMP, involving families in HIV/AIDS prevention, and supporting HSI as it leads these efforts. In the section below, we further highlight specific tensions as well as offer recommendations to those contemplating similar initiatives.

Challenges

Individually, and as a group, we have experienced many conflicts in our efforts to place CHAMP under HSI's leadership. Heuristically, these tensions can be grouped into four broad categories: (a) a struggle to balance a collaborative process with achievement of concrete project outcomes; (b) transfer of the scientific principles and practices underlying CHAMP; (c) transplanting of community leaders to a new organizational culture; and (d) negotiating of multiple logistics related to moving the program to a new setting.

Balancing a collaborative process with outcome goals. At various points in our planning we felt stuck, unable to achieve significant milestones in transferring the program. At one of these junctures, we stopped to reflect and, in particular, to identify barriers in our process. Two individuals who served as *"process observers"* during planning meetings conducted interviews with a majority of constituents, including agency staff, researchers, and community leaders. A pervasive theme that emerged from these conversations was the differential weights individuals placed on achieving *process* and *outcome* goals in decision-making.

For example, relationships within CHAMP have been constructed based on the core value of "working collaboratively." For many of us, this meant adopting an open and inclusive posture in planning. In our view, a collaborative posture ensured that everyone's "voice" would be

FIGURE 1. Habilitative Systems Incorporated (HSI) Internal Agency Committee Structure

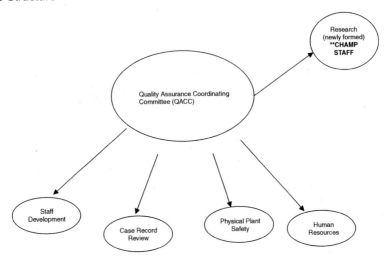

**Newly developed oversight committee that will include CHAMP staff

FIGURE 2. Habilitative Systems Incorporated (HSI) External Governance Board Structure

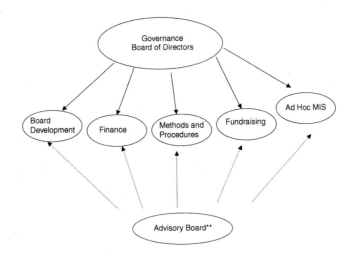

**CHAMP Advisory board member incorporated here

heard and a consultative approach would be used in decision-making. Although we all ascribed to this value in theory, in practice there were tensions. Community leaders, in particular, who often voiced feeling "less powerful" than researchers, questioned the way in which decisions were made and ideas were prioritized. In essence, there was a schism between the goal of inclusiveness and democracy in decision-making on the one hand, and achieving of benchmark tasks, on the other.

The act of reflecting on and illuminating our individual values and styles, and re-affirming a commitment to both process and outcome goals, was helpful in diminishing tensions such that planning could proceed. Although our attempts to balance these goals are ongoing, we recognized that the two are not mutually exclusive. Collaborative conversations contain symbolic features, such as attention to the structure of conversations, indicating whose voices and views are prioritized. Time spent to reflect on these features of discussions can be worthwhile. However, collaborative conversations can co-exist with urgency and accountability around task accomplishment, thus simultaneously emphasizing the achievement of critical project milestones.

Transferring the scientific basis of CHAMP. In moving CHAMP to HSI, we actually are transferring a scientific approach to HIV/AIDS prevention that is centered in community knowledge and leadership. This includes a process for ensuring that the HIV/AIDS preventive intervention can be refined with community input to match the population and agency dynamics. But the CHAMP intervention is delivered as a component of prevention research. Accordingly, evaluation of the intervention's impact is a critical consideration. We have utilized an experimental research design with randomization of families to intervention and comparison conditions. Data are collected from youth and parents, and complex data analytic techniques are used to determine the longitudinal impact of the intervention in decreasing HIV/AIDS risk exposure (McKay et al., 2000; Paikoff et al., 1995). All of these aspects underlie the empirical base of CHAMP and must be transferred along with its tangible resources. Transfer of these scientific aspects has been more difficult that we first envisioned.

First, community leaders are not currently equipped to conduct full-scale evaluations of the intervention. Whereas they grasp the basic tenets of a research study, community members are unfamiliar with more technical aspects of research, such as data analytic strategies and procedures. Second, unlike the CHAMP research lab, HSI is not a research facility and its primary mission is broader than HIV/AIDS prevention. Issues such as design of a randomized trial, program fidelity, analysis of complex datasets, and longitudinal follow-up of intervention participants is not part of the normative terrain of the agency's operation. Finally, HSI is not accustomed to the regular dissemination–through publications and presentations–of research findings and process papers related to the interventions they develop, implement, and evaluate within their organization.

Transplanting community leaders. It should be clear from prior discussions that we view community leaders as the bearers of CHAMP technology. However, we made the decision to mentor/train community leaders within the university walls without full appreciation of how its culture would affect their work styles and aspirations. We also did not consider the impact of a move on their career goals, aspirations, and quality of life.

In our view, the culture of our academic lab within the University varies significantly from the culture of the agency. Our lab has been comprised of research faculty, full-time academic staff, civil servants, and graduate student workers. Overall, we maintained flexible working hours in a relatively unstructured setting in which work was mostly self-directed. Wider university values also trickled down to the lab, such as pursuit of educational opportunities as a route to social mobility. Thus, community leaders have been encouraged to taking advantage of the university's many opportunities for learning and self-advancement. Finally, as employees of a grant-funded initiative, CHAMP employees received an attractive compensation and benefit package.

Although appealing, many of the above features are idiosyncratic to the organizational culture of a large, state-funded university. A relatively small community agency like HSI, with limited financial resources, cannot offer the volume and range of opportunities a university can offers its employees. Further, like many other community agencies, HSI's workplace may be structured with more hierarchical working relationships and lower priority for self-direction in determining and prioritizing daily tasks. Thus, community leaders' move from the University involves an adjustment to a new organizational culture. In and of itself, this is not problematic. But, as is evident from the list of questions discussed above, community leaders have many anxieties about how the moving to the agency will impact their lives. For example, community leaders raised questions about their status within HSI's hierarchy, their level of pay and benefits, their opportunities to work autonomously, and other intangibles such as educational opportunities to help promote career growth. Notably, many of these issues may affect their day-to-day lives and future aspirations.

Our approach to resolving perceived discrepancies in organizational cultures has been to talk about differences openly, as well as to hold HSI accountable to the highest standards of ethical practices in terms of work climate and provision of opportunities for community leaders. At the same time, we acknowledge that the culture and practices of a grant-funded university lab seldom represent the "real world." Although we are still uncertain as to how community leaders will weather the transition, we are optimistic that their best interests will remain paramount in our process.

Attending to multiple logistical tasks. The genesis of the transfer idea to the final stage when staff and resources moved to the agency has taken several years. The process has involved many individuals working on multiple and varied tasks over time. Although the process has unfolded in phases, each stage has generated a large number of logistical tasks–and the volume of work has been daunting. Maintaining continuity as priorities shift and key players leave our initiative also has been challenging. We have found it helpful to focus not only on the "endgame" of transfer, but also on the critical milestones pointing to a growing knowledge- and asset-base that would be transferred to the agency. For example, the relatively tedious tasks involved in blending academic and community ideas into an intervention helped us to refine a process model for collaborative program development that we have been able to use in later stages with greater efficiency. This knowledge will be passed on to the agency. Similarly, the years spent mentoring and training community leaders in major aspects related to running CHAMP has paid off in their expanded leadership capacity, also transferred to the agency.

Notwithstanding our accomplishments related to transferring the program, we learned many lessons that will shape our future efforts, particularly efforts to build international coalitions to conduct HIV/AIDS prevention research in developing regions. We summarize some of our observations and recommendations below.

Recommendations

First, HSI came on board six years after CHAMP began its mission of HIV/AIDS prevention; yet, it may have been helpful to involve the agency from the inception of the CHAMP research program, even prior to crafting the first grant application. Notably, the latter approach has been described by Baptiste (2000; 2003), Voisin et al. (2006) and Bell et al. (2000) in the Caribbean and South Africa studies. Second, we have lost valuable opportunities to systematically observe and evaluate our transfer processes. We have struggled to find adequate methods for collecting process-level, qualitative data. We have been dependant on retrospective accounts to document our transfer approach, and while these data are useful, direct observation (e.g., via audiotapes, videotapes, and/ or process logs) may have captured the nuances of the rich collaborative transactions related to transfer. Third, whereas we have begun discussions of long-term sustainability of the program, the reality is that it will take time to find an appropriate level of funding to maintain the program at HSI. We advise others to embed this consideration into early planning stages, perhaps two-three years prior to moving the program to a new setting. Fourth, we are in the post-transfer stage of our planning, but the roles of academic researchers in the agency's efforts to lead CHAMP are as yet unspecified. We left this task to the later stages of our process but if it were to take place earlier, it might facilitate a smoother transition. Finally, whereas community collaborative HIV/AIDS prevention is meaningful, the work contains many ambiguities. One of these is the question: Is this a better way to conduct HIV/AIDS prevention? This is the question that all on CHAMP are committed to answering.

CONCLUSION

We believe that our approach to HIV/AIDS prevention departs from more traditional prevention research initiatives in both the *depth and breath* of the community's involvement in shaping CHAMP from its inception. Community input has shaped the "message"–that is, the ideas and opinions that determined the intervention's structure and content. Community members have been the "messengers"–delivering the intervention to youth and families in their neighborhoods (McKay et al., 2000; Baptiste et al., 2006). Finally, community members will oversee implementation as the entire initiative is housed within an agency, which itself is a stable "citizen" of the community. All of these aspects enhance the likelihood that CHAMP will be sustained over time.

NOTE

1. During the initial 5-year CHAMP study all research activities at the University were suspended due to alleged IRB violations. Some carry-over tasks related to re-consenting all former research subjects under new and improved new IRB procedures.

REFERENCES

Baptiste, D., Bhana, A., Petersen, I., McKay, M., Voisin, D., Bell, C., & Martinez, D.D. (2006) "Community Collaborative Youth focused HIV/AIDS prevention in South Africa and Trinidad: Preliminary Findings." *J. Pediatric Psychology,* 119(6): 1224-35.

Baptiste, D., Paikoff, P., McKay, M., Madison, S., Bell., C., Coleman, D., & The CHAMP Board. (2005). Collaborating with an urban community to develop and deliver an HIV/AIDS Prevention program for Black youth. *Behavior Modification.* 29, 370-416.

Baptiste, D.R. (2000). *The Trinidad and Tobago HIV Prevention Project.* NIMH-funded Minority Supplement Proposal. Available from the first author, University of Illinois, Chicago.

Baptiste, D.R. (2003). *Family Intervention for Caribbean Youth HIV/AIDS Risks.* NIMH-funded Career Development Award (K01) Proposal. Available from the first author at the University of Illinois, Chicago.

Bell, C.C., Bhana, A., Paruk. B., McKay, M. M., Mock, L., & Baptiste, D. (2000). *The CHAMP/South Africa Community Collaborative HIV/AIDS Project.* NIMH Grant Proposal. Available from the first author at the Community Mental Health Council, (CMHC), Chicago

Bhana, A., Petersen, I., Mason, A., Mahintsho, Z., Bell, C., & McKay, M. (2004). Children and youth at risk: Adaptation and pilot study of the CHAMP (Amaqhawe) programme in South Africa," *African Journal of AIDS Research* (AJAR) 3(1): 33-41.

Centers For Disease Control and Prevention (2000). The Prevention Marketing Initiative. *www.cdc.gov/hiv/projects/pmi* (last updated Oct 17, 2000).

Domitrovich, C. E. & Greenberg, M.T. (2000). The study of implementation: Current findings from effective programs that prevent mental disorders in school-aged children, *Journal of Educational and Psychological Consultation, 11,* 193-221.

Elias, M. J. (1997). Reinterpreting dissemination of prevention programs as widespread implementation with effectiveness and fidelity. In R. P. Weissberg (Ed.) *Healthy Children 2010: Establishing preventive services.* Thousand Oaks, CA: Sage, 253-289.

Everhart, K. & Wandersman, A. (2000). Applying comprehensive quality programming and empowerment evaluation to reduce implementation barriers. *Journal of Educational and Psychological Consultation, 11,* 177-191.

Galbraith, J., Ricardo, I., Stanton, B., Black, M., Feigelman, S., & Kaljee, L. (1996). Challenges and rewards of involving community in research: An overview of the "Focus on Kids" HIV risk reduction program. *Health Education Quarterly,* 23, 383-394.

Glisson, C. (2002). The organizational context of children's mental health services. *Clinical Child and Family Psychology Review,* 5, 233-253.

Goark, C.J. & McCall, R.B. (1996). Building successful university-community human service agency collaborations. In C.D. Fisher J.P. Murray, & I.E. Sigel (eds.), *Applied developmental science: Graduate training for diverse disciplines and educational settings* (pp. 28-49). Norwood, NJ: Ablex.

Habilitative Systems Incorporated (HSI) (2003). *Annual Report 2003*. Available from HSI: 415 South Kilpatrick Street, Chicago, IL 60644.

Hatch, J., Moss, N., & Saran, A., Presley-Cantrell, L., & Mallory, C. (1993). Community research: Partnership in black communities. *American Journal of Preventive Medicine*, 9, 27-31.

Heller, K (1990). Social and community intervention. *Annual review of Psychology*, 41, 141-168.

Jensen, P., Hoagwood, K., & Trickett, E. (1999). Ivory towers or earthen trenches? Community collaborations to foster "real world" research. *Applied Developmental Psychology*, 3(4), 206-212.

Kellam, S. G. & Langevin, D. J. (2003). A framework for understanding "evidence" in prevention research and programs. *Prevention Science*, 4 (3), 137-153.

Kelly J.A., Heckman T.G., Stevenson L.Y., Williams P.N., Ertl T., Hays R.B., Leonard N.R., O'Donnell, L., Terry, M.A., Sogolow, E.D., & Neumann, M.S. (2000). Transfer of research-based HIV prevention interventions to community service providers: Fidelity and adaptation. *AIDS Education and Prevention*, 12(Suppl. A), 87-98.

Madison, S., McKay, S & the CHAMP Collaborative Board (1998). *Parents on the Move*. Funded grant proposal, Center For Urban Educational Research and Development (CUERD). Available from the second author at Mount Sinai Hospital, New York.

Madison, S. M., McKay, M. M., Paikoff, R. L., & Bell, C.C. (2000). Basic research and community collaboration: Necessary ingredients for the development of a family-based HIV prevention program. *AIDS Education and Prevention*, 12, 281-298.

McKay, M., Paikoff, R., Baptiste, D., Bell, C., Coleman, D., Madison,S., McKinney, L. & CHAMP Collaborative Board (2004). Family-level impact of the CHAMP Family Program: A community collaborative effort to support urban families and reduce youth HIV risk exposure. *Family Process 43*(1): 79-93.

McKay, M., Baptiste, D., Paikoff, R.; Madison, S., & CHAMP Collaborative Board. Preventing HIV Risk Exposure in Urban Communities: The CHAMP Family Program. (2000), 67-87. In W. Pequegnat & Szapocznik (Eds). *Working with Families in the Era of HIV/AIDS*. Sage: CA.

McKay, M.M., Paikoff, R.L., Bell, C.C., Madison, S. M., & Baptiste, D.R. (1999). *Community Partnerships to Prevent HIV/AIDS-New York & Chicago*. NIMH- funded Grant Proposal. Available from the first author at Mount Sinai Hospital. NY.

Neumann, M.S. & Sogolow ED. (2000). Replicating effective programs: HIV/AIDS prevention technology transfer. *AIDS Education and Prevention*, 12(Suppl. A), 35-48.

Neumann, M.S., Sogolow, E.D., & Holtgrave, D.R. (2000). Introduction: Supporting the transfer of HIV prevention behavioral research to public health practice. *AIDS Education and Prevention*, 12(Suppl. A), 1-3.

Olds, D. L. (2002). Prenatal and infancy home visiting by nurses: From randomized trials to community replication. *Prevention Science*, 3 (3), 153-172.

Paikoff, R. L., Parfenoff, S.H., Greenwood, G. L., & McCormick, A. (1997). Parenting, parent-child relationships, and sexual possibility situations among urban African American preadolescents: Preliminary findings and implications for HIV prevention. *Journal of Family Psychology*. 11, 11-22.

Paikoff, R. L. (1995). Early heterosexual debut: Situations of sexual possibility during the transition to adolescence. *American Journal of Orthopsychiatry.* 65, 389-401.

Paikoff, R. L. & McKay, M., Bell, C. et al. (1995). *Family-based intervention to prevent HIV risk exposure for urban adolescents.* NIMH-funded grant proposal. Available from the first author at the University of Illinois, Chicago.

Paruk, Z., Peterson, I., Bhana, A., Bell, C., & McKay, M. (2002). A Focused Ethnographic Study to Inform the Adaptation of the NIMH Funded CHAMP Project in South Africa. In Manfredi R (Ed). *XIV International AIDS Conference.* Bologna, Italy: Monduzzi Editore S.P.A.

Pequegnat. W. & Szapocznik, J. (Eds.). (2000). *Working with Families in the Era of HIV/AIDS.* CA: Sage Publications.

Rotheram-Borus, M.J., Rebchook, G.M., Kelly, J.A., Adams, J., & Neumann, M.S. (2000). Bridging research and practice: Community-researcher partnerships for replicating effective interventions. *AIDS Education and Prevention,* 12(Suppl. A), 49-61.

Roussos, S, T. & Fawcett, S. B. (2000). A review of collaborative partnerships as a strategy for improving community health. *Annual Review of Public Health,* 21, 369-402.

Schensul, J.J. (1999). Organizing community research partnerships in the struggle against AIDS. *Health Education & Behavior,* 26, 266-283.

Schoenwald, S.K. & Hoagwood, K. (2001). Effectiveness, transportability, and dissemination of interventions: What Matters When? *Psychiatric Service,* 52, 1190-1197.

Spoth, R. L., Kavanagh, K. A., & Dishion, T. J. (2002). Family-centered preventive intervention science: Toward benefits to larger populations of children, youth, and families. *Prevention Science,* 3 (3), 145-151.

Swisher, J.D. (2000). Sustainability of prevention. *Addictive Behaviors,* 25, 965-973.

Stevenson, H.C., & White, J.J. (1994). AIDS prevention struggles in ethno-cultural neighborhoods: Why research partnerships with community based organizations can't wait. *AIDS Education and Prevention,* 6, 126-139.

Voisin, D., Baptiste, D., Martinez, D., & Henderson, G. (2006). Exporting a US-HIV/AIDS prevention program to a Caribbean-island nation: Lessons from the field. *International Social Work,* 49(1): 75-86.

doi:10.1300/J200v05n03_02

Understanding the African American Research Experience (KAARE): Implications for HIV Prevention

Dara Kerkorian
Dorian E. Traube
Mary M. McKay

SUMMARY. Despite recognition that the African American population is underrepresented in studies of health and mental health treatment and prevention efforts, few investigations have systematically examined barriers to African American research participation. Without their participation, treatment and prevention strategies designed to curtail the spread of HIV in their communities will be bound to achieve less than optimal outcomes. Based on the assumption that successful recruitment

Dara Kerkorian, PhD, and Mary M. McKay, PhD, are affiliated with the Mt. Sinai School of Medicine. Dorian E. Traube, CSW, is affiliated with the Columbia University School of Social Work.

Address correspondence to: Mary M. McKay, PhD, Professor of Social Work in Psychiatry & Community Medicine, Mount Sinai School of Medicine, One Gustave L. Levy Place, New York, NY 10029 (E-mail: mary.mckay@mssm.edu).

The contributions of Carl C. Bell, MD, Sybil Madison-Boyd, PhD, Donna Baptiste, PhD, Doris Coleman, MSW, and CHAMP Collaborative Board members and participants are especially recognized.

Funding from the National Institutes of Mental Health Grant # 5T32MH014623-24 is gratefully acknowledged.

[Haworth co-indexing entry note]: "Understanding the African American Research Experience (KAARE): Implications for HIV Prevention." Kerkorian, Dara, Dorian E. Traube, and Mary M. McKay. Co-published simultaneously in *Social Work in Mental Health* (The Haworth Press, Inc.) Vol. 5, No. 3/4, 2007, pp. 295-312; and: *Community Collaborative Partnerships: The Foundation for HIV Prevention Research Efforts* (ed: Mary M. McKay, and Roberta L. Paikoff) The Haworth Press, Inc., 2007, pp. 295-312. Single or multiple copies of this article are available for a fee from The Haworth Document Delivery Service [1-800-HAWORTH, 9:00 a.m. - 5:00 p.m. (EST). E-mail address: docdelivery@haworthpress.com].

Available online at http://swmh.haworthpress.com
doi:10.1300/J200v05n03_03

of African Americans requires knowledge of (a) their beliefs about research, (b) their perceptions of the research process and researchers, (c) their motivations to participate, and (d) the historical and social factors that may be the source of at least some ambivalence, the current study undertook semi-structured interviews with 157 African American, low-income mothers residing in a large urban community where they and their children were at high risk for HIV. Given the sensitive nature of the research topic, members of the community were trained to conduct the interviews. Qualitative and quantitative analyses of the interview content suggest that despite having been consented, many participants (a) are not aware of their rights under informed consent and (b) lack knowledge of how the research will be used. Despite this and the subtle suspicion of White researchers held by some, many decide to participate for altruistic reasons. The implications for recruitment of participants in general and African Americans in particular into HIV prevention studies are discussed as are the implications for service providers directly or indirectly involved in the development and delivery of these interventions. doi:10.1300/J200v05n03_03 *[Article copies available for a fee from The Haworth Document Delivery Service: 1-800-HAWORTH. E-mail address: <docdelivery@haworthpress.com> Website: <http://www.Haworth Press.com>*

KEYWORDS. Examine barriers to participation, implications of recruitment, implications for service, providers, under representation of African American population, low-income mothers ar high risk

Research aimed at creating and testing preventative interventions in social work or allied professions depends on the recruitment of participants from the communities and populations for which these interventions are intended. Additionally, ethical conduct of research calls for sensitivity to the needs and circumstances of ethnically diverse populations (Gil and Bob, 1999; Fisher, Hoagwood, Boyce, Duster, Grisso et al., 2002). Noting the under-representation of African Americans in psychosocial research and with the ultimate goal of devising strategies to encourage African American enrollment in research projects, the current study aims to identify impediments to recruiting African American research participants and to understand their experiences as participants in research.

To date, few studies have addressed the issue. Of those that have, the majority have considered the under-representation of African Americans in medically-oriented research, particularly clinical trials (e.g., Gorkin, Schron, Handshaw, Shea, McKinney, Branyon et al., 1996; Roberson, 1997; Green, Partridge, Fouad, Kohler, Crayton, and Alexander, 2000). Based on reviews of the literature or extrapolation from publications on cultural competence (Shavers-Hornaday, Lynch, Burmeister, and Torner, 1997; Dennis and Neese, 2000; Alvidrez and Arean, 2002), the feedback of focus groups (Freimuth, Quinn, Thomas, Cole, Zook, and Duncan, 2001), or evaluations of samples of less than 75 participants (Freedman, 1982; Freimuth, Quinn, Thomas, Cole, Zook, and Duncan, 2001), most have suggested that social, political, and historical factors and widely held beliefs and attitudes about research impede African Americans adults from participating in health-oriented projects.

Salient themes in this body of literature have included the impact of knowledge of the Tuskegee Syphilis Study (Brawley, 1998; Shavers, Lynch, and Burmeister, 2000), African American distrust of White researchers and institutions (Corbie-Smith, Thomas, and St. George, 2002), the importance of culture-specific recruitment strategies (Bonner and Miles, 1997; Ashing-Giwa, 1999), and motivations to participate (Sengupta, Strauss, DeVillis, Quinn, DeVillis, and Ware, 1999).

These studies have yielded conflicting and often surprising results. For example, when asked in one study if knowledge of Tuskegee influenced decisions to participate in a clinical trial, interviews with thirteen African American women suggested that it would not (Freedman, 1998). In another study, African Americans were significantly more likely than Whites to say that knowledge of Tuskegee caused them to be less trustful of the researchers, but were not more likely than Whites to cite the event as a deterrent to participation (Shavers, Lynch, and Burmeister, 2000). Others (Bonner and Miles, 1997; Ashing-Giwa, 1999) have concluded that culturally compatible recruitment strategies, while important, do not guarantee increased enrollment among African Americans and urge exploration of additional impediments. In a few existing studies, explanations of African Americans' decisions to participate have included altruism (Sengupta, Strauss, DeVillis et al., 2000; van Stuijvenberg, Suur, de Vos, Tijiang, Steyerberg, Derksen-Lubsen, and Moll, 1998) and volunteerism (Corbie-Smith, Viscoli, Kernan, Brass, Sarrel, and Horwitz, 2003).

While this research provides insights into African Americans' thinking regarding research, the hypothetical or actual context of the clinical trial or medical research typically differs dramatically from the contexts of psychosocial research where participants are not being confronted with the possibility of death or negative health consequences. Unfortunately, a relatively limited number of studies address recruitment or the participation of African Americans in research on health-related behaviors, psychosocial issues, or interventions. Examples include studies of recruitment of African Americans into research on a smoking cessation program (Woods, Harris, Mayo et al., 2002), a HIV-prevention program, and mental health (Thompson, Neighbors, and Munday, 1996; Alvidrez and Area, 2002). Each of these studies raise questions about the generalizability of findings regarding research participation in medical settings to research participation in studies concerned with psycho-social issues or behavior change. Discussions of the recruitment and experiences of African American research participants in the social work literature (Hatchett, Holmes, Duran, and Davis, 2000) are especially rare.

The current study adds to the literature pertaining to African American research participation in several ways. First, it addresses African Americans' thoughts about and knowledge of research and research participation outside the medical context. Second, to increase the reliability and validity of results, it draws upon a socio-economically homogeneous group of 157 African American individuals from a large mid-western city, utilizes a semi-structured interview and trained African American interviewers from the participants' community, and relies upon both quantitative and qualitative analysis. Finally, all members of the sample were parents of children under eighteen years of age and had agreed to participate and to allow their children to participate in this study.

METHOD

The authors of this study employed grounded theory. This approach, rather than beginning with a hypothesis to test, develops concepts based on the data and hypotheses grounded in the data (Charmaz, 1990; Glaser and Strauss, 1967; Strauss & Corbin, 1990). The approach, therefore, highlights the perspective of the client and, in doing so, remains consistent with a full range of social work values and values in the field of psychosocial research (Arnoff and Bailey, 2003). Quantitative analyses supplemented this approach and served as a useful source of contrast and comparison.

Measures

The basic study instrument, the Research Information Questionnaire, consisted of 15 open-ended questions meant to tap previous experience with research, attitudes about research activities, barriers to participation (Stevenson, 1994), and understanding of previous research events in African American communities (e.g., The Tuskegee Syphilis Experiment). The questions typically called for brief explanations of (a) the participants' reasons for participating and (b) their attitudes and perceptions related to the research endeavor. Because of the sensitive nature of the interview questions, all interviews were conducted by trained members of the community to reduce the likelihood that participants would censor their responses.

DATA COLLECTION PROCEDURES

Sample

The sample for the KAARE project consisted of 157 adult caregivers who were selected to participate in the Chicago HIV and Adolescent Mental Health Project (CHAMP), a multiple family group program aimed at increasing family communication to reduce the risk of children contracting HIV. The sample was randomly drawn from schools located adjacent to or on Chicago public housing projects and within 11 blocks of each other. These schools serve elementary school children and are 99% African American. Approximately 70% of families are supported by Public Assistance; 75% are single, female-headed households; 63% of adult caregivers had not worked in the last year. Selection of these schools from which to draw the sample of adult caregivers allowed the authors to draw a relatively homogeneous sample, to help control for factors of community, poverty, and ethnicity.

Informed consent was obtained from all participants following IRB approval of the protocol from the University of Illinois, Chicago. The protocol entailed reading the informed consent aloud with participants and answering questions. In addition, interviewers asked a set of questions to insure that participants understood.

DATA ANALYSIS

The researchers reviewed the completed interviews, identified response patterns distinct to each question, and a developed a preliminary coding scheme that would allow for quantitative analysis of the data and permit detection of general trends that could inform the qualitative review. The inter-rater reliability, based on a two way random effects inter class correlation, revealed an alpha value of .85.

The researchers adopted Campbell's (1978) mixed methods approach to analyze the data based on the belief that it is important to express qualitative perspectives, methods, perceptions, and conclusions while also communicating findings that are at least partially amenable to quantitative representation and, therefore, quantitative analysis.

The coded interviews and the complete qualitative responses to each question were entered into an SPSS database. Qualitative analysis involved isolating the text that corresponded to each question, noting common themes, and interpreting the responses against the backdrop of the scaled response created for the quantitative analysis. This approach enhanced the possibility of distinguishing participants' explicit and implicit responses.

The first step in the quantitative analysis involved calculating the frequencies of responses as coded through the qualitative analysis. Then, correlations and multiple regressions were used to determine the relationship between motivations to participate in research and the tensions between community residents and outside researchers. Because variables measuring the understanding of the research experience were dichotomous, one-way ANOVAs and logistic regressions were employed to determine the relationship between the motivation to participate in research and knowledge of the research process.

RESULTS

Univariate Results

Motivations to participate in research. Nearly one in four participants maintained that they would not agree to be in a research study if they would not get anything out of it. While many did not expound on their negative responses, far more indicated that they expected to learn something as a result of participation or to contribute to the welfare of their children and/or community. None cited money or in-kind reimbursement as a motivation. Interestingly, those saying that they would agree to be in a research study, regardless of what they would receive in return, implied that they were motivated by what they assumed to be intrinsic to the research participation experience: learning something or contributing to the welfare of others. The remainder of those who replied "yes" conditioned their participation on the nature of the study itself. One individual's comments, "just verbal, not physical, no medicine, no needles," summed up the general rationale of these participants.

Tensions between community residents and outside researchers. The overwhelming majority of participants claimed that being interviewed by someone who was not from their neighborhood would not be a problem (83.4%, $n = 132$). Reasons varied. Some said they thought it would be easier to talk to an interviewer from outside the neighborhood. Others' responses were consistent with the statement, "It will be okay; a researcher is just a researcher." The minority of participants, asserting that they would be less comfortable with an interviewer who did not reside in the neighborhood, almost unanimously cited the interviewer's lack of familiarity with the neighborhood as the reason for their uneasiness.

Participants were similarly indifferent to being interviewed by a White researcher. 92.4% ($n = 145$) said they would feel comfortable being interviewed by a White researcher. While some simply said that it wouldn't bother them and implied that the White researcher was the equivalent of the interviewer from outside the neighborhood, many specifically noted that they were "not racist," "not prejudice," or "it does not matter of the color of your skin." Others attributed this comfort with the White interviewer to characteristics that distinguished them as individuals.

> *It wouldn't make a difference because I am biracial.*
> *I was brought up Christian.*

A few implied that the race of the interviewer did not matter because "help come from Black or White," the research was being conducted "for a good cause," or interviewers were just "here to do a job."

Seventy-two percent ($n = 113$) of respondents believed that African American's can be treated fairly by White researchers. Those who did not trust White researchers cited reasons including:

> *We've never been treated fairly.*
> *They (White researchers) are the devil. I can't trust these people.*

> *White people think they are all that and treat black people like slaves.*

Similarly, roughly two-thirds (*n* = 103) of participants did not believe that Whites would use information any differently than Blacks. Their explanations can be captured in three categories: (1) Whites and Blacks are really no different, (2) the subject of the research threatened the White community as well; racism was not the focus of the study, and (3) Whites who are researchers are different. The third of participants who expected that Whites would utilize the data differently suggested that Whites, not sharing the same worldview, would misinterpret, or less often twist, the words of Black participants. A small subset answered that the White researcher's use of the data "depends on" the individual interviewer, his/her professional affiliation, or the purpose of the research.

When asked about their views regarding the possibility of research hurting their community, 72% (*n* = 113) said that research could not hurt their community. Most participants replied that research would not be used to hurt people because their own responses were intended to help people or would not include information that could implicate or harm someone else.

Another group asserted that research would not be harmful because its aim was to help the people and community or because it was confidential. When elaborating on their responses, the nearly one-third of participants who said that they thought research could be hurtful, cited lapses in confidentiality and the nature of information that people gave to researchers as the reason. Overall, in answering this question, participants did not refer to research as an impersonal, objective process. Rather, their responses quite consistently concerned the individual effects of what they said or what researchers divulged, rather than the nature or results of the scientific investigation itself, as the potentially hurtful consequence of research.

Knowledge of the research process. For the purpose of this study, knowledge of the research process refers to the extent to which participants are knowledgeable about the purpose of the study, clear about the expectations associated with participation, and accurate about the risks and benefits associated with the proposed study prior to deciding to involve themselves.

Twenty one percent (*n* = 33) were unaware that a researcher must obtain written consent before a person can participate in a research study:

> *It would depend on the nature of the research as long as it is not negative [they don't need to know they are participating].*

[They don't need to consent] because there is a lot they can be done to help African Americans. Some of them have a lot of problems.

Participants with knowledge of the informed consent process cited the following reasons for its importance:

Too much has happened to us already.
It's illegal not to get their consent.
So Black people will know what White people are saying about them.

When asked if they worried that a researcher was not informing them of all the information they needed to know before they consented to the study, 45.2% ($n = 71$) said they had some level of concern. Those who answered "no" seemed to fall into one of two groups. The first group who said they would not worry about the researcher disclosing important information about the research suggested that they did not worry because they trusted the researcher. These participants often conveyed a willingness to "suspend" judgment or belief in the researchers' good intentions:

I wouldn't worry 'cause I'm hoping they're telling the truth.

The second group, conveying more suspicion and a greater sense of control, said they would not worry because their participation would be contingent upon having their own set of questions satisfactorily answered by the researchers.

The participants who said "yes," they would worry about the researchers' divulgence of all necessary information usually explained that they did not trust people as a general rule. Fewer suggested that, if one was not suspicious of the research and did not ask questions, he/she was acting irresponsibly. Just five singled out researchers as people not to be trusted.

Participants' responses to the question about their concerns about their information being kept private closely resembled their explanations of why they would or would not worry about being told everything they needed to know about the research. 42.7% ($n = 67$) said that they did worry that all information was not being kept private. However, more ($n = 78$) simply chose to take their chances and believe what they were told:

[I don't worry] because it's supposed to be confidential.

Others were not concerned about privacy because they controlled their responses as in:

I wouldn't tell nothing that I would be scared for somebody else to see.

The majority of those who stated that they did have concerns about privacy, like those who worried about being told everything they needed to know, implied that they generally viewed others with skepticism. Fewer of them distinguished the characteristics of the research environment with its easily accessible information that might get lost or viewed by unauthorized eyes as the basis of their concerns or the sensitivity of the information they provided. Most of these individuals regarded "leaks" of information as inevitable. For some, the sensitivity of the subject matter affected their concerns.

When asked what they thought researchers would do with the information they were given, participants often referred to specific aspects of the research endeavor–"analyze it," "compare it," "study it," "combine it with other information." The majority "[did] not know," were not sure, or "hoped" that researchers would use all of the data. In fact, more participants skeptically predicted that researchers would do nothing with the information than draw upon it to improve the community or people in general.

To tap into the participants' knowledge of the history of the African American experience within the context of research, questions were included about their knowledge of the Tuskegee Project. Thirty-five participants had heard of Tuskegee. Of these, ten correctly noted that the Tuskegee experiment involved Black men and syphilis, fourteen remarked only on the study's focus on syphilis, four mentioned only that the experiment involved Black men, and the remainder associated it with sexually transmitted diseases, did not know, or did not respond at all. Four of the 35 respondents had learned about Tuskegee from the television movie, "Miss Evers Boys." Just three of the 35 provided explanations of the Tuskegee Experiment that accurately captured what occurred. While a few mentioned that the cure for syphilis or the "disease" had been withheld, just one individual noted that the subjects in the study were not aware of their role in the experiment. Refer to Table 1 for a summary of descriptive statistics.

Bivariate Results

Motivations to participate in research. At the bivariate level, Pearsons correlations revealed that there was a positive relationship between the belief that information from research could be used to help people and that African Americans can be treated fairly by Whites ($r = .17$, $p < .05$).

Tensions between community residents and outside researchers. A negative relationship existed between the belief that White researchers will use information differently and feelings about researchers who are not from the neighborhood ($r = -.15$, $p < .05$). This relationship indicates that the more comfortable individuals were with the researcher not being from their neighborhood, the less likely they were to believe that a White researcher would use information differently than a black researcher. Conversely, those who were not comfortable with the "outside" researcher tended to believe that Whites would utilize the information differently than African Americans.

Knowledge of the research process. Numerous relationships existed between the variables measuring knowledge of the research process. Pearson's correlations revealed a relationship between the belief that White researchers will use information differently than black researchers and the fear that researchers do not tell participants all pertinent information about the study ($r = .16$, $p < .05$). The fear that researchers do share pertinent information with participants was also associated with the worry that information from the study is not kept confidential ($r = .21$, $p < .01$). Results from an analysis of variance showed that people who had heard of Tuskegee also believed that research could be hurtful to them or their neighborhood ($F = 5.95$, $p < .05$) and that White researchers would use the information differently than African American researchers ($F = 3.72$, $p < .05$), but that they would still be willing to participate in a research study even if they would not benefit directly ($F = 6.40$, $p < .01$). Table 2 describes these bivariate relationships.

Multivariate Results

Motivations to participate in research. Logistic regression revealed that when controlling for the fear that White researchers will do something different with research data than black researchers and the fear that the research could harm their neighborhood, people who had heard of Tuskegee were significantly more likely to participate in research even if they did not personally gain from it ($Exp(B) = 2.165$, $p < .05$).

TABLE 1. Univariate Analysis

Variable	Percentage	n	n missing
Fear researcher is not sharing all information about the study	45.2	71	
Would participate even if there was no personal benefit	67.5	106	
Worry that information is not private	42.7	67	2
Comfortable speaking to a researcher	88.6	139	2
Research can hurt my neighborhood	24.8	39	2
Comfortable with a researcher not from the neighborhood	83.4	132	
Research information can be used to help people	86.0	135	
Comfortable with White researchers	92.4	145	
White researchers will use information differently than black researchers	10.8	17	
Had heard of Tuskegee	22.3	35	2
Research should be done with African Americans without their knowledge	5.7	9	4
African Americans can be treated fairly by White researchers	72.0	113	6
People can be involved in a study without written consent	21.0	33	11

TABLE 2. Bivariate Analysis

Motivation to participate in research variable	r
Information could be used to help people(x)	.17*
African Americans can be treated fairly by Whites	
Tensions between community residents and outside researchers	**r**
Feelings if researcher is not from the community(x)	−.15*
Whites will use information different than black researchers	
Knowledge of the research process	**r**
Fear that information is not private(x)	.21**
Worry that researcher is not sharing all information	
Worry that researcher is not sharing all information(x)	.16*
Whites will use information different than black researchers	

*p < .05, ** p < .01

Tensions between community residents and outside researchers. Multiple regression analysis indicated that when controlling for comfort of being asked questions by a researcher, people who worried the information they provided would not be kept private also worried that the researcher was telling them all the information they needed to know about the study (F = 5.60, p < .01). Refer to Table 3 for a complete description of the multivariate analysis.

DISCUSSION

Motivation and Trust

The majority (67.5%) of respondents' comments suggested that they would agree to participate in research studies if, in doing so, they would learn something or would help their children or the African American community. Even higher percentages indicated they would have no problem answering questions posed by an interviewer from outside the neighborhood (83.4%) or who were White (92%). Both the willingness to participate without assurance of tangible gain and the level of comfort with non-community interviewers were surprising given that substantial, albeit smaller, numbers conveyed some level of distrust. For example, 12.3% (n = 17) did not think African Americans could be treated fairly by Whites, 10% (n = 14) believed that Whites would use the data differently, 43% (n = 59) expressed at least some concerns about the researchers' divulgence of all important information about the research, and 41.3% (n = 57) worried about researchers maintaining confidentiality.

TABLE 3. Multivariate Analysis

Ordinary Least Squares Regression "Privacy of information provided"			
Variable	B	SE B	β
Comfortable speaking to a researcher	−.13	.07	−.15
Fear researcher is not sharing all information about the study	.09	.03	.21**
R^2=.07, Adj. R^2 = .05, df = 154, F = 5.30, p <.01			

Logistic Regression "Heard of Tuskegee"			
Variable	B	SE B	Wald χ^2	Odds Ratio
Whites will use information differently than black researchers	.21	.14	2.47	1.24
Research can hurt the community	.21	.13	2.56	1.23
Would participate in research even if no personal gains	.77	.40	3.72	2.17*

*p < .05, **p < .01

While the univariate analyses generally portray African Americans as trusting of researchers and Whites, bivariate analyses imply that, for at least a subset of the African American population, racial tensions or distrust are associated with negative views of research. African Americans who believed that African Americans could not be treated fairly by Whites were more likely to support the view that research information could be used to hurt people. Likewise, those believing that Whites researchers would use information differently were more inclined to worry that all pertinent information about the research was not being shared and less inclined to be comfortable with a researcher from outside the community.

In explaining why research could not be used to harm their communities, most participants suggested that, by giving well-intended answers or by refraining from divulging potentially hurtful information, they were preventing this from happening. Implicitly, such comments indicate that many participants maintained a sense of what could be said without risking someone else's welfare and, at the same time, suggest that, in spite of professing their trust in researchers and their altruistic motivations, many may be guarded and/or unconsciously self-censor.

Knowledge of Research

Forty-five percent of the current sample worried that a researcher might not share important information about the research, nearly 43% worried about privacy, and 21% thought that one could be involved in a study without his/her permission. These results highlight the extent to which current approaches to informed consent may be inadequate or inappropriate. Misinformed or uninformed, prospective participants may elect not to enroll, those enrolled may censor what they say, and many may engage in research without a clear understanding of its potential risks, their rights as participants, and its purpose.

Participants' vague depictions of what researchers actually do with the information (e.g., "study it") and the more common response of "I don't know" also speak to how little is understood about the research endeavor.

Tuskegee

Those who had heard of Tuskegee tended to be more cognizant of the potential of research to hurt individuals or communities and to be more likely to believe that Whites could use information differently. However, even with this awareness of the potentially harmful effects of research and the sense that Whites will use data differently than African Americans, those who knew of Tuskegee appeared more willing to participate in research without any direct benefit.

IMPLICATIONS

The study's findings draw attention to (a) the visceral nature of distrust that may exist between the African American community and outside White investigators and (b) the lack of accurate knowledge regarding research in general and informed consent in particular. These results have clear implications for social work researchers and clinicians.

First, the results underscore the need to remain attuned to racial tensions and distrust that, unacknowledged, may lead to sub-optimal treatment and prevention interventions. Without such sensitivity, researchers increase the likelihood that some groups of African Americans, possibly those most disenfranchised and in need of services, will remain un-represented and/or reluctantly engage in clinical research projects. Although participants in the current study were more likely to deny a preference for African American researchers or interviewers, their qualified explanations suggest otherwise. Indeed, speaking with a community-based interviewer who represented a White researcher, may not have been, by itself, enough to keep participants from censoring their comments.

Second, both researchers and clinicians must take steps to assure that African Americans, presented with opportunities to join clinical research projects, truly understand their rights and the potential risks and rewards of participating. Far too many in the current study lacked accurate information about basic aspects of informed consent, confidentiality, and other aspects of typical research protocols. Clarifying the terms of recruitment and the goals and nature of the research process, while certainly an ethical responsibility, may also assuage misgivings about divulging sensitive information and empower participants in ways that make them more inclined to sustain enrollment in a project and become involved in future research.

Ultimately, by empowering those they aim to assist, clearly specifying their intentions and how and why they aim to achieve them, and acknowledging the distinct perspectives of potential research participants, social work researchers and clinicians will mitigate distrust, enrich the quality of research they produce, and enhance the fidelity of interventions.

In the words of one participant:

[Research data from African Americans] may give other researchers a better idea on how to do things because everybody mind is not the same.

In focusing on a homogeneous stratum of the African American population, the current study offers insights regarding one group's knowledge and perceptions of psychosocial research participation and permits some comparison with similar surveys of more heterogeneous or older African American samples. However, to validate the study's conclusions about the perceptions and knowledge of one group of African Americans, future research on the topic should include more diverse groups of African Americans and other ethnic-minorities. Additionally, the study's findings that participants lacked basic information about research protocol and outcomes highlight the need to explore the knowledge of research participants from other ethnic-minority groups as well as whites.

REFERENCES

Advani, A.S., Atkeson, B., Brown, C.L., Peterson, B.L., Fish, L., Johnson, J.L., Gockerman, J.P., & Gautier, M. (2003). Barriers to participation of African American patients with cancer in clinical trials: A pilot study. *Cancer*, 97 (6),1499-1506.

Alvidrez, J., & Area, P.A. (2002). Psychosocial treatment research with ethnic minority populations: Ethical considerations in conducting clinical trials *Ethics and Behavior*, 12 (1), 103-116.

Ashing-Giwa, K. (1999). The recruitment of breast cancer survivors into cancer control studies: A focus on African American women. *Journal of National Medical Association*, 91 (5), 255-260.

Bonner, G.J., & Miles, T.P. (1997). Participation of African Americans in clinical research. *Neuroepidemiology*, 16 (6), 281-284.

Brawley, O.W. (1998). The study of untreated syphilis in the Negro male. *Journal of Radiation Oncology, Biology, Physics.* 40(1), 5-8.

Campbell, D. T. (1978). Qualitative knowing in action research. In M. Brenner, P. Marsh, and M. Brenner (Eds.), *The Social Contexts of Method* (pp. 184-209). London: Croom Helm.

Charmaz, K. (1990). "Discovering" chronic illnesses: Using grounded theory. *Social Science in Medicine*, 30, 1161-1172.

Corbie-Smith, G., Thomas, S.B., & St. George, D.M. (2002). Distrust, race, and research. *Archives of Internal Medicine*, 162, 2458-2463.

Corbie-Smith, G., Viscoli, C.M., Kernan, W.N., Brass, L.M., Sarrel, P., & Horwitz, R.I. (2003). Influence of race, clinical, and other socio-demographic features on trial participation. *Journal of Clinical Epidemiology*, 56 (4), 304-309.

Dennis, B.P., & Neese, J.B. (2000). Recruitment and retention of African American elders in community-based research: Lessons learned. *Archives of Psychiatric Nursing*, 14 (1), 3-11.

Fisher, C.B., Hoagwood, K., Boyce, C., Duster, T., Frank, D.A., Griss-Levine, R.J., Macklin, R., Spencer, M.B., Takanishi, R., & Trimble, J.E. (2002). Research ethics for mental health science involving minority children and youths. *American Psychologist*, 57 (12), 1024-1040.

Fowler, B.A. (2002). An outsider's experiences in conducting field research in an African American community. *Journal of Black Nurses Association*, 13(1), 31-37.

Freedman, T.G. (1998). Why don't they come to Pike Street and ask us? Black American women's health concerns. *Social Science and Medicine*, 47 (7), 941 947.

Freimuth, V.S., Quinn, S.C., Thomas, S.B., Cole, G., Zook, E., & Duncan, T. (2001). African Americans' views on research and the Tuskegee Syphilis Study. *Social Science and Medicine*, 52, 797-808.

Glaser, B & Strauss, A.L. (1967). *The discovery of grounded theory*. New York: Aldine De Gruyter.

Gorkin, L., Schron, E.B., Handshaw, K., Shea, S., Kinney, M.R., Branyon, M., Campion, J., Bigger, J.T., Sylvia, S.C., Duggan, J., Stylianou, M., Lancaster, S., Ahern, D.K., & Follick, M.J. (1996). Clinical trial enrollers vs. nonenrollers: The Cardiac Arrhythmia Suppression Trial (CAST) Recruitment and Enrollment Assessment in Clinical Trials (REACT) project. *Controlled Clinical Trials*, 17 (1), 46-59.

Green, B.L., Partridge, E.E., Fouad, M.N., Kohler, C., Crayton, E.F., & Alexander, L. (2000). African American attitudes regarding cancer clinical trials and research studies: Results from focus group methodology. *Ethnicity and Disease*, 10 (1), 76-86.

Hatchett, B.F., Holmes, K., Duran, D.A., & Davis, C. (2000). African Americans and research participation: The recruitment process. *Journal of Black Studies*, 30 (5), 664-675.

Roberson, N.L. (1994). Clinical trial participation: Viewpoints from racial/ethnic groups. *Cancer*, 74 (9), 2687-2791.

Sengupta, S., Strauss, R.P., DeVellis, R., Quinn, S.C., DeVellis, B., & Ware, W.B. (2000). Factors affecting African American participation in AIDS research. *Journal of Acquired Immune Deficiency Syndromes*, 24 (3), 275-284.

Shavers, V.L., Lynch, C.F., Burmeister, L.F. (2000). Knowledge of the Tuskegee study and its impact on the willingness to participate in medical research studies. *Journal of National Medical Association*, 92(12), 563-572.

Shavers-Hornaday, V.L., Lynch, C.F., Burmeister, L.F., & Torner, J.C. (1997). Why are African Americans under-represented in medical research studies? Impediments to participation. *Ethnic Health*, 2(1-2), 31-45.

Strauss, A., & Corbin, J. (1990). *Basics of qualitative research*. Newbury Park, CA: Sage Publications.

Stevenson, H.C., & White, J.J. (1994). Aids prevention struggles in ethnocultural neighborhoods: Why research partnerships with community based organizations can't wait. *AIDS Education and Prevention*, 6(2), 126-139.

Thompson, E.E., Neighbors, H.W., Munday, C., & Jackson, J.S. (1996). Recruitment and retention of African American patients in clinical research: An exploration of response rates in an urban psychiatric hospital. *Journal of Consulting and Clinical Psychology,* 6 (5), 861-867.

van Stuijvenberg, M., Suur, M.H., de Vos, S., Tjiang, G.C., Steyerberg, E.W., Derksen-Lubsen, G., & Moll, H.A. (1998). Informed consent, parental awareness, and reasons for participating in a randomized controlled study. *Archives of Disease in Childhood,* 79 (2), 120-125.

Woods, M.N., Harris, K.J., Mayo, M.S., Catley, D., Scheibmeir, M., & Ahluwalia, J.S. (2002). Participation of African Americans in a smoking cessation trial: A quantitative and qualitative study. *Journal of the National Medical Association,* 94 (7), 609-618.

doi:10.1300/J200v05n03_03

Voices from the Community: Key Ingredients for Community Collaboration

Lydia M. Franco
Mary McKay
Ana Miranda
Nealdow Chambers
Angela Paulino
Rita Lawrence

SUMMARY. When community members are allowed to participate in the planning and implementation process of a program, they are empow-

---

Lydia M. Franco, MSSW, and Mary McKay, PhD, LCSW, are affiliated with the Mount Sinai School of Medicine. Ana Miranda, Nealdow Chambers, Angela Paulino, BS, and Rita Lawrence, BSN, are affiliated with the CHAMP-New York Collaborative Board.

Address correspondence to: Lydia Franco, MSSW, Child and Adolescent Outpatient Psychiatry, Mount Sinai Medical Center, One Gustave L. Levy Place, Box 1228, New York, NY 10029 (E-mail: lydia.franco@mountsinai.org).

CHAMP-NY is the result of a collaborative effort involving the Mount Sinai School of Medicine, Morris Heights Health Center, elementary and junior high schools, parents, and social service agencies in the Bronx, New York community.

CHAMP-NY is supported by the National Institute of Mental Health Research on AIDS (RO1 MH63622).

[Haworth co-indexing entry note]: "Voices from the Community: Key Ingredients for Community Collaboration." Franco, Lydia M. et al. Co-published simultaneously in *Social Work in Mental Health* (The Haworth Press, Inc.) Vol. 5, No. 3/4, 2007, pp. 313-331; and: *Community Collaborative Partnerships: The Foundation for HIV Prevention Research Efforts* (ed: Mary M. McKay, and Roberta L. Paikoff) The Haworth Press, Inc., 2007, pp. 313-331. Single or multiple copies of this article are available for a fee from The Haworth Document Delivery Service [1-800-HAWORTH, 9:00 a.m. - 5:00 p.m. (EST). E-mail address: docdelivery@haworthpress.com].

313

ering themselves and their community. The CHAMP Family Program uses a collaborative programming approach with a focus on building the capacities of community members to deliver a family-based HIV prevention program. The CHAMP Program has a Collaborative Board that oversees all aspects of the research project. Using an empowerment framework, this article explores Community Board members' perspectives on their experience in working on CHAMP. Recommendations to researchers in the form of ten key ingredients for community collaboration are presented. The key points primarily focus on building trust with the community, recognizing community strengths, developing skills, building intragroup relations, and involving the community as partners from the beginning to the end. *doi:10.1300/J200v05n03_04* *[Article copies available for a fee from The Haworth Document Delivery Service: 1-800-HAWORTH. E-mail address: <docdelivery@haworthpress.com> Website: <http://www.HaworthPress.com>*

KEYWORDS. Community collaboration, community empowerment, family-based HIV prevention program, recognizing and developing community strengths, community as partners

The term "community" is often used in public health, social work, and other related disciplines, but what does it really mean? In previous literature, community was defined "as a group of people with diverse characteristics who are linked by social ties, share common perspectives, and engage in joint action in geographical locations" (MacQueen et al., 2001). We often define communities through broad descriptive categories such as race (e.g., African American community), class (e.g., the low-income community), sexual orientation (e.g., gay community), neighborhood (e.g., the Bronx community), profession (e.g., medical community), and many more. It is within these "communities" that we, as researchers, programmers, and administrators, identify social issues and attempt to address them.

A growing emphasis has been placed on community collaboration within the research and programmatic fields, especially when addressing major public health issues. However, what is often referred to as "community" are representatives of community-based agencies situated within a geographic area or who address a specific issue (Harper & Salina, 2000; Schmitz, 1999; Walsh, 2002; Tiamiyu & Jenks, 2001).

Although community-based agencies play an important and vital role within the community, many times you do not find collaboration with community members themselves–the very same people you are trying to help. Community member participation may be relegated to advisory positions and only included after the program has been designed. Ideally, a diverse mix of people from the community and those representing related community agencies should be present from the conception of the program. In addition to researchers, each group can bring to the table a number of valuable perspectives and resources.

When community members are allowed to participate fully in the program planning and implementation process, they are not only empowering themselves, but also the community in which they live. Members are then able to work together and create change through this process. In community psychology research, empowerment at the community level is "collective action to improve the quality of life in a community and to the connections among community organizations (Perkins & Zimmerman, 1995). It is also described as "the process of gaining influence over conditions that matter to people who share neighborhoods, workplaces, experiences, or concerns" (Fawcett, Paine-Andrews, Francisco, & Schultz, 1995). By not incorporating those who are most affected by the problem, researchers may be disempowering the community (Labonte, 1994)–and creating ineffective interventions. Through participation and collective action, individuals are also empowered through increased access to social power, relationships among individual members, active participation, and subsequent reflection on their involvements in the group (Speer & Hughey, 1995).

Himmelman (2001) distinguishes collaborative empowerment coalitions from betterment coalitions as the first includes grassroots leadership development and an increase in the ownership and power of those who are affected by the coalition's activities. He further explains that people and communities in collaborative empowerment coalitions are not just targets of institutional intervention, but are those who control the purpose and process. Betterment coalitions usually begin outside of the community through university researchers or other larger institutions. However, most collaborations occur in-between these two models of community coalitions (Fawcett et al., 1995). Similarly, disease prevention efforts generally begin outside of the community with a top-down programming approach where issues are defined by health researchers and they later seek to involve community groups (Laverack & Labonte, 2000). However, there are existing planning frameworks that can help prevention and health-oriented researchers who work in this top-down approach to incorporate community empowerment goals (Laverack & Labonte, 2000).

CHAMP: A UNIQUE COLLABORATIVE PROGRAM

With funding from the National Institute of Mental Health, the CHAMP (Collaborative HIV-Prevention and Adolescent Mental Health Project) Family Program was constructed by a team of university-based researchers and community parents (McCormick et al., 2000; Madison, McKay, Paikoff, & Bell, 2000). The main focus of CHAMP is to build the capacities of community members to deliver a family-based HIV prevention program targeting pre-adolescent youth and their families living in inner-city United States communities (Chicago and New York) and within countries hardest hit by the HIV/AIDS epidemic (South Africa and Trinidad). Through a series of multiple family group education workshops, CHAMP involves youth (9 to 11 years of age) prior to the onset of sexual activity, but in close proximity to the beginning of early adolescence. Furthermore, the program includes a family-based approach to support families, enhance family protective processes, and increase parenting skills as urban families raise children in inner-city environments where risks and psychosocial stressors are often elevated.

CHAMP uses a collaborative programming approach to address difficulties in prior HIV prevention research efforts within urban communities, such as low rates of participation, community apprehension about the appropriateness of the HIV prevention programs for children, and mistrust of researchers and program staff (Madison et al., 2000; McKay et al., 2007). Previous efforts to transport empirically supported prevention programs to a larger number of urban communities have encountered numerous obstacles (i.e., insufficient school and community resources, poor community participation, and suspicions of outside researchers) (Dalton, 1989; Galbraith et al., 1996; Thomas & Quinn, 1991). Furthermore, from negative experiences with projects such as the Tuskegee Syphilis Study, people of color often have misgivings about participating in health promotion and prevention projects. Therefore, it is clear that community-based HIV prevention programs targeting urban communities are likely to fail if they do not use collaborative interventions (Aponte, Zarski, Bixenstene, & Cibik, 1991; Boyd-Franklin, 1993; Fullilove & Fullilove, 1993; Secrest, Lassiter, Armistead, Wychoff, Johnson, Williams, & Kotchick, 2004; Fullilove, Green, &

Fullilove, 2000; Schensul, 1999) or neglect to design and implement programs which do not appreciate stressors, scarce contextual resources, or community core values (Boyd-Franklin, 1993; McLoyd, 1990; Sanstand, Stall, Goldstein, Everett, & Brousseau, 1999).

In each of its sites, the CHAMP Program has a Collaborative Board comprised of urban parents, school staff, representatives from community-based agencies, and university-based researchers. The Board oversees all aspects of the research project, including planning, imple- mentation, and evaluation. In addition to CHAMP, the Board also oversees other related research projects that focus on family-based prevention and intervention services for school age urban youth and their families. Through participation on the Board and various sub-committees, community members have real decision-making power and direction of the research project is shared between researchers and community members (Madison et al., 2000; McKay et al., 2007). As the members master the skills necessary to develop, implement, and evaluate programs, it is hoped that they will be able to sustain the program after federal funding has ended. Moreover, the community will have full ownership of CHAMP as it transfers from a university research project to a community program housed within a community agency.

WHAT DO COMMUNITY MEMBERS SAY?

Interestingly, research writing is similar to the top-down health promotion approach that was discussed above. We discuss theories and what other academics have said about a topic, but we often do not have the opportunity to hear what the participants have to say, in their own words. The nature of collaboration is that it is often long and challenging work. Although the CHAMP Family Program has had a number of achievements in its ten years of existence, it has also faced many challenges. The purpose of this paper is to give voice to the community members who are vital to the community collaborative model and lead the program. We will discuss their individual experiences with the program, how effective it has been, and what advice they would provide to other researchers who may be forging into the community collaborative world.

METHODS

Using an empowerment framework, this article will explore Community Board members' perspectives on their experience in working on the CHAMP-New York Family Program. There will be three main areas for exploration: (1) how community members became involved in the program, (2) what their experience was like, and (3) what advice would they give to other researchers who want to develop programs in the community.

Data Collection Procedures

The procedures for collecting the data were similar to how the community manages all its projects. The author presented the concept of the article to the entire Collaborative Board at one of its bi-weekly meetings. A request was made to the whole group to create a sub-committee of about six members who would volunteer to participate in developing this article. The group was coordinated by the first author who was a social work intern completing a field placement as part of the CHAMP Family Program. These members agreed to meet over a series of weeks. The first group meeting focused on developing a set of key points for all researchers to know. A second group meeting was scheduled to document each member's personal experiences as Board members.

Each meeting was semi-structured and was guided by a set of open-ended questions that focused on the members' experiences (i.e., How did you become involved in the program? What do you feel you have contributed to the program? How effective has this type of program been in preventing HIV?). The set of questions were asked of one participant at a time but the whole group had the opportunity to comment.

Process notes taken by the first author of this article were used as the basis of its content. Following each meeting, the notes were analyzed for themes and condensed into a succinct list of key points. The individual case profiles of the members were also analyzed and transcribed into a case study format. Once both of these tasks were completed, the author presented the list of key points to all the group members and the appropriate case study profile to each individual for verification of accuracy. After development of the article, it was presented to the entire Collaborative Board for review and approval. During this review, it was determined that not all members' perspectives were included. The first and third author then conducted separate individual interviews with four more members. The article was then presented again to the Collaborative Board for a final review and approval.

Participants

There are 34 Collaborative Board members in the CHAMP-New York Program of which 28 are members from the local community. The community members are primarily African American and Latino. The majority of the community members are female with only two male members. They live within a low-income, inner-city community with high rates of poverty and overlapping psychosocial stressors, including community violence, substance abuse, and HIV infection. The participant group for this article consisted of ten members–two male and eight female; four Latinos and six African Americans. All but two group members are parents.

RECOMMENDATIONS FOR PROGRAMMERS AND RESEARCHERS

The CHAMP Board sub-committee identified 10 key ingredients for successful community collaboration (see Figure 1). The basis for these points arose through the members' reflection of their experiences with CHAMP from the first time they were approached. Most of these factors are interrelated, but they were identified separately to emphasize their importance according to the members.

1. *Don't enter our community without doing your homework.* Learn about our culture and how the community works before you approach us. For example, be aware that the Bronx has high rates of HIV.
2. *You have to earn our trust.* The community has been used many times before by other researchers or program developers. Community members may also be wary of people with degrees and titles (e.g., PhD., Social Worker, etc.) based on previous negative experiences. Generally, you need to be honest about the program you are trying to implement. Don't plan on bringing in a program and just leave after your money is gone. Plan ahead and work with us to leave good programs within the community. Also, take the time to get to know us. Show you are concerned for us and listen to us–don't do all the talking. Lastly, make sure

to use a common language that we can all understand or explain the terms you use.

3. *Put in your time in the community.* Spend time in the community. Do not just come for meetings and run right out. You need to spend time here to get to know us and show that you are not afraid of being here.

4. *Have full participation of community members within the program.* Community members can and should be involved in all planning and decision-making related to the program. Community members can serve on committees and Boards. A second piece to having full participation is to support and encourage community members to work together. Although we live in the same community, we come from different backgrounds and experiences. We need to be able to understand each other and come to the table to work on these problems together. Furthermore, you must support these members with ongoing training, such as leadership, budgeting, understanding research, conflict resolution, team-building, etc.

5. *Recognize our strengths.* Do not come in assuming that community members do not have a lot to offer. Do not assume that all community members are uneducated. Every community is filled with a diverse array of people with different backgrounds and experiences. With these strengths, community members can enrich your program and expose you to new ideas.

6. *Have the community involved from the beginning.* Approach the community with an open-mind and willingness to incorporate new ideas into your plan. Don't just present your ideas, but ask the community to be collaborators in the planning of the program.

7. *Be compassionate and understanding when working with community members.* Really listen to the community members and do not act shocked when negative things happen in the neighborhood.

8. *Be on time.* Our time is just as valuable as yours. Don't assume that we have nothing to do.

9. *We want your help for our children and families, but WE MUST BE INVOLVED!* Many researchers and program developers don't take the time to teach us how to do this work. We are not here to just sign consent forms. We can learn and pass the information on to our friends. Also, share your findings with us so that the community can benefit from this information too.

10. *When working with other agencies, make sure those agencies are truly collaborative.* We have to transfer our program into the community to keep it alive after our funding ends. We have been working with a local community center for many years. They were even on our Board, but now that we are in this transfer process, we are realizing that the agency is having a lot of problems incorporating our collaborative model. [The members often feel marginalized and feel that they have lost some decision-making power over the program.] Some agency employees often refer to us as "those people" and they assume that we are dumb. We learned that we have to work for what we want or accept what's given to us. We decided not to become our own organization. Now, we have to figure out a way to work with this agency but we are not sure what will happen to CHAMP.

DISCUSSION

Each of the key ingredients for collaboration reflects the members' own experiences on CHAMP. Many of them focus on building a relationship with the researchers and describe a process of mutual understanding and acceptance. Many of the members' initial apprehension in working with the researchers can be reflected through their personal comments. Ms. A. illustrates her initial reaction to being approached by the principal investigator:

FIGURE 1. Ten Key Ingredients for Community Collaboration Developed by the CHAMP-NY Collaborative Board

Key Ingredients for Community Collaboration
(1.) Don't enter our community without doing your homework.
(2.) You have to earn our trust.
(3.) Put in your time in the community.
(4.) Have full participation of community members within the program.
(5.) Recognize our strengths.
(6.) Have the community involved from the beginning.
(7.) Be compassionate and understanding when working with community members.
(8.) Be on time.
(9.) We want your help for our children and families, but WE MUST BE INVOLVED!
(10.) When working with other agencies, make sure those agencies are truly collaborative.

> *Ms. A. has been with CHAMP for six years. She is African American, married, and a mother of six children. She was a school aide when she first heard of CHAMP. She was introduced to the researcher by a counselor at her school. She initially didn't know what the researcher's motives were and did not agree to participate when first approached by her. She didn't trust her. She also did not want her son to talk to her. She continued to say no even through the phone calls and the offer of a stipend but the researcher was very persistent. She decided to let her son be interviewed but only after she coached him. She was concerned that they "would pick my child's brain." They were both nervous about this first meeting which took place during her lunch break. After the interview and speaking with the researcher, she saw how they could use the information they were collecting and how it could benefit the community. She stayed with "Parents on the Move" which later became CHAMP-NY. Ms. A. has had a good experience as a member of the CHAMP Board and she learned a lot about HIV and helping the community.*

Ms. A. showed great concern about what the researcher would actually do to her child and what the repercussions may be on her family. This initial mistrust was assuaged as both groups began to get to know each other. Similarly, Ms. B. explains her own apprehensions:

> *Ms. B. has been with CHAMP for 3 years. She is African American, married, and a mother of three children. She has lived within the community for 23 years. She was recruited into CHAMP by two other Board members. When she came to CHAMP, she learned about the AIDS epidemic and how it was affecting her community. She could also see that there were a lot of young girls having children and not protecting themselves. Initially, she didn't trust the researchers because of a previous negative experience with university researchers trying to implement another program. They had never asked for their permission to use them as part of a thesis project and it left her wondering, "What is the purpose of this work?" After meeting the researchers, she felt that some were ignorant towards their issues but also saw that some were very fair-minded. She decided to stay on and began working with the families. She saw the impact of the program and how they were helping children—and changing lives. It took her a little while to get accustomed to the Board and how it works but did see the ne-*

cessity for it. She feels that the Board works more like a family now.

From the above descriptions, one can see that prior negative experiences with researchers can inhibit participation by community members. Some previous literature on recruitment attributes this apprehension to the legacy of major unethical research projects, such as the Tuskegee Syphilis Study (Dalton, 1989; Madison et al., 2000; Stevenson, Davis, Weber, Weiman, & Abdul-Kabir, 1995; Thomas & Quinn, 1991) and ideological models of blame and deficit such as those in The Moynihan Report and *The Bell Curve* (Hatchett, Holmes, Duran, and Davis, 2000). Interestingly, Hatchett and colleagues (2000) have found that African Americans are not necessarily involved in research because of these historical impacts, but because they have not been asked for their involvement. This can be seen through the experiences of other Board members who may have been apprehensive about the program, but wanted to help address the high rates of HIV in the community.

Ms. M. has been with CHAMP for three years. She is an African American, married, mother and has lived within the community for 20 years. She became involved with CHAMP through a neighbor. A year before, she had learned about the program, but she felt that she still needed more information. As time went on, she spoke with a couple of the Board members who worked at her school. She then attended a Board meeting where she sat in and observed. At this meeting, they were discussing the expansion of the program into South Africa and Ms. M. was concerned by knowing how much AIDS had spread worldwide. She also was concerned with how many people were affected by AIDS within their local community. As a Board member, she worked to recruit families into the program. She has stayed with the program because of the importance of educating the community about HIV/AIDS.

For Latino members of CHAMP, their initial encounter with the Board and the researchers were very important. Although some of them had previous experiences with other community programs, the manner in which they were approached and welcomed is what helped to keep them involved. Mr. P., a Latino, married father who has lived in the community for nine years, had a positive first impression of the researchers because they welcomed and encouraged him to participate.

For Ms. J., a young Latina woman who has been with CHAMP for four years, was unsure about participating in the program until a university intern helped her to understand the process. The importance of the encounter and relationship in recruiting Latino participants in research had been a focus of other research (Albert, 1996; Marin & Marin, 1991; Miranda, Azocar, Organista, Munoz, & Lieberman, 1996; Skaff, Chesla, Mycue, & Fisher, 2002). When working with Latino participants, researchers need to keep in mind cultural values that govern interactions and relationships so that they do not inadvertently alienate them.

Nevertheless, other members' initial reason for participating was the monetary incentive. Although this initial reason may have brought them into the group, they stayed because of the collaborative nature and importance of the work for the community.

Ms. K. has been with CHAMP for six years. She is African American and a single mother of three children. She has lived in the community for 21 years. She became involved after her son brought home a letter describing the program. She describes that the $20 stipend was the real incentive for coming to the meeting. After she got there, she liked the program and the interactions with other families. As a nurse, Ms. K. was used to working with researchers, doctors, and other medical professionals. From her experience, she felt that all researchers need to be taught how to approach the community or else they can do more damage than good. Oftentimes, many researchers come into a community, get what they want, and leave which creates mistrust within the community. She feels more empowered as a Board member and enjoys doing something good for the community.

Further exploration of challenges in minority recruitment really boils down to the lack of cultural competency on the part of researchers who do not understand the communities in which they work. This is reflected in practically all of the Collaborative Board's recommendations for researchers listed above. Additionally, Ms. B. would like to change some researchers' views of the community and help them to realize that community members are just as capable: "They need to realize that they should treat us the same way they want to be treated." Without this understanding, researchers will not be able to develop true collaborative partnerships. By not "doing your homework" and being open-minded, you may be alienating the very same people you are trying to reach. In effect, researchers may be disempowering the community by not using culturally appropriate methods of recruitment and collaboration.

A second important emphasis by the Board was placed on full participation by all members in planning, decision-making, and evaluation. Laverack and Labonte (2000) describe participation as basic to community empowerment. It is in these groups that community members can analyze and act on important community issues. With participation, come skills of leadership, problem assessment, and resource mobilization–all of which are vital organizational elements necessary in collaboration for effective community empowerment (Laverack & Labonte, 2000). In order to do this, researchers must recognize the strengths of the community members (Key Ingredient 5) who can bring a variety of personal and professional experiences to the table. Additionally, members' educational and training needs should be assessed in order to determine what skills should be developed that will help the members and the Board (Key Ingredients 6 and 9). One of the basic premises of collaboration is 'with knowledge, comes empowerment.' If members are lacking any skills that are necessary for doing the work, a mechanism could be put into place where the members can receive ongoing training. Ms. K. illustrates this through her views of the program's job descriptions:

> . . . all, including higher-level, positions should be open to the community members. Although we may not be able to be the Principal Investigator because of the need for a doctoral degree, all other managerial positions should be equally open to the community members regardless of education level. The CHAMP program is unique because the community is doing the programmatic work. The Board members are more trusted in the community because their kids are in the same schools and they would not allow anyone to hurt their kids with a bad program.

An important component to encouraging full participation by all members is also recognizing that the group may need ongoing support in order to build intragroup relations (Key Ingredient 4). Although the members may live within the same community, they may come from different cultures, backgrounds, and experiences. As with any group or team, the members need the space and time in which to get to know and understand each other. Collaborative Boards go through a great deal of problem-solving, planning, and idea generation that takes a lot of discussion and teamwork to be able to come to effective resolutions. Oftentimes, conflicts may arise or some members may feel left out of the process. Mr. P. illustrates this key point through his observations:

> *. . . although there is a lot of discussion in the Board meetings, it seems like the decisions have already been made ahead of time. Sometimes, Mr. P. feels that not everyone has a say in the decision-making or that some people may be afraid to speak up. Oftentimes, he finds that issues are presented too late and that decisions need to be made too quickly without enough time to really discuss and analyze it. He also feels that members have different levels of commitment or interest in the program and that the group is not as united as it used to be.*

Mr. P.'s frustrations with the Board are similar to what most teams who work together go through. A couple of Board members who share the same concerns offer the following suggestions:

> *Ms. J. advises researchers to ensure that all members recruited to the program are truly interested in moving the community forward. It may be helpful to have a screening process whereby you can make sure that everyone can bring something to the table. She advises that problems should be brought to the entire group for discussion and resolved soon after they occur instead of allowing them to linger. It will help everyone to work better together.*

Ms. T., a Latina single mother, offers the following perspective:

> *"It is very important that we learn from each other. If we are going to serve the community, we need to recognize and learn that we each have different talents, and we can only move forward if we respect each other." Ms. T. suggests developing an orientation and mentoring program for all new members of the Board to help them understand the process and build teamwork.*

Despite the challenges, it is vital that community members continue to do the programmatic work and take over the managerial positions for the program in addition to being on the Collaborative Board. The CHAMP-NY Program has been looking at ways to develop a Leadership Institute whereby members will receive a variety of training, such as GED, grant-writing, team-building, and budgeting classes, that will enable them to continue to work together effectively and lead the program once it is transferred to the community.

Full community participation also means involving members from the beginning planning phase (Key Ingredient 6). Although health promotion models often use a top-down approach where researchers are presenting their ideas and plans to the community, a more effective approach is to include the community beforehand. When you are interested in addressing a community issue, it is necessary to work with the community to determine what interventions would work best to address this problem. Ms. O. advises researchers that, "it is important to get support of the community when implementing any new programs. They need to embrace and respect the community." Mr. R., a father who has lived within the community for eleven years adds that "CHAMP is a unique program because of its Collaborative Board. We are able to do more than other programs and work more effectively as well." Researchers need to be willing to incorporate community ideas into their programs. The CHAMP-NY program uses a model developed from Hatch, Moss, Saran, Presley-Cantrell, and Mallory (1993) that illustrates a process that may begin with a less intense form of collaboration but ends with true partnerships between community and researcher in shared decision-making (Madison et al., 2000). Ms. T. explains, "CHAMP is a unique program because it is adaptable to the ideas of the community members." Furthermore, researchers can also use Laverack and Labonte's (2000) framework for incorporating community empowerment goals within a health promotion program. These methods incorporate a non-linear and multi-directional way of incorporating community and researcher needs within a program.

Lastly, within a collaborative model, community members sit side-by-side with researchers and community agencies. The understanding is that anyone who sits at this table believes in community participation. The CHAMP-NY Board is in the process of transferring from a research project to a community program housed within a community agency. The CHAMP Board members have faced a number of challenges in incorporating their program model into the agency's existing structure. From this experience, the Board feels that collaborative boards need to ensure that all agencies they work with are truly collaborative (Key Ingredient 10). With such an emphasis on community empowerment and decision-making, the Board is now seeing that agencies are not equipped to include such a non-hierarchical structure. Additionally, Board members have also found that community-based agencies may not be as willing to embrace the community as one would think. Mr. R. feels that the Board members made CHAMP what it is and that they would lose ownership once it was embodied within the local agency. Furthermore, Ms. K. is not completely happy with the transfer process because she feels that they are unable to advocate for themselves within this larger agency. Ms. K is one of the few Board members who works within an office in the agency and finds that agency staff looks down upon and marginalizes the Community Board members. With this process are concerns of the long-term effects of the transfer on the effectiveness of the program. The Board is working with the agency on a temporary basis as they try to work out some of these concerns. Many of the members understand that transferring to an agency means having to fit within its structure. However, it is important to remember that in collaborative partnerships, the real power does still lay with the Board and they are able to redefine the terms of the relationship with the agency as necessary. One option may be to incorporate the Board into is own non-profit organization. Mr. C. does feel that it would have been better to run the program themselves and not to transfer it to a community agency. He would have preferred to have been better trained in program administration so that they could become their own organization.

CONCLUSION

From the experiences of the Board members in the CHAMP-NY Family Program, we can see that a collaboration model is not without its significant benefits and challenges. However, one can not deny the sense of empowerment that members feel from participating in such a model. Over and over again, the members also discussed how fulfilled they felt in educating their fellow community members and seeing the impact of the program. What they found was that families enjoyed the program so much that they did not want to leave and many of these workshop participants later became involved within the programmatic structure. This sense of empowerment did not only come from being able to help your neighbor, but also by having access to social power through participation in the collaborative programming process. Mr. P. in particular is extremely thankful to CHAMP for helping to build his knowledge about HIV, research, and public speaking–"Even though I do not have a high school diploma, I can now speak about HIV in professional academic fields." Similarly, Ms. H. has lessened her fear of public speaking since she has been a workshop facilitator. With the development of the program, Board members have since been able to enlarge their networks and have access to additional resources. Many of the members have even moved into programmatic positions in other public health-related fields.

Researchers must understand that community members are more than sources of data and targets of interventions, but can instead become an integral part of the research process with some training. Although researchers may be reluctant to lose some of their administrative control, these types of collaborative partnerships with community members and community-based agencies can create better research quality and applicability, greater public support, and help other empowerment applications in the community (Perkins, 1995). By empowering communities to learn and do this work themselves, they are better able to alleviate a number of social problems that may arise. Furthermore, they are able to maintain the work in the community once the researchers move on to another project. Over time, this will create a more self-sufficient community, whereby we will see that social problems, such as the high rates of HIV, can be alleviated.

This article focused only on one collaborative model within the HIV prevention field. Although the experiences of the members and their suggestions are very valuable and coincide with prior literature, it is important to continue analyzing the effects of empowerment and the community collaborative model in addressing major community issues. Only with continued commitment on the part of researchers, can this model be perfected and disseminated so as to help all communities. In Ms. M's words, "It is important that researchers understand that community members are bright people who can contribute a lot to the program. Spend some time in the community. Take the time to show community members that you care and that you are bringing a program that will stay within the community."

REFERENCES

Albert, R. D. (1996). A framework and model for understanding Latin American and Latino/Hispanic cultural patterns. In D. Landis & R.S. Bhagat (Eds.), *Handbook of Intercultural Training*. Thousand Oaks, CA: Sage Publications.

Aponte, H.J., Zarski, J., Bixenstene, C., & Cibik, P. (1991). Home/community-based services: A two-tier approach. *American Journal of Orthopsychiatry, 61* (3), 403-408.

Boyd-Franklin, N. (1993). Race, class, poverty. In F. Walsh (Ed.), Normal *Family Processes*. New York: Guilford.

Dalton, H.L. (1989). AIDS in blackface. *Daedalus, 118* (3), 205-227.

Fawcett, S.B., Paine-Andrews, A., Francisco, V.T., & Schultz, J.A. (1995). Using empowerment theory in collaborative partnerships for community health and development. *American Journal of Community Psychology, 23* (5), 677-698.

Fullilove, M.T. & Fullilove, R.E. (1993). Understanding sexual behaviors and drug use among African Americans: A case study of issues for survey research. In D.G. Ostrow & R.C. Kessler (Eds.). *Methodological Issues in AIDS Behavioral Research.* (pp. 117-132). New York: Plenum Press.

Fullilove, M.T., Green, L., & Fullilove, R.E. (1999). Building momentum: An ethnographic study of inner-city redevelopment. *American Journal of Public Health, 89* (6), 840-845.

Galbraith, J., Stanton, B., Feigelman, S. Ricardo, I., Black, M., & Kalijee, L. (1996). Challenges and rewards of involving community in research: An overview of the "Focus on Kids" HIV risk reduction program. To be published in *Health Education Quarterly, 23*(3): 383-94.

Harper, G.W. & Salina, D.D. (2000). Building collaborative partnerships to improve community-based HIV prevention research: The University-CBO Collaborative Partnership (UCCP) Model. *Journal of Prevention & Intervention in the Community, 19* (1), 1-20.

Hatch, J., Moss, N., Saran, A., Presley-Cantrell, L., Mallory, C. (1993). Community research: Partnership in Black communities. *American Journal of Preventive Medicine, 9*, 27-31.

Hatchett, B.F., Holmes, K., Duran, D.A., Davis, C. (2000). African Americans and research participation: The recruitment process. *Journal of Black Studies, 30* (5), 664-675.

Himmelman, A.T. (2001). On coalitions and the transformation of power relations: Collaborative betterment and collaborative empowerment. *American Journal of Community Psychology, 29* (2), 277-285.

Labonte, R. (1994). Health promotion and empowerment: Reflections on professional practice. *Health Education Quarterly, 21*, 253-268.

Laverack, G. & Labonte, R. (2000). A planning framework for community empowerment goals within health promotion. *Health Policy and Planning, 15*(3), 255-262.

MacQueen, K.M., McLellan, E., Metzger, D.S., Kegeles, S., Strauss, R.P., Scotti, R., Blanchard, L., & Trotter, R.T. (2001). What is community? An evidence-based definition for participatory public health. *American Journal of Public Health, 91*(12), 1929-1938.

Madison, S.M., McKay, M.M., Paikoff, R., Bell, C. (2000). Basic research and community collaboration: Necessary ingredients for the development of a family-based HIV prevention program. *AIDS Education and Prevention, 12* (4), 281-299.

Marin, G. & Marin, B.V. (1991). Research with Hispanic populations. Newbury Park: Sage Publications.

McCormick, A., McKay, M.M., Wilson, M., McKinney, L., Paikoff, R., Bell, C., Baptiste, D., Coleman, D. Gillming, G., Madison, S., & Scott, R. (2000). Involving families in an urban HIV preventive intervention: How community collaboration addresses barriers to participation. *AIDS Education and Prevention, 12* (4), 299-208.

McKay, M., Hibbert, R., Lawrence, R., Miranda, A., Paikoff, R., Bell, C., Madison, S., Baptiste, D., & Coleman, D. (2007). Creating mechanisms for meaningful collaboration between members of urban, minority communities and university-based HIV prevention researchers. *Social Work in Mental Health* 5(1/2): 183-197.

McLoyd, V. C. (1990). The impact of economic hardship on Black families and children: Psychological distress, parenting, and socioemotional development. *Child Development, 61*, 311-346.

Miranda, J., Azocar, F., Organista, K.C., Munoz, R.F., & Lieberman, A. (1996). Recruiting and retaining low income Latinos in psychotherapy research. *Journal of Consulting and Clinical Psychology, 64*, 868-874.

Perkins, D.D. (1995). Speaking truth to power: Empowerment ideology as social intervention and policy. *American Journal of Community Psychology, 23* (5), 765-795.

Perkins, D.D., & Zimmerman, M.A. (1995). Empowerment theory, research, and application. *American Journal of Community Psychology, 23* (5), 569-580.

Sanstad, K.H., Stall, R., Goldstein, E., Everett, W., & Brousseau, R. (1999). Collaborative community research consortium: A model for HIV prevention. *Health Education and Behavior, 26* (2), 171-185.

Schensul, J.J. (1999). Organizing community research partnerships in the struggle against AIDS. *Health Education and Behavior, 26* (2), 266-284.

Schmitz, C.L. (1999). Collaborative practice in low-income communities: University, agency, public school partnerships. *Social Thought, 19* (2), 53-67.

Secrest, L.A., Lassiter, S.L., Armistead, L.P., Wyckoff, S.C. et al. (2004). The Parents Matter! Program: Building a successful investigator-community partnership. *Journal of Child and Family Studies, 13* (1), 35.

Skaff, M.M., Chesla, C.A., Mycue, V., & Fisher, L. (2002). Lessons in cultural competence: Adapting research methodology for Latino participants. *Journal of Community Psychology, 30* (3), 305-323.

Speer, P.W., & Hughey, J. (1995). Community Organizing: An ecological route to empowerment and power. *American Journal of Community Psychology, 23* (5), 729-749.

Thomas, S.B. & Quinn, S.C. (1991). The Tuskegee syphilis study, 1932-1972: Implications for HIV education and AIDS use education programs in the black community. *American Journal of Public Health, 81* (11), 1495-1505.

Tiamiyu, M.F., & Jenks, J. (2001). Health related support groups for youths and the role of university-community collaboration. *Journal of Multicultural Nursing & Health, 7* (3), 26-33.

Walsh, D.S. (2002). Emerging strategies in the search for effective university-community collaborations. *Journal of Physical Education, Recreation & Dance, 73* (1), 50-54.

doi:10.1300/J200v05n03_04

Preventing HIV/AIDS Among Trinidad and Tobago Teens Using a Family-Based Program: Preliminary Outcomes

Donna R. Baptiste
Dexter R. Voisin
Cheryl Smithgall
Dona Da Costa Martinez
Gabrielle Henderson

Donna R. Baptiste, PhD, is affiliated with the Institute For Juvenile Research, University of Illinois at Chicago. Dexter R. Voisin, PhD, and Cheryl Smithgall, MA, are affiliated with the University of Chicago, School of Social Service Administration. Dona Da Costa Martinez, MA, and Gabrielle Henderson, MA, are affiliated with The CHAMP-TT Collaborative Board, Family Planning Association of Trinidad and Tobago.

Address correspondence to: Donna R. Baptiste, PhD, Institute For Juvenile Research, Department of Psychiatry, University of Illinois at Chicago, 1747 West Roosevelt Road, Room 155 (MC747), Chicago, IL 60608 (E-mail: dbaptiste@psych.uic.edu).

The authors thank the FPATT, CHAMP-TT staff, and Community Advisory Board for their extraordinary work on the project. The authors are also very grateful to the families in Trinidad and Tobago who participated in their research.

The Collaborative HIV/AIDS Prevention and Adolescent Mental Health Project of Trinidad and Tobago (CHAMP-TT) was supported by a supplement to a National Institute of Mental Health, Office of AIDS Research grant (5RO1-MH55701).

[Haworth co-indexing entry note]: "Preventing HIV/AIDS Among Trinidad and Tobago Teens Using a Family-Based Program: Preliminary Outcomes." Baptiste, Donna R. et al. Co-published simultaneously in *Social Work in Mental Health* (The Haworth Press, Inc.) Vol. 5, No. 3/4, 2007, pp. 333-354; and: *Community Collaborative Partnerships: The Foundation for HIV Prevention Research Efforts* (ed: Mary M. McKay, and Roberta L. Paikoff) The Haworth Press, Inc., 2007, pp. 333-354. Single or multiple copies of this article are available for a fee from The Haworth Document Delivery Service [1-800-HAWORTH, 9:00 a.m. - 5:00 p.m. (EST). E-mail address: docdelivery@haworthpress.com].

333

SUMMARY. This paper describes a family-based HIV/AIDS prevention project currently underway in Trinidad and Tobago–an English speaking twin-island nation in the Caribbean. The project involves a partnership between U.S.-based researchers and a social service agency on the Islands. It describes the development and adaptation of the intervention and reports preliminary outcomes from a pilot intervention (*n* = 32). Findings indicate high participant retention; statistically significant pre to posttest changes in HIV/AIDS knowledge and awareness; parent/youth discussions at home; condom self-efficacy; and parental monitoring. Findings are discussed within the context of collaborative HIV/AIDS prevention research. doi:10.1300/J200v05n03_05 *[Article copies available for a fee from The Haworth Document Delivery Service: 1-800-HAWORTH. E-mail address: <docdelivery@haworthpress.com> Website: <http://www.HaworthPress.com> © 2007 by The Haworth Press, Inc. All rights reserved.]*

KEYWORDS. International collaboration, HIV/AIDS prevention, adolescents, family education, Trinidad and Tobago, Caribbean

INTRODUCTION

The Caribbean region ranks highest in adult Human Immune-Deficiency Virus and Acquired Immune-Deficiency Syndrome (HIV/AIDS) cases in the Americas, and second only to sub-Saharan Africa. The majority of cases are among individuals ages 15-44 years and females ages 15-19 years, revealing a distinct pandemic profile (Camera et al., 2003). In 2000, Caribbean and international agencies drafted a strategic plan targeting priority areas to defeat HIV/AIDS in the region. Preventing transmission of the virus among young people is a major focus of this plan and a recommended strategy is development and delivery of "Health and Family Life Education Programmes" (Caribbean Task Force on AIDS, 2000, p. 15). We describe our attempts to work along these lines in the Republic of Trinidad and Tobago (T & T).

In this paper, we describe our collaborative HIV/AIDS prevention initiative that is currently underway in T & T aimed at reducing adolescent HIV/AIDS risk exposure. Our initiative involves a partnership between researchers connected to the Collaborative HIV/AIDS Adolescent Mental Health Projects (CHAMP) based at the University of Illinois at Chicago (UIC), and the Family Planning Association of Trinidad and Tobago

(FPATT), a local social service agency on the islands. We outline the family-education intervention that was developed to address youth HIV/AIDS problems and present preliminary outcome data from the pilot with a small sample (*n* = 32) of youth and their parents. We discuss findings in relation to the goals of our initiative that includes: (1) creating a strong cross-national coalition to conduct a randomized efficacy trial, (2) adapting the US-based CHAMP family intervention for T&T, (3) assessing the feasibility of recruiting and retaining an adequate sample and (4) evaluating the potential impact of intervention components on individual and family-level variables.

Adolescent HIV/AIDS Trends in T & T

In T & T, adolescents and young adults make up the majority of all new HIV/AIDS cases and these reported cases may only represent about 50% of *actual* infections (CAREC, 2002). Female adolescents seem most vulnerable. Although there are equal numbers of male and female adolescents on the islands, females are three to seven times more likely to be infected than males (Camera et al., 2003) Factors linked to adolescent trends in T & T are similar to those found in the US and in other parts of the world. These include early sexual debut, multiple partners, and low condom use. For example, a study of 1200 adolescents, ages 14-20 years, on these islands reveals that 46% were sexually active by age 16; more than 40% had more than one partner; and only 47% consistently used condoms during sexually-activity (PAHO/Ministry of Health, 1998; UNICEF/, UNAIDS/WHO, 2002). Thus in T & T, a risk matrix of low detection, low condom use, and sex with multiple partners indicate vulnerability among the youth population who need information, education, and support to alter risk trajectories (Caribbean Task Force on AIDS, 2000; PAHO/Ministry of Health, 1998).

These disturbing trends have influenced T & T's governmental and non-governmental organizations (NGOs) to implement outreach programs to youth in and out of schools via various media. The majority of HIV/AIDS prevention programs and interventions target youth *individually* to increase their awareness about the virus; to influence them to make less risky sexual choices; and to educate them about prevention (World Bank, 2000). While families, particularly parents, are also considered to be important to helping youth along these same lines, we found no programs or interventions that specifically involved youth in conjunction with parents/caregivers in HIV/AIDS education and prevention activities.

Considering a Family-Education Approach

In the US, involved parents are considered to play a key role in helping youth to decrease risky sexual activities and by extension, HIV/AIDS exposure (Pequegnat & Szapocznik, 2000). Having community members play a driving role is the basic premise guiding CHAMP's (Collaborative HIV Prevention and Adolescent Mental Health Project) research programs (Paikoff, McKay, & Bell, 1994; McKay, Paikoff, Bell, Baptiste, & Madison, 2000). In exporting the CHAMP family-based approach to T & T, we speculated as to whether a family-education intervention could have a significant impact. We found no intervention outcome data to answer this question, but survey data and theoretical treatises pointed to a pivotal role for families in prevention. Harris-Hastick et al. (2001) discuss HIV/AIDS interventions for Caribbean youth and suggest that along with information and awareness campaigns and sexuality education targeting youth directly, approaches targeting family networks are also important. Similarly, Roopnarine et al. (2000) acknowledge a diversity of family configurations in the Caribbean, but highlight parent-child relationships and overall family support as important to positive youth outcomes.

In T & T, parents appear to be heavily involved in the lives of their adolescents (PAHO/Ministry of Health, 1998). But, open conversations about sex and sexuality are proscribed in many homes and also in schools (Voisin & Remy, 2001). For example, in a recent study of youth ($n = 675$) in Tobago, 53% reported being sexually active by age 16, but a significant majority indicated that they found it extremely difficult to talk to parents about sexuality and contraception (FPATT, 2000). We believe our research provides missing empirical links, specifically between parental involvements in youth HIV/AIDS risk reduction. We briefly introduce CHAMP and the FPATT and how we partnered to produce a family-education intervention to address adolescent HIV/AIDS problems on the islands.

COLLABORATIVE HIV/AIDS PREVENTION ADOLESCENT MENTAL HEALTH PROJECT (CHAMP)

CHAMP involves high-intensity partnerships with community members in Chicago neighborhoods that have significant youth HIV/AIDS prevalence rates. In US-based CHAMP studies, researchers and members of affected communities have combined their ideas and energies to design, deliver, and test family-based preventive interventions for youth and their parents/caregivers. Researcher-community partnerships have been operationalized through the formation of a community advisory Board comprised of researchers, community members, school staff, and community-agency personnel. Madison et al. (Preventing HIV/AIDS Among Trinidad and Tobago Teens Using a Family-Based Program: Preliminary Outcomes 2002) describe the community collaborative approach guiding CHAMP programs in the U.S. Baptiste et al. (2005) describe how researchers and community members collaborated to develop the intervention's theoretical framework and activities. Mckay et al. (2004) document the intervention's impact on individual and family-level constructs.

THE CHAMP FAMILY INTERVENTION

Briefly, the CHAMP intervention is developmentally-grounded, targeting youth before and during the pubertal transition. The intervention adopts a *family-education* approach in that parent/caregivers attend sessions with their youngsters. The intervention is designed to strengthen family-level characteristics such as parental monitoring, parent/child communication about sensitive topics, discipline, conflict-resolution, and support. It also targets young teens' social problem-solving abilities, such as recognition of risk, refusal, and assertiveness in handling peer pressure to engage in risky sexual activities (Baptiste et al., 2005).

Goals of the intervention are met through discussing *sexual possibility situations* that are likely to occur for the majority of youth in this age range. A sexual possibility situation refers to a time and place when adolescents are alone, without adult supervision, in which a sexual encounter may be possible (Paikoff et al., 1995). The intervention focuses on the important role of parents in providing information, structure and values to help youth to cope with sexual possibility situations in their peer and friendship relationships. Additionally, the intervention provides parents/caregivers and youth with information on puberty, HIV/AIDS, and safer-sex behavior and suggests that parents continue these discussions in a non-combative way with their teens.

We encourage a three-step approach to decision-making to prevent HIV/AIDS risk exposure. Youth are encouraged to *ABSTAIN* from intercourse as a way of deterring risk exposure. Youth are also encouraged to *DELAY* sexual activity until they are older and are able to make more responsible decisions about sexual partners. If abstaining and delaying does not work, youth are further encouraged to *PROTECT* themselves from HIV/AIDS risk exposure through safer-sex behavior, particularly proper use of a condom (Baptiste et al., 2005). Figure 1 describes the CHAMP intervention model.

THE FPATT

The FPATT, a non-governmental organization (NGO), has a 50-year history of service to the local community. FPATT advocates "planning for a family" as an element of social change in the society and many of its activities are developed along these lines. Well-qualified medical and nursing provide high quality service (e.g., awareness and skill-building programs on sexually transmitted infections (STI) prevention, sexuality and interpersonal relationships, domestic violence, incest, and rape) in three clinics, in addition to a mobile unit that visits disadvantaged communities on the islands. CHAMP researchers contacted the FPATT to collaborate on a proposal for funding related to the transfer of

FIGURE 1. Conceptual Model of Family and Individual Factors Influencing HIV/AIDS Risk Exposure

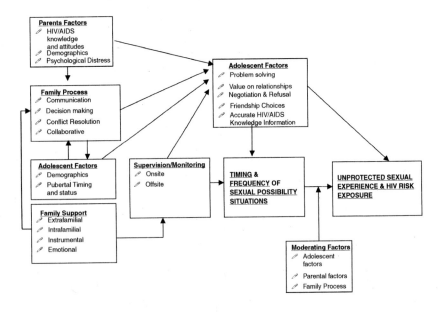

an HIV/AIDS prevention program that would be culturally adapted for the country.

Initial conversations between researchers and agency leaders centered on assessing the compatibility of missions and interests with regard to HIV/AIDS. We viewed CHAMP's primary mission as being consistent with the FPATT's, which is to provide sexual and reproductive health education to youth to help them to protect themselves from all sexually transmitted infections (STIs), including HIV/AIDS. FPATT also articulated an aspect of its mission: to involve families in STI prevention targeting youth and to train its staff to conduct prevention research (FPATT, 2001). Once researchers and the agency agreed to partner, major tasks were to secure funding, hammer out details of the partnership and establish norms and expectations for building a research coalition. The researcher-agency relationship developed over 12-months prior to submission of the first grant proposal and involved extensive dialogue and negotiation.

ADAPTING THE CHAMP INTERVENTION FOR TRINIDAD AND TOBAGO

The FPATT retained the idea of community involvement in the initiative and created a 15-member Board comprised of individuals involved in HIV/AIDS prevention activities or who worked in youth-centered fields in T&T. Researchers were also considered *de facto* Board members and received proceedings via e-mail, phone calls, and memos. The Board met monthly (or more often in subcommittees) and their initial work was to assess the goodness-of-fit of the CHAMP curricula and materials; to adapt it for youth and families on the island; to recruit suitable facilitators to implement an intervention pilot; to develop guidelines for implementation and program fidelity; to select representatives for dissemination (e.g., travel to conferences) and to plan for long-term direction of the research program.

We adapted the CHAMP family intervention for the local setting over three phases (Baptiste, Martinez & the CHAMP-TT Board, 2003). First, the advisory Board was sub-divided into three focus groups to review CHAMP curricula and materials to make recommendations for revisions. This information was used to develop a first revised version. Second, facilitators were recruited by the Board to receive training in preparation to deliver the intervention to families. Facilitators reviewed and role played each session and based on their feedback, we drafted a second revised version of the intervention Third, local families, including early adolescent youth and parents/caregivers evaluated the intervention and we used this information to develop a third revised version. This version was disseminated to members of the Board for additional review. Board members selected the program name, assessed its overall suitability, and the level of social and cultural themes relevant to islands. This yielded the fourth revised version of the family-education intervention, titled CHAMP-Trinidad and Tobago (CHAMP-TT) that will be assessed via a randomized efficacy trial in the second stage of our initiative. Baptiste, Martinez and the CHAMP-TT Board (2003) and Voisin, Baptiste, Martinez and Henderson (2006) provide a detailed description of adaptation procedures, intervention revisions, and challenges.

Overall, we have been surprised by the low number of changes that were suggested by local collaborators to retool the US intervention for the islands. We attribute this to our phased approach to adaptation, including a review stage in which Board members and facilitators evaluated the material. Many of these individuals were parents raising young adolescents. They provided important insights about aspects of the CHAMP intervention that should be changed to better suit local families. We also believe that historical and contemporary influences of Western and more specifically, American culture, in the local setting, international travel, trade, and other components of globalization have created cultural links between US and local youth that made many ideas and topics in the U.S. CHAMP intervention suitable for the islands. Next, we describe the CHAMP-TT intervention and also provide some preliminary data on its impact on family and individual-level variables.

THE CHAMP-TRINIDAD AND TOBAGO INTERVENTION (CHAMP-TT)

The CHAMP-TT intervention is delivered in a family-group format that includes multiple family discussions, parent/youth breakout groups, and individual family-discussions. The intervention addresses entire family needs, as well as specific needs of youth and parents that can potentially impact family climate and relationships. For parents/caregivers these include getting support from other parents, discussing strategies to help their youth negotiate sexual issues, discussions about their own sexual risk behavior, and opportunities to evaluate their parenting styles and practices. For youth, these needs include developing peer supports, social problem-solving skills to assist in recognizing different types of risk situations, and improving negotiation and self-assertion skills to deal with peer pressure situations.

Family groups meet for 12 sessions each lasting approximately two hours. Every session will be structured comparably: (1) a warm up component with multiple families together, (2) separate parent and youth breakout discussions to prepare for a family discussion, (3) individual family meetings to exchange ideas on session topics and to make an action plan around it, and (4) wrap-up component focused on linking the topic to HIV/AIDS prevention. Detailed components of the CHAMP-TT intervention are outlined in Table 1.

PILOT DESIGN

We conducted an intervention pilot with a small convenience sample of early adolescent youth and their parents ($n = 32$) utilizing a simple one-group (family-education intervention) pre to post-test research design. This pilot was aimed at refining our ability to recruit and retain families and preliminarily assessing of the intervention's impact on proximal family-level constructs (i.e., parental monitoring; and frequency of parent/child discussions of sensitive topics at home) and risk-related constructs (i.e., perceived self-efficacy in condom-use and HIV/AIDS knowledge and awareness).

PARTICIPANTS

In September 2002, project staff visited 2nd form classrooms (equivalent to US 6th/7th grades) in two schools and distributed permission forms ($n = 150$) for youth to take home to parents. Parents who returned signed forms indicating interest ($n = 117$) were invited to attend one informational meeting held at their respective school. Those who attended ($n = 75$) received additional information about the pilot and a random sample of 16 families (8 from each school) were selected by lottery from among those eligible. Families were eligible if they had an adolescent between the ages of 11 to 13 enrolled in one of two selected public schools situated in high HIV/AIDS sero-prevalent counties in Trinidad. Parents had to be adult caregivers, over the age of 18 and living in the home and fulfilling parenting responsibilities towards the targeted youth. Total participants were 32 (16 targeted youth with 16 parents/care-

TABLE 1. Overview of the CHAMP-TT Curriculum

SESSION TOPIC	SESSION OBJECTIVES	PARENT GROUP ACTIVITIES	YOUTH GROUP ACTIVITIES	FAMILY INTERACTION TASKS
Session 1: *Introduction to CHAMP-Trinidad and Tobago (CHAMP-TT)*	• To get introduced to CHAMP-TT • To get acquainted with other families • To talk about why CHAMP-TT works with youth and parents • To complete consent documents	• Parents set up guidelines for parent discussions • Parents identify risks for youth in their neighborhoods	• Youth discuss guidelines for youth discussion groups • Youth identify risky behaviors that make parents worry	• Families list how families can protect youth against risks, including HIV/AIDS • Families list how participation in CHAMP-TT can improve relationships at home • Families complete consents
Session 2: *Paperwork!*	• To discuss research aspects in CHAMP-TT • To complete pre assessment data	• Complete Pre-Assessments	• Complete Pre-Assessments	None
Session 3: *Talking and Listening*	• To identify important aspects of good parent/child communication • To link good parent/child communication to decreasing HIV/AIDS risk	• Parents discuss enablers and barriers to good communication with their youth • Parents practice handling discussions around sensitive topics • Parents identify how good communication is linked to preventing HIV/AIDS risks	• Youth discuss enablers and barriers to good communication with their parents • Youth practice raising sensitive topics with parents • Youth practice strategies to improve communication with parents	• Families list how communication strengthens • Families list communication weaknesses • Families list strategies to improve communication • Families list how good communication is linked to preventing HIV/AIDS
Session 4: *It's a Sexy World!*	• To discuss sexual media messages • To understand how media messages influence risk behavior among youth • To discuss how families can combat media messages	• Parents discuss how messages about sex in music, TV shows, movies affect adolescents • Parents review lyrics of a popular Calypso to track messages about sex • Parents practice strategies to help adolescents combat media influences	• Youth discuss how messages about sex in music, TV shows, movies influence their choices • Youth review messages in lyrics of Calypso's to track messages about sex • Youth list "counter messages" to respond to those in songs	• Family exchange ideas about media messages • Families come up with plan to deal with media messages, especially in music and music videos
Session 5: *Growing Up: Dealing with Peer Pressure*	• To discuss data about sexual behavior • To help kids practice dealing with peer pressure situations • To discuss how peer pressure is related to preventing HIV/AIDS	• Parents review data on youth's sexual behavior • Parents list peer pressure situations that youth encounter • Practice talking to kids about Peer pressure situations	• Youth identify peer pressure situations for young adolescents • Youth learned practice steps to making a good decision in peer pressure situations	• Families discuss different peer pressure scenarios that youth experience • Families plan ways to help youth deal with peer pressure situations • Families complete process measures
Session 6: *Growing Up: Preparing for Adolescence*	• To discuss puberty • To discuss romantic feelings that adolescents develop • To prepare youth to deal with romantic feelings • To link puberty and romantic feelings to HIV/AIDS risk	• Parents discuss puberty information • Parents identify romantic feelings that adolescents experience • Parents practice talking to youth about romantic puberty and romantic feelings	• Youth make a list of questions about puberty • Youth pretend to be an expert panel helping each other with questions about romance	• Families discuss youth list of puberty questions and parents provide answers • Families discuss youth's romantic feelings • Families list how discussions of puberty and romantic feelings can help prevent HIV/AIDS

SESSION TOPIC	SESSION OBJECTIVES	PARENT GROUP ACTIVITIES	YOUTH GROUP ACTIVITIES	FAMILY INTERACTION TASKS
Session 8: *Understanding HIV/AIDS*	• To increase families' knowledge and awareness about HIV/AIDS • To explain how HIV/AIDS is transmitted and prevented • To demonstrate proper use of a condom	• Parents discuss myths about HIV/AIDS • Parents talk about HIV/AIDS transmission and prevention • Parents prepare to demonstrate condom use to youth	• Youth discuss myths about HIV/AIDS • Youth talk about no, low, and high risk behaviors • Youth prepare for a condom demonstration	• Families discuss how condom, properly used, can prevent HIV/AIDS • Parents demonstrate proper use of a condom to youth • Youth practice proper use of a condom • Complete process measures
Session 9: *Respect yourself and others!*	• To discuss the importance of respecting self and others • To discuss ways to show respect for boys and girls • To discuss how having self respect is connected to prevention HIV/AIDS	• Parents discuss ways to improve youth self-respect • Parents list how their youth can show respect for different sexual peers • Parents discuss messages girls need to handle pressure against sex	• Youth list dos and don'ts about respecting self and others • Youth list ways for girls to show respect for boys • Youth list ways for boy to show respect for girls • Youth list ways girls should show self-respect in dealing with boys	• Families discuss youth list of dos ad don'ts regarding respect • Families list ways they can show more respect for each other • Families discuss how respect is connected to HIV/AIDS
Session 10: *Keeping Track of Teens*	• To understand what sexual possibility situations are • To discuss the importance of supervising/ monitoring sexual possibility situations • To discuss how sexual possibility situations are linked to HIV/AIDS risks	• Parents List sexual possibility situations for youth in the home ad out of the home • Parents know ways to help youth deal with sexual possibility situations • Identify discussion strategies to monitor growing teenagers	• Youth list sexual possibility situations that they have been in • Youth lists strategies to handle sexual possibility situations • Youth practice handling these situations	• Families discuss youth's sexual possibility situations with parental suggestions for how youth should handle them • Families list rules and consequences for regarding youth's friends, activities, and whereabouts • Families discuss how parental monitoring protect youth from HIV • Families complete process measures
Session 11: *More Paperwork!*	To remind families about the value of collecting data • To discuss how families' participation will help CHAMP-TT to know if the program works • To collect post assessment data	• Complete Post-Assessments	• Complete Post-Assessments	• None
Session 12: *Celebrating Safe and Healthy Families!*	• To list of lessons learned in CHAMP-TT • To develop a family mission statement to combat HIV/AIDS • To celebrate the end of the CHAMP-TT Program	• Parents list lessons learned in CHAMP . • Parents discuss how information can help prevent HIV/AIDS	• Youth list of lessons learned in CHAMP • Youth discuss how information can help prevent HIV/AIDS	• Families create and share their mission statement against HIV/AIDS • Families receive certificates of participation • Parents complete follow-up contact paperwork

givers). The Institutional Review Boards at University of Illinois at Chicago, University of Chicago, and CAREC approved all study procedures and each family member completed consent documents.

FACILITATORS' TRAINING

All facilitators were T & T nationals recruited by the local advisory Board based on at least one of three criteria: (a) involvement in HIV/AIDS education, (b) participation in youth outreach or family education, and/or (c) parenting an early adolescent. Prior to conducting the pilot, facilitators received 40 hours of training to build skills and competencies related to the pilot. Training focused on issues as understanding family systems, adolescent development, HIV/AIDS prevention, puberty, consent procedures, data collection, group discussion skills and team work. A team of four facilitators conducted each of the twelve intervention sessions and collected assessment data. In addition, while the pilot was underway, facilitators met weekly for two hours for added training.

MEASURES

The CHAMP-TT assessment battery included measures from the original CHAMP battery that were adapted for local families (McKay, Paikoff, Bell, Baptiste & Madison, 2000). These paper/pencil measures were self-administered and completed by parents and youth during sessions two and eleven of our twelve-session intervention. Parents and youth completed measures separately and privately and facilitators provided help in understanding instructions and to those with reading difficulty.

Demographics. Parents/caregivers provided family demographics on marital status, age, education, income, household size and the like.

Attendance. Facilitators kept attendance records for each family by session number and date, individuals attending (e.g., mother, father, targeted child).

Frequency and comfort with parent/child in-home discussions. Parents and youth completed a 14-item measure on how often they talk at home about sensitive topics such as alcohol, drugs, HIV/AIDS, having sex, and puberty and comfort level with such discussions (Guerra & Tolan, 1991; Paikoff et al., 1995). Frequency of discussion and comfort level were both scored on a 4-point scale ranging from "a lot" to "we don't talk about this." A higher score on both parent and youth measures indicated increased frequency and comfort in discussions at home. This scale had satisfactory internal levels of inter-item reliability (Cronbach's alpha for youth pre-test items = .85, Cronbach's alpha for parents pre-test items = .78 with 3 items omitted).[1]

Knowledge and awareness about HIV/AIDS. Knowledge and awareness about HIV/AIDS was assessed via an 18-item scale (Paikoff et al., 1995). Caregivers and youth were asked their understanding about how HIV/AIDS is transmitted (e.g., "can you get HIV/AIDS from being bitten by a mosquito?). Response categories for the knowledge and awareness items were "true," "false" or "not sure." For each respondent, a score equaling total correct responses was used to assess confident and accurate knowledge.

Condom Self-Efficacy. A 21-item scale was used to assess parent and youth condom self-efficacy (e.g., "how confident are you about using a condom every time you have sex," Paikoff et al., 1993). Items are scored on a 5-point scale ranging from "not sure at all" to "very sure." Parents and youth also were asked about their efficacy in using condoms in situations involving sex (e.g., "if someone liked you and wanted to have sex with you?"). This scale had adequate inter-item reliability (Cronbach's alpha for youth pre-test items = .78, Cronbach's alpha for parents pre-test items = .95 with 1 item omitted).[2]

Parental monitoring. Caregivers and youth completed a 13-item scale assessing the level of parental knowledge and awareness of youth's whereabouts, friends and activities (e.g., "after school child is expected to be at a certain place by a certain time," Gorman-Smith et al., 1996). Responses were coded on a 4-point scale ranging from "always true" to "always false." Higher scores indicate greater parental supervision and monitoring. This scale had adequate internal levels of inter-item reliability (Cronbach's alpha for youth pre-test items = .81, Cronbach's alpha for parents pre-test items = .72).

DATA ANALYSIS

All data were analyzed using SPSS 12.0. Univariate analyses were used to describe the overall sample. Bivariate analyses were used to compare mean change from pretest to posttest and statistical significance of those changes using paired samples *t*-tests for each scale item. Participants who did not complete both pre and posttests were excluded from paired sample t-tests. Thus, the maximum number of parents with complete pre and post data was 13 and the maximum number of youth with pre and post data was 12. As statistical significance is difficult to achieve with such a small sample size, we were also interested in the direction of change from pretest to posttest and whether overall scales had face validity for participants. Cronbach alphas were computed for all continuous scales in order to test the psychometric properties of these scales with this sample. In addition we compared pretest and posttest item means for each item in order to determine which aspect of the variable construct was potentially being affected by the intervention.

RESULTS

Demographics. Table 2 provides an overall description of the sample that was comprised of 32 participants (16 parents and 16 youth). Parents were 12 mothers and 4 fathers, who were all biological parents with a mean age of 43.1 years. More than two-thirds of parents were married, 64% were working outside the home, and around 14% were receiving some form of governmental assistance. Targeted youth were mostly female ($n = 12$) and mean age of all youth was 12.5 years. The sample was religiously diverse reflecting most major religious persuasions in the general population of the islands, except one. Notably, the Hindu religion was not represented.

Attendance. Families averaged 91% attendance over 24 sessions (i.e., 2 groups $\times$ 12 sessions) and all families originally selected were retained in the pilot. Parent/caregivers and youth participated mostly as dyads, one parent attending with one targeted youth. However, 18% of families brought along either a younger or older sibling in the 11 to 13 age range but sibling data were not included in our analyses.

Frequency and comfort with parent/child discussions at home. See Table 3. On average, at pretest youth indicated that they talked about most topics with their parents somewhere between "once in a while" and "often" and that they were "somewhat comfortable" to "comfortable" in most discussions. At pretest, youth rated discussions about having sex as being "somewhat uncomfortable" to "somewhat comfortable." The changes in frequency of discussion were statistically significant for two items completed by youth: an increased frequency of discussions about HIV/AIDS ($p < .02$) and a decreased frequency of discussions about gangs ($p < .02$). No observed changes in comfort level with these discussions were observed. Parents' pretest responses were similar to youth's in

TABLE 2. Sample Characteristics (*n* = 32)

Demographic Item	
Parents/Caregivers	12 females, 4 males
Average Age	43.1 years
Married	71.4%
Completed Education Beyond High School Level	28.6%
Working Outside the Home	64%
Religion	Catholic- 33%
	Islam- 25%
	Protestant-Evangelical-33%
	Indigenous -8%
Receiving Government Assistance	14.3%
Youth	14 females, 2 males
Average age	12.5 years

TABLE 3. Frequency and Comfort with Parent/Child Discussions at Home

	Child				Parent			
How often do you talk about...	*n*	Pre-test Mean	Mean Change	*p*-value	*n*	Pre-test Mean	Mean Change	*p*-value
alcohol	11	2.50	.00	.99	10	3.09	−.70	.09
drugs	12	4.00	−.08	.80	11	3.18	−.55	.14
HIV/AIDS	12	2.67	.83	.025	11	2.73	.09	.85
having sex	12	3.91	.58	.09	11	2.64	.18	.71
sexually transmitted diseases	12	2.33	.50	.11	10	2.64	.09	.85
gangs	12	3.64	−.83	.025	10	2.67	−1.33	.01
puberty	12	2.33	.17	.64	8	3.09	.45	.14
How comfortable are you talking about...								
alcohol	11	2.64	−.27	.19	11	2.73	−.50	.14
drugs	11	2.25	−.27	.28	11	4.00	−.60	.08
HIV/AIDS	11	3.45	.00	.99	9	4.00	−.30	.39
having sex	11	2.33	.36	.31	10	3.70	−.70	.07
sexually transmitted diseases	11	3.70	.00	.99	10	3.80	−.60	.08
gangs	9	3.00	−.33	.52	9	3.90	−1.29	.05
puberty	11	3.09	.45	.24	10	4.00	−.30	.19

1 = very uncomfortable, 2 = somewhat uncomfortable, 3 = somewhat comfortable and 4 = very comfortable. A positive change score indicates movement toward increased frequency of or comfort with the discussions from pre-test to post-test.

that frequency of discussion was reported to be somewhere between" once in a while" and "often." Parents generally reported being "very comfortable" with these discussions. Parents reported a statistically significant change in decreased frequency of discussions about gangs ($p < .01$) with a decreased comfort level regarding those discussions ($p < .05$).

Parental monitoring. Parents' average pre-test response suggested that they perceived themselves as providing a high level of monitoring of youth. No statistically significant changes in parents' responses from pre-test to post-test were observed for parents. Youth also responded at pretest that most of the items were "usually" or "always" true, suggesting a high level of monitoring. Findings on the parental monitoring items for youth were mixed. Youth reported an increase of parents expecting them to be at a certain place at a particular time ($p < .02$); a decrease in parents monitoring their television watching ($p < .03$); a decrease in knowing their best friends ($p < .03$); a decrease in being in bed at a certain time during school nights ($p < .04$); a decrease in going out after school without asking parents ($p < .02$); a decrease in parents knowing in advance of adult supervision during activities ($p < .05$); a decrease in talking to their friends' parents prior to them spending the night ($p < .02$); a decrease in doing places without telling parents ($p < .04$); and increase in adult monitoring when at a friend's house ($p < .04$).

Knowledge and awareness about HIV/AIDS. There were significant changes in parents' and youths' knowledge and awareness of HIV/AIDS from pre to posttest scores. On average, youth answered 47 percent of the items correctly on the pre-test and 72 percent of the items correctly on the post-test. This increase in the proportion of items they could correctly respond to was statistically significant on a paired samples t-test ($p < .001$). Parents answered 78 percent of the items correctly on the pre-test and 84 percent of the items correctly on the post-test. The increase in accurate knowledge of HIV/AIDS transmission risk factors was also statistically significant for the parents ($p < .04$).

Condom self-efficacy. As shown in Table 4, youth generally showed a movement towards an increased level of confidence on the post-test for 9 of the 21 items, and parents showed an increase level of confidence for 17 of the 14 items. Among this mostly female youth sample, participants reported statistically significant increases in condom self-efficacy on three items at posttest: correctly putting on a condom ($p < .02$), using a condom and enjoying the experience ($p < .02$), and going to a clinic to obtain condoms ($p < .001$). Parents also reported a statistically significant increase in using a condom and enjoying the experience ($p < .002$).

TABLE 4. Condom Self-Efficacy

		Child				Parent		
	n	Pre-test Mean	Change	Paired t test p-value	n	Pre-test Mean	Change	Paired t test p-value
Put on a condom so it won't slip or break	12	2.25	1.50	.023	13	3.00	.54	.28
Use a condom and enjoy the experience	9	2.42	.78	.023	12	3.67	.58	.002
Bring up using a condom with your boy/girl friend	11	4.00	.00	.99	12	4.85	.00	.99
Ask your boyfriend or girlfriend about their past sexual experiences	11	3.67	.09	.779	13	4.54	−.08	.84
Use a condom every time you decided to have sex	12	4.33	.08	.857	10	3.45	.60	.31
Insist on using a condom even if your boyfriend or girlfriend did not want to	11	4.17	−.45	.360	11	4.00	.91	.11
Get the money needed to buy condoms from a store	12	3.58	.50	.256	11	4.18	.55	.33
Go to a store and buy condoms	11	2.92	.82	.223	11	4.45	.36	.37
Go to a clinic and get condoms	11	2.25	1.82	.001	11	4.18	.36	.51
Carry a condom with you in case you needed to use it	9	3.83	.22	.738	8	3.67	1.13	.14
Refuse alcohol offered to you at a party	12	4.42	.00	.99	9	4.40	.56	.28
Refuse marijuana offered to you at a party	12	4.75	−.17	.689	7	5.00	.00	†
Use a condom during sex after you have had alcohol	10	3.75	−.60	.382	5	3.89	.57	.36
Use a condom during sex after you have had marijuana	9	3.75	−.56	.468	9	4.11	.40	.70
How sure are you that you would not have sex if you don't want to	11	4.08	−.18	.77	6	4.55	.33	.50
How sure are you that you could get him or her to agree to use condoms	12	4.50	−.33	.43	6	4.44	.00	.99
How sure are you that you would decide to not have sex until you had a condom	12	4.67	−.58	.15	6	4.00	.88	.18
If you wanted to use a condom how sure are you that your partner would decide not to have sex with you	12	2.50	−.58	.18	6	2.44	.33	.67
How sure are you that you would have safe sex if you were teased by your partner	12	3.42	.58	.38	3	3.67	.89	.17
If your partner refused to use a condom how sure are you that you would not have sex	11	4.33	−1.09	.10	4	4.56	.11	.83
If you wanted to have sex with someone and you had been drinking or smoking marijuana how sure are you that you would make sure you used a condom	12	3.50	−.41	.53	4	4.38	.33	.68

† This item had no response variance therefore a standard error could not be computed and no p-value was produced.
1 = Not sure at all, 5 = Very sure; A positive change score indicates increased confidence from pretest to posttest.

DISCUSSION

This is the first study involving a cross-national partnership between US researchers and a social service agency in T & T to design and deliver a *family-education intervention* to address youth HIV/AIDS problems on the islands. Preliminary findings indicate that we have built a robust partnership. Strong attendance was noted in advisory Board meetings (80% over 18 meetings) and local partners have been significantly involved in customizing the CHAMP family intervention for the islands and in conducting an intervention pilot. This has led to increased knowledge related to developing family-based interventions among agency staff, Board members, and facilitators. The agency's leadership has begun discussions of how a family-based approach to decreasing youth's vulnerability to STIs might be incorporated into its existing programming structure. We believe that institutionalizing this intervention into the agency's mission, hierarchy, standard operations, and budget is a potential strategy to ensure its continuity and sustainability (O'Loughlin et al., 1998).

We were also encouraged by high attendance and retention among pilot participants. This suggests that we can potentially recruit and retain the larger sample needed for our NIMH-funded randomized efficacy trial that will begin in the near future (Baptiste, Martinez, & The CHAMP-TT Board, 2003). A more robust research design including a larger sample ($n = 250$) and random assignment to intervention and control conditions will enable us to overcome many of the methodological and statistical limitations we encountered in our small pilot of the intervention.

While collective findings related to the intervention's impact on individual and family level constructs may well be an artifact of our simple design and small sample, we found the information useful. Both parents and youth report significant improvements in HIV/AIDS knowledge and awareness and this information is a basic building block to decreasing HIV/AIDS risk. At home parent/child discussions of sensitive issues such as HIV/AIDS, having sex, and STI also appeared to move in a positive direction which is promising, given that many youth indicate difficulty talking to parents about these sensitive issues (FPATT, 2001). Moreover, our predominantly female adolescent sample reported increased readiness to secure condoms at clinics and properly use a condom. This is an important finding as these young females appear to be engaging in increased health protection behavior within a context with high HIV prevalence (Camera et al., 2003).

However, we were surprised by the mixed findings on parental monitoring, in conjunction with both youth and parents reporting decreased conversations about and gangs. In T & T "gangs" generally refer to peers who endorse negative norms. Given these findings we speculate that some of the items may not have been correctly interpreted by the participants or that some aspects of the parental monitoring curriculum would need to be retooled But, we were struck by the finding that these same youth indicated decreased confidence on items related to negotiating condom use in the midst of sexual behaviors (e.g., "deciding to not have sex until you have a condom," "getting a partner to agree to use a condom"). We speculate that at posttest, youth may be more aware of the complexities of negotiating condom-use with partners and a decreased level of confidence.

LESSONS

We learned valuable lessons in developing our cross-national coalition and a detailed discussion of them can be found in Voisin, Baptiste, Martinez & Henderson (in review). In brief, several steps emerged as significant in building our partnership. These include: (1) selecting a mature host agency with a strong infrastructure such as the FPATT's, (2) aligning the missions, interests, and agenda of both researchers and the participating agency in the early stages of work, (3) developing explicit norms for communication and negotiations; (4) using culturally competent mediators to anchor the initiative and to build trust, (5) carefully establishing roles and responsibilities and giving the local agency maximum say in determining the course of the initiative, (6) respecting the local employment climate in hiring, staffing, compensations, and the like, and (7) reconciling the role of the specific initiatives (e.g., HIV/AIDS prevention) within the overall mission of the participating agency. Additionally, partnerships such as ours may also struggle with trust-building in post-colonial nations; reconciling science and service missions; ensuring human subject protections in developing country settings; and embedding mutuality and balance in researcher-agency relationships (Voisin, Baptiste, Martinez & Henderson, 2006).

CONCLUSION

Without a vaccine, reducing the spread of HIV/AIDS in regions hardest hit like the Caribbean will require innovative prevention approaches to mount a credible response to the virus. This may involve an unprecedented level of international inter-agency partnerships to channel resources to affected regions (Caribbean Task Force on AIDS, 2000). We hope that insights provided from our collaboration will assist other HIV/AIDS prevention alliances. Ultimately, we are all affected by the virus and hopefully our combined efforts can eventually defeat it.

NOTES

1. For parents, items regarding comfort level talking about alcohol, drugs, and gangs all had zero variance and were removed from the scale analysis.
2. Table 7 lists the individual items and detailed results are discussed later. Regarding scale reliability, the item "refusing marijuana offered to you at a party" had zero variance and was removed from the scale.

REFERENCES

Baptiste, D., Paikoff, P., McKay, M., Madison, S., Bell, C., Coleman, C., & the CHAMP Board. (2005). Collaborating with an urban community to develop an HIV/AIDS prevention program for black youth and families. *Behavior Modification.* 29(2): 370-416.

Baptiste, D., Martinez, D., & The CHAMP-TT Collaborative Board. (2003). Family Interventions for Caribbean Youth HIV/AIDS Risks. Funded NIMH grant proposal submitted to the National Institutes of Mental Health (NIMH), Office of AIDS Research. Available from the first author.

Camera, B., Lee, R., Gatwood, J., Wagner, H., Cazal-Gamelsy, R., & Boisson, E. (2003). The Caribbean HIV/AIDS epidemic epidemiological status: Success stories–A summary. *CAREC Surveillance Report (CSR) Supplement, Vol 23:1* Caribbean Epidemiology Center (CAREC): Port of Spain, Trinidad.

Caribbean Task Force on AIDS. (February, 2000). The Caribbean regional strategic plan of action for HIV/IADS-1999-2004. Available at https://www.paho.org

Caribbean Epidemiology Center. (2002). *Quarterly AIDS surveillance reports submitted to CAREC's Epidemiology Division by CAREC member countries.* Port-of-Spain: Trinidad.

Family Planning of Trinidad and Tobago (FPATT) (September 2000). *The sexual health needs of youth in Trinidad and Tobago: Summary report.* Port of Spain, Trinidad: FPATT.

Gorman-Smith, D., Tolan, P. H., Zelli, A., & Huesman, L. R. (1996). The relation of family functioning to violence among inner-city minority youth. *Journal of Family Psychology, 10*, 115-129.

Gurerra, N. G. & Tolan, P.H. (1991*). Metropolitan Area Child Study (MACS).* Grant Proposal. Available from the second author at University of Illinois at Chicago.

Harris-Hastick, E. F. & Modeste-Curwen, C. (2001). The importance of culture in HIV/AIDS prevention in Grenada. *Journal of HIV/AIDS Prevention & Education for Adolescents & Children*, 4, 5-22.

Jack, N. (2002). HIV/AIDS in Caribbean adolescents and children. *Journal of HIV/AIDS Prevention and Education for Adolescents and Children, 4* (2/3), 23-40.

Madison, S.M., McKay, M. M., Paikoff, R. L., & Bell, C.C. (2000). Basic research and community collaboration: Necessary ingredients for the development of a family-based HIV prevention program. *AIDS Education and Prevention, 12*, 281-298.

McKay. M., Baptiste, D., Paikoff, R., Madison, S., & CHAMP Collaborative Board. (2000). *Preventing HIV Risk Exposure in Urban Communities: The CHAMP Family Program.* In W. Pequegnat & Szapocznik (Eds). *Working with families in the Era of HIV/AIDS.* Sage: CA.

McKay, M., Bell, C., Paikoff, R, L., Baptiste, D. & Madison, S. (2000). Community partnerships to decrease adolescent HIV/AIDS risks. NIMH-funded grant proposal. Available from the first author at the Mount Sinai University hospital.

McKay, M., Taber-Chasse, K., Paikoff, R., Baptiste, D., & Paikoff, R. (2004). Family-level impact of the CHAMP family program: A community collaborative effort to support urban families ad reduce HIV/AIDS risk exposure. *Family Process.*

O'Loughlin, J., Renaud, L., Richard, L., Gomez, L., & Paradis, G. (1998). Correlates of the sustainability of community-based heart health promotion interventions. *Preventative Medicine, 15*, 522-536.

Pan American Health Organization (PAHO) & The Ministry of Health, Trinidad and Tobago (June 1998). *Adolescent Health Survey.* Available from the Ministry of Health, Trinidad and Tobago. Port-of-Spain.

Pan American Health Organization (PAHO). (2001). *Health in the Americas.* Geneva: World Health Organization.

Paikoff, R. L. (1995). Early heterosexual debut: Situations of sexual possibility during the transition to adolescence*. American Journal of Orthopsychiatry.* 65, 389-401.

Paikoff, R., McKay, M., & Bell, C., (1994) The Chicago HIV prevention and adolescent mental health project (CHAMP) family-based intervention. National Institute of Mental Health, office on AIDS and William T. Grant Foundation funded grants.

Pequegnat. W. & Szapocznik, J. (Eds.). (2000). *Working with Families in the Era of HIV/AIDS.* CA: Sage Publications.

Roopnarine, J., Clawson, M., Benetti, S., & Lewis, T. (2000). Family structure, parent-child socialization, and involvement among Caribbean families. In A. Comunian, & U. Gielen (Eds), *International perspectives on Human Development* (pp. 309-329). Pabst Science Publishers: Lengerich, Germany.

Trinidad and Tobago National Surveillance Unit. (2002). *Quarterly Reports of the Trinidad and Tobago National Surveillance Unit-August 2001.* Port-of-Spain, Trinidad: Ministry of Health Trinidad and Tobago. Available at http://www.carec.org

UN/AIDS/WHO. (2002). *Report o the global HIV/AIDS epidemic.* Joint United Nations Programme on HIV/AIDS, World Health Organization.

UNICEF/UNAIDS/WHO. (2002). *Young people and HIV/AIDS: Opportunity in crisis*. United Nation Children's Fund. Available at http://www.unicef.org

Voisin, D., & Remy, M. (2001). Psychocultural factors associated with HIV infection among Trinidad and Tobago adolescents. *Journal of HIV/AIDS Prevention and Education for Adolescents and Children, 4* (2/3), 65-82.

Voisin, D., Baptiste, D., Martinez, D., & Henderson, G. (2006). Exporting a US-HIV/AIDS prevention program to a Caribbean-island nation: Lessons from the field. *International Social Work, 49*(1): 75-86.

Voisin, D. (2002). Family ecology and HIV sexual risk behaviors among African American and Puerto Rican males. *American Journal of Orthopsychiatry, 72 (2)*, 294-302.

Whitaker, D. J., & Miller, K. S. (2000). Parent-adolescent discussions about sex and condoms: Impact on peer influences of sexual risk behavior. *Journal of Adolescent Research, 15*(2), 251-273.

World Bank. (2000). *HIV/AIDS in the Caribbean: Issues and options*. Report no. 20491-Lac. Washington, DC: World Bank.

doi:10.1300/J200v05n03_05

Adapting a Family-Based HIV Prevention Program for HIV-Infected Preadolescents and Their Families: Youth, Families and Health Care Providers Coming Together to Address Complex Needs

Mary McKay

Megan Block

Claude Mellins

Dorian E. Traube

Elizabeth Brackis-Cott

Desiree Minott

Claudia Miranda

Jennifer Petterson

Elaine J. Abrams

Mary McKay, PhD, is Professor of Social Work in Psychiatry & Community Medicine, Mount Sinai School of Medicine. Megan Block, MPH, Claude Mellins, PhD, and Elizabeth Brackis-Cott, PhD, are affiliated with New York State Psychiatric Institute, HIV Center for Clinical and Behavioral Studies. Dorian E. Traube, CSW, Claudia Miranda, MSW, and Jennifer Petterson, MSW, are affiliated with the Columbia University School of Social Work. Desiree Minott, MPH, is affiliated with Harlem Hospital Center, Columbia University. Elaine J. Abrams, MD, is affiliated with Harlem Hospital Center, Columbia University.

Address correspondence to: Mary M. McKay, PhD, Professor of Social Work in Psychiatry & Community Medicine, Mount Sinai School of Medicine, One Gustave L. Levy Lane, New York, NY 10029 (E-mail: mary.mckay@mssm.edu).

The authors acknowledge the significant contributions of participating families and consultants.

Funding from the New York State Psychiatric Institute, HIV Center for Clinical and Behavioral Studies Grant (P30 MH43520) is gratefully recognized. Dorian Traube is currently a pre-doctoral fellow at the Columbia University School of Social Work supported by a training grant from the National Institutes of Mental Health (5T32MH014623-24).

[Haworth co-indexing entry note]: "Adapting a Family-Based HIV Prevention Program for HIV-Infected Preadolescents and Their Families: Youth, Families and Health Care Providers Coming Together to Address Complex Needs." McKay, Mary et al. Co-published simultaneously in *Social Work in Mental Health* (The Haworth Press, Inc.) Vol. 5, No. 3/4, 2007, pp. 355-378; and: *Community Collaborative Partnerships: The Foundation for HIV Prevention Research Efforts* (ed: Mary M. McKay, and Roberta L. Paikoff) The Haworth Press, Inc., 2007, pp. 355-378. Single or multiple copies of this article are available for a fee from The Haworth Document Delivery Service [1-800-HAWORTH, 9:00 a.m. - 5:00 p.m. (EST). E-mail address: docdelivery@haworthpress.com].

doi:10.1300/J200v05n03_06

SUMMARY. This article describes a family-based HIV prevention and mental health promotion program specifically designed to meet the needs of perinatally-infected preadolescents and their families. This project represents one of the first attempts to involve perinatally HIV-infected youth in HIV prevention efforts while simultaneously addressing their mental health and health care needs. The program, entitled CHAMP+ (Collaborative HIV Prevention and Adolescent Mental Health Project-Plus), focuses on: (1) the impact of HIV on the family; (2) loss and stigma associated with HIV disease; (3) HIV knowledge and understanding of health and medication protocols; (4) family communication about puberty, sexuality and HIV; (5) social support and decision making related to disclosure; and (6) parental supervision and monitoring related to sexual possibility situations, sexual risk taking behavior and management of youth health and medication. Findings from a preliminary evaluation of CHAMP+ with six families are presented along with a discussion of challenges related to feasibility and implementation within a primary health care setting for perinatally infected youth. doi:10.1300/J200v05n03_06 *[Article copies available for a fee from The Haworth Document Delivery Service: 1-800-HAWORTH. E-mail address: <docdelivery@haworthpress.com> Website: <http://www.HaworthPress.com> © 2007 by The Haworth Press, Inc. All rights reserved.]*

KEYWORDS. Perinatally-infected preadolescents and their families, family communication, challenges with feasibility and implementation, parental supervision and monitoring, social support and decision making

As a result of improvements in HIV medical treatment, increasing numbers of perinatally-infected children are surviving into adolescence and beyond. Yet these youth continue to live with a stigmatizing, still potentially fatal, chronic illness (Havens, Mellins, & Hunter, 2002; Lindegern, 2001; Grosz, 2001). They must cope with the numerous health care demands of the illness as well as the effect of HIV on normative developmental processes, including puberty, growth, peer relations, and sexuality. Furthermore, given the epidemiology of pediatric HIV, the majority of perinatally infected children are born into families who have struggled with poverty, inner-city stressors, drug use, and often previous loss due to parental HIV. Thus, this is a population at high risk for poor behavioral and mental health outcomes.

To date, few studies have examined the emotional and behavioral sequelae of perinatal HIV infection in older youth, although a few studies indicate that younger children present with high rates of mental health problems (Havens, Whitaker, Ehrhardt et al., 1994; Mellins et al., 2003) and clinical reports indicate that as perinatally HIV-infected children reach adolescence, sexual behavior and substance use emerge as significant issues (Ledlie, 2000; Havens and Ng, 2001). Involvement in sexual and drug risk taking behavior not only threatens the safety and well being of the HIV-infected child, but also poses a significant public health threat for transmission of the virus. Corresponding with the limited literature on behavioral outcomes of perinatal HIV infection, few efficacy-based interventions have been developed to decrease risk taking behavior and improve the mental health and well-being of perinatally HIV-infected youth and their families.

This article describes a family-based HIV prevention and mental health promotion program specifically designed to meet the needs of perinatally-infected preadolescents and their families. The process by which youth, adult caregivers, health care providers and HIV prevention scientists came together to adapt an existing evidence-based HIV prevention program will be detailed here. Issues specific to this population, including HIV as a stigmatizing disease, communication about HIV within and outside the family, adherence to medical treatment, child and parental mental health issues, are discussed. The preliminary impact of the program and related feasibility and implementation challenges are presented and next steps for research and program development are detailed.

NEED FOR PSYCHOSOCIAL INTERVENTIONS FOR PERINATALLY HIV-INFECTED YOUTH

Pediatric HIV

Nationally, more than 13,502 children less than 13 years of age are living with HIV infection (CDC, 2000) with the vast majority of these children exposed perinatally and growing up in inner city environments, such as New York City (NYC). Corresponding with the epidemiology of HIV disease in women, the majority of HIV-infected children in NYC are African American (55%) and Latino (35%), living in poverty, and affected by parental substance use (NYC DOH, 2004). Fortunately, antiretroviral therapies, when used effectively during pregnancy and the birth process, have significantly diminished the risk of mother-to-child transmission of HIV (Cooper, 2002), virtually eradicating pediatric HIV for future generations. However, use of HIV antiretrovirals, as well as other medications that prevent opportunistic infections has resulted in decreased morbidity and mortality for children with established HIV disease (De Martino, 2000; Epstein, Little, & Richman, 2000). Thus, increasing numbers of perinatally infected children are surviving into their teens and beyond, yet needing to incorporate a stigmatizing, chronic illness into their development and transition through adolescence.

Stigma Associated with Perinatal HIV Infection and Disclosure

Perinatally infected adolescents must confront the social ramifications of having a chronic stigmatized disease. Complicating their adjustment is the fact that many youth are not told about their illness until they enter their second decade of life (Mellins et al., 2002; Wiener, Battles, & Heilman, 1998). Caregivers are often afraid of the negative consequences of disclosure including child distress, child anger at parent for infecting them, and inappropriate disclosure to others (Havens, Mellins, Pilowsky, 1996; Mellins et al., 2002). For youth who do know their diagnosis, there are complicated decisions related to disclosure of serostatus that may impact friendships, relationships with sexual partners, and the risk for HIV transmission. For HIV-infected children, caregiver concerns about disclosure of child HIV status to the child may be one of the most significant barriers to adequate parent-child communication around sexuality, drug use, and adherence. Limited parent-child communication is of concern given that several studies have found that youth with more frequent and open parent-child communication have better psychological adjustment, (Amerikaner, Monks, Wolfe, & Thomas, 1995) as well as delayed sexual activity, fewer partners, and more use of contraception (Baumeister, Flores, & Marin, 1995; Fox & Inazu, 1980; Klein & Gordon, 1990; Kotchick et al., 1999; Miller et al., 1998; O'Sullivan et al., 1999; Pick & Palos, 1997).

Antiretroviral Adherence

To achieve viral suppression, combination antiretroviral therapy often requires multiple daily doses of three or more medications over an indefinite period. These therapies have created challenges for both youth as well as their adult caregivers (Mellins et al., 2003; Chesney et al., 2000). Adherence has emerged as a major treatment obstacle. Pediatric adherence is complicated by issues of volume, taste, and repeated, potentially unpleasant, child-caregiver encounters related to adherence. HIV-infected youth frequently have irregular daily schedules due to school, after-school activities, and medical appointments. This, coupled with the desire to lead as normal a life as possible may make it very difficult for youth to adhere to strict medication regimens. In addition, there are numerous adherence challenges for the adult caregivers of these youth including remembering frequent doses, accurately identifying varied pills and liquids, integrating multiple medications into daily activities, and maintaining privacy (Byrne et al., 2002).

Unfortunately, even brief episodes of non-adherence to ART can permanently undermine treatment and lead to reduced efficacy of and increased resistance to medications (Patterson et al., 2000). In addition, many older perinatally-infected children, during early days of antiretroviral treatment, received monotherapy before the importance of combination treatment was understood. Thus, many perinatally infected adolescents are living with multidrug resistant HIV that not only impairs the health of the youth, but can also be transmitted to others through sexual and drug use behaviour. This grim reality becomes a serious public health issue as youth approach adolescence, a time of increased experimentation with sexual behavior and drug use. For HIV-infected youth, engaging in any type of risk behavior increases opportunities for transmission of HIV (including ART-resistant strains of the virus) to others. The fact that perinatally infected children are now becoming adolescents in relatively large numbers presents a public health concern that warrants immediate attention, particularly in NYC, home to over 20% of the HIV-infected women and children in the U.S. (Centers for Disease Control, 2002; NYC Department of Health, 2002).

Mental Health Needs and Functioning of Perinatally Infected Children

Studies of children with other chronic debilitating diseases have shown increased rates of mental health problems, including depression or social withdrawal (Abrams, 1990; Grosz, 2001; Havens, 2001; Mellins, 2001). Perinatally HIV infected youth may be at particularly high risk for mental health problems given the high rates of co-morbid mental health and substance use disorders in HIV-infected women, the potential inheritability of these disorders, and the stressful family and social environments often associated with parental mental illness and substance abuse (Havens, Mellins, & Ryan, 1997). Clinical reports indicate that adolescents with perinatal HIV infection are presenting with:

(1) serious mental health difficulties, including mood, anxiety, and behavioral problems, and (2) high-risk sexual behaviors and substance use (Abrams, 1990; Grosz, 2001; Havens, 2001; Mellins, 2001). Furthermore, emotional and behavioral difficulties, including social problems, anxiety, depression, as well as other disorders associated with impulse control problems and affective dysregulation, potentially related to the neurological and cognitive sequelae of HIV, have been found in 12 to 44% of younger HIV-infected children (Abrams & Nicholas, 1990; Corsi et al., 1991; Mellins et al., 2003; Tardieu et al., 1995).

In summary, the potential for stigma and disclosure issues, difficulties with adherence to multiple medications, and mental health problems may place HIV-infected youth at high-risk for multiple behavioral difficulties as they age. However, the authors know of no efficacy-based interventions that target the unique needs of perinatally HIV-infected youth and their families, as the youth approach adolescence. Thus, the authors developed a new program, CHAMP+ (Collaborative HIV Prevention and Mental Health Project-Plus), based on models of family-based prevention developed for other populations of inner city adolescents. The program and preliminary evaluation of CHAMP+ presented here is an important opportunity to further understand the needs of perinatally infected youth and their families and examine issues related to feasibility, implementation, and impact of prevention programs that target unique risk factors and attempt to bolster protective influences in this population.

DEVELOPMENT OF CHAMP+

The Original CHAMP Model and Consumer Involvement

The Collaborative HIV-Prevention and Adolescent Mental Health Family Program (CHAMP) served as a template for the intervention developed for perinatally HIV-infected youth, CHAMP+. The original CHAMP Family Program was developed in response to the increasing need to reduce urban adolescent HIV exposure in inner-city populations. CHAMP's original goal was to increase understanding of sexual development and HIV risk within the urban context, while applying that understanding of development to an intervention program (Paikfoff, 1997; McKay et al., 2000). The content and structure of the CHAMP Family Program were influenced by research findings and a collaborative partnership. A longitudinal study conducted with 315 urban, African American early adolescents and their families provided the empirical basis and conceptual framework for the intervention (Paikoff, 1997). In addition, the development of the CHAMP intervention program was shaped by a collaborative partnership between urban community parents, school staff, and university-based researchers.

Creating culturally sensitive interventions through collaboration with consumers is necessary in light of increasing evidence that HIV prevention programs designed for urban minority youth have faced significant obstacles to involving participants (Dalton, 1989; Gustafson et al., 1992; Stevenson & White, 1994). Specifically, Stevenson and White (1994) identified obstacles to the implementation of HIV prevention programs that include: (1) denial of the epidemic in minority communities related to stigma; (2) distrust of majority cultural institutions; and (3) myths/beliefs regarding AIDS contraction, transmission and origin. Also, cultural concerns arise when research on health problems that disproportionately affect minority communities are investigated by "outsiders" (Dalton, 1989; Thomas & Quinn, 1991). Involving consumers in research can effectively help researchers address many of these issues (Hatch et al., 1993; Madison et al., in press). One particularly effective model is to have community members take a driving role, with research staff to develop programs of research and services to meet consumer needs (Hatch et al., 1993). This model was used in the development of the original CHAMP family program. More specifically, consumers and health care providers were integrally involved in the program' in its design, oversight and preliminary testing.

The primary goals of the original CHAMP Family Program curriculum are to: (1) foster discussion of *sexual possibility situations*; (2) make links between family processes and children's participation in sexual possibility situations (in particular, stressing family communication, rule setting, monitoring, support, and provision of clear values); and (3) increase caregiver and youth understanding of puberty and HIV/AIDS in order to prepare families for the coming changes of adolescence. CHAMP is delivered via multi-level group modalities, which include both multiple family sessions and parent/child group sessions (McKay et al., 2000; Madison, McKay et al., 2000).

Given the goals of promoting communication and support both within and between families, the idea of combining families into groups is a logical format for program delivery. In addition to entire family needs, however, children and parents within families have individual needs as well. For parents, these needs include support from other parents, and frank discussion of strategies for supervision and monitoring, as well as chances to discuss information and communication strategies separately from their children. For children, these needs include developing peer supports, as well as social problem skills to assist in recognizing different types of risk situations, and negotiation/self-assertion skills to deal with such situations. Thus, a combination of multiple family sessions and parent/child sessions are used. Based upon the previous research related to risk and protective influences for urban youth, as well as findings from the CHAMP Family Study (see Paikoff, 1997 for summary), a theoretical model guiding the development of the original CHAMP Family Program was created (see Figure 1). In depth descriptions of the CHAMP model, program, and preliminary results of large clinical trials evaluations have been presented elsewhere (see Madison et al., 2000; McKay, Chasse et al.; 2004).

Creating CHAMP+ Curriculum

A collaboration was forged between HIV-infected early adolescents, their adult caregivers, pediatric HIV primary care providers, and university-based HIV prevention scientists in order to adapt the CHAMP Family Program to address the complex needs of children with perinatally-acquired HIV. The collaborative partnership took place in 2002 at an urban pediatric AIDS center, Harlem Hospital Center, an area that especially mirrors the complexities of the HIV/AIDS epidemic in NYC. Following the model of consumer involvement used in previous adaptations of CHAMP, consumers (five caregivers of perinatally HIV-infected youth and three HIV+ teenagers) met with university-based research staff for a period of six months to: (1) identify salient issues related to HIV, family life, and youth development and risk; (2) review existing CHAMP Family Program to assess appropriateness of content, format, etc.; and (3) develop new intervention content based upon perceived needs. Simultaneously, research staff met with HIV health care providers at the hospital to gather input related to programmatic content and feasibility of integrating a test of CHAMP+ into the hospital's service delivery system. These health care providers have worked with the families they serve for 10-12 years and are, therefore, very familiar with the strengths and needs of the families.

Information gathered from the collaborative partnership, including the constant involvement of consumers, was critical to the adaptation and development of CHAMP into the new intervention program. Although the format of the original CHAMP program was maintained, additional sessions were added to CHAMP+ and changes were made to

FIGURE 1. CHAMP Family Program Theoretical Model

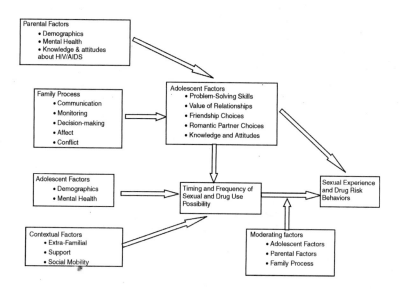

programmatic content. Key changes that were made to the CHAMP theoretical model and program include consideration of: (1) the impact of HIV on the family; (2) loss and stigma associated with HIV disease; (3) HIV knowledge and understanding of health and medication protocols; (4) family communication about puberty, sexuality and HIV; (5) social support and decision making related to disclosure; (6) parental supervision and monitoring related to sexual possibility situations and sexual risk taking behavior; and (7) parental supervision related to helping youth manage their health and medication. CHAMP+ programmatic content was also revised to encompass family level issues such as death of a parent or HIV status of the parent. Key changes were then made to the CHAMP theoretical model (Figure 2).

CHAMP+ Family Curriculum and Program

CHAMP+ aims to intervene with families by targeting specific child, parent, and family factors within the context of HIV. The program relies on theories of community collaboration while also utilizing a strength and family-based approach. The goal of the program is to increase family communication while creating an environment that supports and encourages families to raise healthy children.

FIGURE 2. CHAMP+ Theoretical Model

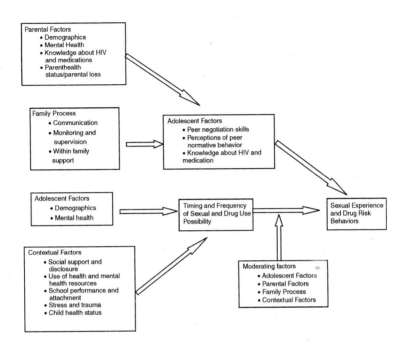

The family-based curriculum focuses on communication skills, relationship maintenance skills (negotiation and refusal skills), social support, and HIV education. Children and caregivers learn these skills by participating in a variety of interactive activities, discussions, role-plays, and games, etc. The curriculum is appropriate for both youth and caregivers; it is developmentally appropriate for preadolescent HIV-infected children, and also appropriate for the varied caregiver/child relationships (i.e., biological, kin, or adoptive caregivers).

CHAMP+ PILOT STUDY

Methods

Setting. The CHAMP+ Family Program was pilot-tested over 10, two-hour sessions at Harlem Hospital's Family Care Center. The sample included children receiving their HIV primary care at Harlem Hospital's Family Care Center and their respective caregivers. The Family Care Center at Harlem Hospital is a comprehensive care and research program that has been providing multidisciplinary medical, psychological, and social services to HIV-infected and affected children and their families since 1986. Currently there are approximately 130 children, ages newborn to 21 years of age, who are infected with HIV/AIDS in care. The populations reflect the larger population of perinatally HIV-infected children in NYC (NYC Department of Health HIV/AIDS Surveillance, 2003).

Recruitment. Families were recruited based on the study's eligibility requirements. In order to participate in the CHAMP+ Family Program, caregivers had to be the legal guardian of the child, the biological or adoptive caregiver of the child, and had to have lived with the child for at least one year prior to study commencement. Child eligibility requirements included that the child received his/her HIV primary care at Harlem Hospital Center and that the child had been disclosed his/her HIV+ status prior to study commencement. A total of six families (n = 6 caregiver/child dyads), or 12 participants, were recruited for the CHAMP+ Family Program pilot study. However, one family (caregiver and HIV+ girl) decided not to participate because of the time commitment.

Gender. Although gender was not an inclusion/exclusion criteria, all child participants (n = 5) were male. They were nine to 12 years of age, African American, infected with perinatal HIV, and had been told about their diagnosis. Again, gender was not an inclusion/exclusion criteria, but all caregiver participants (n = 5) were female. They were 39 to 70 years of age, African American, and either the biological (n = 3) or adoptive (n = 2) caregiver of the child. During the introductory intervention session, all participants signed written consent forms informing them of the research study, the possible benefits and risks to participating, and confidentiality. Both the program and debriefing exit-interview (see below) received Institutional Review Board approval.

Procedures. In order to examine issues raised and modifications made to the program during implementation, process notes were taken during sessions by a trained observer. A debriefing exit-interview was developed to evaluate the effectiveness of the CHAMP+ Family Program. A trained graduate student administered the confidential individual interview questionnaires to all child and caregiver participants post-intervention within 2 weeks. Exit interviews consisted of a series of structured questions using Likert scales, as well as a number of qualitative questions assessing issues of program feasibility, participant satisfaction, and perceptions of family change (see Appendix, Exit Interview Questions). Qualitative process notes were collected throughout the planning and implementation phases of the intervention, while in depth qualitative interviews and standardized questionnaires were administered to all participants at the completion of the pilot intervention.

Content analysis involved two raters, trained in qualitative data analysis, separately reviewing process notes and exit interviews to identify (a) barriers to participation, (b) deviation from original *CHAMP+* material, (c) perceptions of family change, and (d) "lessons learned." The first step in qualitative data analysis was to identify the most prominent themes that could reliably be identified by the two raters. The raters reviewed all process notes and qualitative data from the exit interviews and marked phrases and paragraphs containing material relevant to the aims of the process evaluation. Themes were distinguished within those topics and used to develop a coding nomenclature for each question. Discrepancies were resolved by consensus discussion; final codes resulting from that process were then assigned. This coding nomenclature then was used by both raters separately to review and to code all of the qualitative data (process notes and qualitative exit interview questions). The level of rater coding agreement was 88.3%, denoting excellent reproducibility (Rosner, 2000).

Results

The process evaluation of the CHAMP+ Family Program pilot study suggests that overall, the participants perceived their involvement as beneficial. Study findings, based on participants' perception of change as detailed in the post-intervention exit interviews and process notes, showed enhancement of the caregiver/child relationship, increased communication, increased participant self-efficacy regarding family communication, and social network expansion with others affected by HIV. Specific findings are presented below.

Participant Satisfaction

Caregiver/Child Relationship. Results from the exit interviews revealed that 80% (n = 8) of participants felt "closer or more connected" to their caregiver or child after participating in the CHAMP+ Family Program. Results in this section are based on responses to structured questions where participants chose from a Likert scale (see Appendix, Exit Interview Questions). Qualitative findings from the exit interviews also showed that caregivers and children felt more connected after participating in the intervention program, as noted in the following quote from an HIV+ mother:

> [CHAMP+] helped me to get to know my son more and the issues he has. I loved it. My son and I have gotten even closer since [the program].–*HIV+ mother*

Communication. After participating in CHAMP+, 60% (n = 6) of participants reported that the level of communication with their caregiver or child had increased (see Appendix, exit interview question two). For example, during the second CHAMP+ intervention session, caregivers spoke about wanting to "snoop" in order to know what was going on in their child's life. However, by the last intervention session it was evident that caregivers were communicating directly with their children instead of "snooping" to gain information. The majority of participants reported feeling more comfortable discussing sensitive topics with their caregiver or child such as puberty (70%, n = 7), HIV (60%, n = 5), and sex (50%, n = 5). See Appendix, exit interview questions three, four, and five. Qualitative findings from the exit interviews and process notes also revealed that CHAMP+ increased participants' level of perceived communication:

> Communication is definitely a plus, especially for mothers who don't know what or how to ask.–*Caregiver participant*

> I got to express myself.–*HIV+ boy*

> We can talk about those 'boy things' now and he won't get upset, just laughs.–*HIV+ mother*

Self-Efficacy Regarding Communication. Study findings revealed increased self-efficacy among participants in their ability to ask questions or initiate conversation. After participating in CHAMP+, the majority of participants reported feeling more confident that they could ask medical staff an HIV-related question (80%, n = 8). The majority of participants also reported feeling more confident that they could initiate a conversation with their respective caregiver or child if there was something they wanted to talk about (80%, n = 8). See Appendix, exit interview questions six and seven. Qualitative findings from the exit interviews also showed increased self-efficacy among participants. For example:

He's talking more and asks questions about certain things, whereas in the past he wouldn't ask.–*HIV+ mother*

Social Network Expansion. After participating in CHAMP+, participants perceived that their social network with others *affected* by HIV had expanded. Results from the exit interviews revealed that participants felt "closer or more connected" to their family (40%, n = 4) and other CHAMP+ participants (70%, n = 7). See Appendix, exit interview questions eight and nine. Findings also showed social network expansion with others *affected* by HIV among participants:

[The other kids in CHAMP+] all have the same thing, and they know what I mean.–*HIV+ boy*

Its part of a comfortability–we can talk more now and he knows that [other participants] are going through the same things we are, he sees how other moms react.–*HIV+ mother*

Results from the exit interviews also revealed that participants felt "closer or more connected" to CHAMP+ facilitators (80%, n = 8) and the medical staff at Harlem Hospital (80%, n = 8) (see Appendix, exit interview questions 10 and 11). In order to minimize conflict of interest and social desirability of participant response, CHAMP+ staff members were comprised of non-medical personnel. This allowed participants to speak freely without worrying about jeopardizing their child's healthcare. One HIV+ caregiver spoke of the mistrust she felt towards the establishment where she routinely received her medical care:

Have you ever had a doctor tell you like [CHAMP+ facilitator] just did? No, they never give you stats or tell you options. They only tell you to take the regiment.–*HIV+ caregiver*

In conclusion, the exit interview, administered to all participants post-intervention, and the process notes revealed quantitative and qualitative findings related to perceptions of family change and issues related to participant satisfaction.

This group is ringing chimes in my head–been doing good–asking questions.–*Adoptive caregiver*

It really helped me a lot. Things I would never have thought about, it made me think of.–*Adoptive caregiver*

After school he would always ask, Mommy are we going to-day?–*Adoptive caregiver*

Yeah, feeling better about myself.–*HIV+ boy*

Barriers to Participation

Content analysis of the process notes revealed specific barriers to participation in the intervention. Obstacles included both personal and programmatic barriers which are detailed below. It is important to emphasize, however, that even though feasibility related barriers were identified during the CHAMP+ pilot, they did not appear to severely impact participation of families involved in the pilot. As Figure 3 evidences, with the exception of session #3, during which a serious snow storm occurred, family participation rates remained quite high throughout the implementation of the CHAMP+ program. Records of attendance at CHAMP+ Family Program intervention sessions indicated an attendance rate of: session one ($n = 12$), session two ($n = 10$), session three ($n = 4$), session four ($n = 10$), session five ($n = 8$), session six ($n = 10$), session seven ($n = 10$), session eight ($n = 8$), session nine ($n = 6$), and session 10 ($n = 8$).

Participant Personal Barriers

Participant personal barriers to participation included issues related to impaired adolescent and caregiver health, time commitment (a total of six families were recruited, but one chose not to participate due to too big a time commitment), caregiver personal needs, and family health. Given the sub-optimal health status of this population, it was not surprising that impaired health proved to be the most frequent personal barrier to participation in the CHAMP+ Family Program.

Programmatic Barriers

During preparation for the CHAMP+ pilot study, a focused series of meetings between members of the investigative team and health care staff (physicians, nurses, health educators) revealed a number of site-specific barriers, including: (1) space constraints; (2) available time of

FIGURE 3. CHAMP+ Pilot Test Participant Attendance

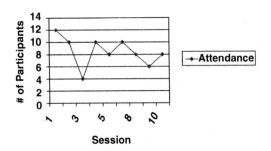

site staff to facilitate the intervention; and (3) need for coordination of refreshments, staffing, and child care materials. Each of these issues was successfully addressed using a solution-focused approach that supported site staff to develop acceptable remedies to each feasibility barrier identified. This approach yielded considerable success as ten sessions of the CHAMP+ program were delivered during the pilot study. However, other programmatic barriers to participation were identified throughout the course of the pilot included issues related to weather, transportation, childcare, and discussion of sensitive topics. Weather appeared as the most frequent programmatic barrier to participation, as the intervention program occurred over the course of the winter and holiday months.

Modifications to the CHAMP+ Family Program Curriculum

Issues of Disclosure and Privacy. Although study findings indicated that the intervention was perceived as beneficial to participants, the process evaluation also revealed several areas where the CHAMP+ Family Program needs to be further tailored to meet the needs of families affected by pediatric HIV. Despite the extensive collaborative and planning stages of CHAMP+, HIV-related issues surfaced continued to emerge during program implementation that resulted in further modification of the intervention protocol. For example, participants continually expressed issues of HIV-related secrecy, disclosure and stigma throughout CHAMP+ Family Program intervention sessions:

No matter how much we talk about it, stigma and people are still there–*Caregiver participant*

People look at us differently because of the virus.–*HIV+ child*

Why isn't he reacting like I did–no emotion (laid back)–I didn't want to face or accept or deal with it until I came here and Dr. A said something–*Caregiver participant*

Recent disclosure was especially significant for this group as one child, who was asked if he had any questions during session 2, asked point blank, "How do you cure HIV, how it happens, and how to stop it?" One caregiver spoke about how telling her child that he was adopted was more of an issue for her than disclosing illness. Another HIV+ caregiver said: "My motto is don't tell nobody."

Qualitative analyses of the process notes indicated that issues of HIV/AIDS-related stigma and disclosure were the most frequently reported issues that arose during program implementation. Since participants clearly needed to express these issues, it was difficult to complete lesson modules. Several sessions thus needed to be altered in order to incorporate such concerns.

Resulting Modifications of CHAMP+ Material. As a result of feedback, existing CHAMP+ curricula were continually modified. Deviation from original curricula was noted, and CHAMP+ programmers modified the delivery of remaining sessions accordingly. For example, the original CHAMP session on 'Talking and Listening' was modified to 'Talking and Listening within the Context of HIV.' In addition, HIV-related content was moved forward in the program, while communication-related content (which was originally planned for earlier sessions) was moved towards the end of the program. Addressing these concerns first, was critical to helping families consider more general parenting and prevention issues.

Besides issues of HIV/AIDS-related stigma and disclosure, certain programmatic content, including parent-child relationships, children's worries/concerns, HIV knowledge, and child sexuality emerged as themes that required revision of the CHAMP+ curriculum.

DISCUSSION

In the pilot study described in this article, a family-based HIV prevention program, CHAMP, provided important intervention design elements for the design and pilot of an intervention for HIV+ preadolescents and their families, entitled CHAMP+. To adapt CHAMP into the CHAMP+ program, issues specific to this population, including HIV as a stigmatizing disease, disclosure of the illness to the child and those within and outside the family, adherence to medical treatment, multiple losses experienced by families and fears about the future were incorporated into the curriculum.

In designing the CHAMP+ pilot project, consumers were involved in roles of critical importance through meetings to design the program. As a result of these meetings, the content of the CHAMP Family Program was changed and additional sessions were added, although the format of program delivery was maintained. The preliminary evaluation of the program revealed that the collaboration between HIV-infected youth, their adult caregivers, pediatric HIV primary care providers, and HIV prevention scientists yielded a program that reflected the special needs of families affected by pediatric HIV. Study findings, based on participants' perception of change as detailed in the post-intervention exit interviews and process notes, showed enhancement of the caregiver/child relationship, increased communication, increased participant self-efficacy, and social network expansion with others affected by HIV.

However, the process evaluation also revealed several areas where the CHAMP+ Family Program needed to be further tailored to meet the needs of families affected by pediatric HIV. More specifically, issues related to HIV stigma, disclosure, and secrecy proved to be of even great importance than anticipated for the study sample. Thus, the overall 'lessons learned' from the process evaluation of the CHAMP+ Family Program was that addressing issues of secrecy, HIV disclosure, and stigma in the early sessions of an intervention are critical to the development of an acceptable preventative intervention for this population. Failure to address these issues prior to the delivery of health promotion messages will undermine any preventative intervention efforts.

Conclusions

The public health implications of the transition of HIV/AIDS from an acute, lethal disease to a sub-acute chronic disease are enormous (Brown, Lourie, & Pao, 2000). Perinatally HIV-infected preadolescents are quickly emerging as a group at risk of engaging in behaviours that jeopardise their own health, and that of others. Programs and services are urgently needed that help perinatally HIV-infected children in making the transition from childhood into adolescence and that engage them in HIV prevention efforts.

A process evaluation of the CHAMP+ Family Program pilot study provided valuable insights related to a possible program structure and process. These preliminary findings will be especially beneficial to programmers seeking to plan, implement, and evaluate HIV preventative interventions with HIV-infected populations of youth and their families. These results suggest that families *affected* by pediatric HIV accepted and identified with a family-based model, implemented in a clinical setting.

However, this was an exploratory, pilot study implemented with only 10 participants (five caregiver/child dyads). Results must be interpreted with caution, as the sample is not large enough to generalize to the larger pediatric HIV population. Clearly, the CHAMP+ Family Program needs to be implemented with a larger sample to determine if the preliminary results are replicable.

Given current estimates and the millions more children projected to be born with perinatally acquired-HIV internationally, particularly in resource poor countries, progressive and innovative approaches to preventative interventions for HIV+ youth are needed. A family-based model such as CHAMP+ that seeks to intervene with perintally HIV-infected youth during the crucial time of adolescence may not only enhance the youths' quality of life, but may also dramatically reduce the spread of HIV/AIDS.

REFERENCES

Abrams, E., Nicholas, S. (1990). Pediatric HIV Infection. *Pediatric Anals, 19*(8), 482-487.

Amerikaner, M., Monks, G., Wolfe, P., Thomas, S. (1995). Family interaction and psychological health. *Journal of Counseling and Development, 72:* 614-620.

Baumeister, L.M., Flores, E., & Martin, B.V. (1995). Sex information given to Latina adolescents by parents. *Health Education Research,* 10: 233-239.

Brooks-Gunn, J. & Furstenberg, F.F. (1989). Adolescent sexual behavior. *American Psychologist,* 44: 249-253.

Byrne, M., Honig, J., Jurgrau, A., Heffernan, S.M., & Donahue, M.C. (2002). Achieving adherence with antiretroviral medications for pediatric HIV disease. *AIDS Reader. 12*(4):151-54, 161

Chesney, M.A., Ickovics, J.R., Chambers, D.B. et al. Self-reported adherence to antiretroviral medications among participants in HIV clinical trials: The AACTG adherence Instruments. AIDS Care 2000;12:255-66.

Centers for Disease Control and Prevention (2002). HIV/AIDS Surveillance report Website: http//www.cdc.gov.

Cooper, E.R., Charurat, M., Mafenson, L. et al. (2002). Combination antiretroviral strategies for the treatment of pregnant HIV-1 infected women and prevention of perinatal HIV-1 transmission. *Journal of Acquired Immune Deficiency Syndrome*, 29(5): 484-94.

Corsi, A., Albizzati, A., Cervini R. et al. (1991). Hyperactive disturbance in the behavior of children with congenital HIV infection. In Abstract of the Seventh International AIDS Conference, Vol 2, Abstract WD 4380. Florence, Italy, June 16-21. 1991.

Dalton, H.L. (1989). AIDS in blackface. *Daedalus*, 118 (3): 205-227,

De Martino, M., Tovo, P.A, Balducci, M., Galli, L., Gabiano, C., Rezza, G., & Pezzotti, P. (2000) Reduction in mortality with availability of antiretroviral therapy for children with perinatal HIV-1 infection. *Journal of the American Medical Association*, 284: 190-197.

Epstein, B.J., Little, S.J., & Richman, D.D. (2000). Drug Resistance among Patients Recently Infected with HIV. *New England Journal of Medicine*, 347(23): 1889-90.

Fox, G.L., & Inazu, J.K. (1980). Patterns and outcomes of mother-daughter communication about sexuality. *Journal of Social Issues*, 36(1): 7-29.

Grosz, J. (2001). Children with HIV infection becoming teenagers. Psychosocial and developmental tasks. Paper presented at *Pediatric AIDS and Mental Health Issues in the Era of Art Conference*, jointly sponsored by NIMH Center for Mental Health research on AIDS and The Office of Rear Diseases, NIH, September 10th, Washington DC.

Gustafson, K.E., McNamara, J.R., & Jensen, J.A. (1992). Informed consent: Risk and benefit disclosure practices of child clinicians. *Psychotherapy in Private Practice*, 10 (4): 91-102.

Hatch, J., Moss, N., Saran, A., Presley-Cantrell, L., & Mallory, C. (1993). Community research: Partnership in black communities. *American Journal of Preventive Medicine*, 9 (6, Suppl): 27-31.

Havens, J.F., Mellins, C.A., & Hunter, J. (2002). *Psychiatric Aspects of HIV/AIDS in childhood and adolescence*. In M. Rutter and E. Taylor (Eds). *Child and Adolescent Psychiatry: Modern Approaches/Fourth Edition*. Oxford, UK Blackwell, 828-841.

Havens, J., & Ng., W. (2001). The Context of HIV/AIDS Infections of Children in the United States. Paper presented at *Pediatric AIDS and Mental Health Issues in the Era of Art Conference*, jointly sponsored by NIMH Center for Mental Health research on AIDS and The Office of Rear Diseases, NIH, September 10th, Washington DC.

Havens, J.F., Whitaker, A.H., Feldman, J.F., & Ehrhardt, A.A. (1994). Psychiatric morbidity in school-age children with congenital human immunodeficiency virus infection: A pilot study. *Journal of Developmental and Behavioral Pediatrics* (Supplement, "Priorities in psychosocial research in pediatric HIV infection"), *15*, S18-S25.

Keller, S. E., Bartlett, J. A., Schleifer, S. J., Johnson, R. L., Pinner, E., & Delaney, B. (1991) . HIV-relevant sexual behavior among a health inner-city heterosexual adolescent population in an endemic area of HIV. *Journal of Adolescent Health*, 12: 44-48.

Klein, M. & Gordon S. (1990). Sex Education. In C.E. Walker, & M.C. Roberts (Eds.). (1990). *Handbook of Clinical Child Psychology* (pp. 933-949). New York: John Wiley and Sons.

Kotchick, B.A., Dorsey, S., Miller, K.S., & Forehand, R. (1999). Adolescent sexual-risk taking behavior in single-parent ethnic minority families. *Journal of Family Psychology*, 31(1): 93-102.

Kranzler EM, Shaffer D, Wasserman G, Davies M. (1990). Early childhood bereavement. *Journal of the American Academy of Child Adolescent Psychiatry*, 29: 513-520.

Ledlie, Susan W. (2000). The psychosocial issues of children with perinatally acquired HIV disease becoming adolescents: A growing challenge for providers. *AIDS Patient Care & Stds*, 15(5), 231-236.

Lindegren (2001). Center for Disease Control Retrieved April 6, 2004 from Website://www.cdc.gov/hiv/projects/perinatal/materials/meeting_summary.htm

Lipsitz, J.D., Williams, J.B.W., Rabkin, J., Remien R.H., Bradbury, M., El-Sadr, W., Goetz, R., Sorrell, S., & Gorman, J. (1994). Psychopathology in male and female intravenous drug users with and without HIV infection. *American Journal of Psychiatry*, 151: 1662-1668.

Lyon, M.E., Silber, T.J., & D'Angelo, L.J. (1997). Difficult Life Circumstances in HIV-infected adolescents cause or effect? *AIDS Patient Care and STDs*, 11: 29-37.

Madison, S., Bell, C. C., Sewell, S. D., Nash, G., McKay, M. M., Paikoff, R. L., & CHAMP Collaborative Board. (in press). Collaborating with communities in intervention and research: Approaching an "ideal" partnership. Manuscript to be published in *Psychiatric Services*.

Madison, S., McKay, M., Paikoff, R., & Bell, C. (2000). Community collaboration and basic research: Necessary ingredient for the development of a family based HIV prevention program. *AIDS Education and Prevention*, 12: 75-84.

McKay, M., Baptiste, D., Coleman, D., Madison, S., McKinney, L., & Paikoff, R. CHAMP Collaborative Board (2000). *Preventing HIV risk exposure in urban communities: The CHAMP family program*. In W. Pequegnat J. Szapocznik (Eds.). *Working with Families in the Era of HIV/AIDS*, Thousand Oaks, CA. pp. 67-87.

Mellins, C.A., Bracks-Cott, E., Dolezal, C., Richards, A., & Abrams, E. (2002). Patterns of HIV status disclosure to perinatally infected HIV-positive children and subsequent mental health outcomes. *Journal of Child Psychology and Psychiatry*, 7:101-114.

Mellins, C.A., Ehrhardt, A.A., & Grant, W.F. (1997). Psychiatric symptomatology and psychological distress in HIV-infected mothers. *AIDS and Behavior*, 1: 233-245.

Mellins C.A., Smith R., O'Driscoll P., Magder, L., Brouwers P., Chase C., Blasini I., Hittleman J., Llorente A., & Matzen E., for the NIH NIAID/NICHD/NIDA-sponsored Women and Infant Transmission Study Group (WITS). (2003). High rates of behavioral problems in perinatally HIV-infected children are not linked to HIV disease. *Pediatrics*, 111: 384-393.

Michaels, D. (1996). The Orphan Project: Estimates of children and youth orphaned by maternal death from HIV/AIDS in New York State. Press release, Albany, New York.

Miller, K., Forehand, R., & Kotchick, B.A. (1998). Adolescent sexual behavior in two ethnic minority samples the role of family variables. *Journal of Marriage and the Family*, 61: 85-98.

Morrison, M.F., Petitto, J.M., Have, T.T., Gettes, D.R., Chiappini, M.S., Weber, A.L., Brinker-Spence, P., Bauer, R.M., & Douglas, S.D. (2002). Depressive and Anxiety Disorders in Women with HIV infection. *American Journal of Psychiatry*, 159: 789-796.

Morrison, M.F., Petitto, J.M., Have, T.T., Gettes, D.R., Chiappini, M.S., Weber, A.L., Brinker-Spence, P., Bauer, R.M., & Douglas, S.D. (2002). Depressive and Anxiety Disorders in Women with HIV infection. *American Journal of Psychiatry*, 159: 789-796.

Murphy, D.A., Moscicki, B., Vermund, S., Muenz, L., and the Adolescent medicine HIV/AIDS Research Network (2000). Psychological distress among HIV+ adolescents in the REACH study: Effects of life stress, social support, and coping. *Journal of Adolescent Health*, 27:391-398.

National Center for HIV, S., and TB Prevention. (2001). *New York: US AIDS Surveillance Report*. Retrieved 10/17/2003, 2003, from *http://www.statehealth facts.kff.org*

New York City Department of Health, Office of AIDS Surveillance (2004). *HIV/AIDS Surveillance update*.

Nicholas, S. W., & Abrams, E.J. (2002). Boarder Babies with AIDS in Harlem: Lessons in Applied Public Health. *American Journal of Public Health*, *92*(2), 163-165.

O'Sullivan, L., Jaramillo, B.M.S., Moreau, D., & Meyer-Bahlburg, H.L. (1999). Mother- daughter communication about sexuality in clinical sample of Hispanic adolescent girls. *Hispanic Journal of Behavioral Sciences*, 21: 447-469.

Paikoff, R.L. (1995). Early heterosexual debut: Situations of sexual possibility during the transition to adolescence. *American Journal of Orthopsychiatry*, 65:389-401.

Paikoff, R.L. (1997). Applying developmental psychology to an AIDS prevention model for urban African American youth. *Journal of Negro Education*, 65, 44-59.

Papola, P., Alvarez, M., & Cohen, H.J. (1994). Developmental and Service Needs of School-Age Children With Human Immunodeficiency Virus Infection: A Descriptive Study. *Pediatrics*, *94*(6), 914-918.

Patterson, D. L., Swindells, S., Mohr, J., Brester, M., Vergis, E. N., Squier, C., Wagener, M. M., & Singh, Z. (2000). Adherence to protease inhibitor therapy and outcomes in patients with HIV infection. *Annals of Internal Medicine*, 1333: 21-30.

Pick, S., Palos, P.A. (1997). Impact of the families on the sex lives of adolescents. *Adolescence*, 30: 667-675.

Regier, D.A., Farmer, M., Rae, D.S., Locke, B.Z., Keith, S.J., Judd, L.S., & Goodwin, F.K. (1990). Co-morbidity of mental disorders with alcohol and other drugs of abuse. *Journal of American Medical Association*, 264: 2511-2518.

Rounsaville, B.J., Foley-Anton, S.F., Carroll, K., & Budde, D. et al. (1991). Psychiatric Diagnosis for Treatment-Seeking Cocaine Abusers. *Archives of General Psychiatry*, 48: 43-51.

Rutter M. (1966). *Children of sick parents*. London: Oxford University Press.

Stevenson, H.C. & White, J.J. (1994). AIDS prevention struggles in ethno cultural neighborhoods: Why research partnerships with community based organizations can't wait. *AIDS Education and Prevention*, 6 (2): 126-139.

Tardieu, M., Mayaux, M.J., Seibel, N., Funk-Brentano, L., Straub, E., Teglas, J., & Blanche, S. (1995). Cognitive assessment of school-age children infected with maternally transmitted human immunodeficiency virus type 1. *Journal of Pediatrics*, 126: 375-379.

Thomas, S.B. & Quinn, S.C. (1991). The Tuskegee syphilis study, 1932 to 1972: Implications for HIV education and AIDS risk education programs in the black community. *American Journal of Public Health*, 81 (11): 1498-1505.

Wiener, L.S., Battles, H.B., & Heilman, N.E. (1998). Factors associated with parent's decision to disclose their HIV diagnosis to their children. *Child Welfare*, 77: 115-135.

doi:10.1300/J200v05n03_06

APPENDIX
Exit Interview

(1) Since participating in CHAMP+, how *connected or close* do you feel to your child/caregiver?
Closer   About the same   Not close

(2) Since participating in CHAMP+, do you feel that the level of communication with your child/caregiver has changed?
More communication   No change   Less communication

(3) Since participating in CHAMP+, how comfortable do you feel discussing topics such as puberty?
More comfortable   The same   Less comfortable

(4) Since participating in CHAMP+, how comfortable do you feel discussing topics such as HIV?
More comfortable   The same   Less comfortable

(5) Since participating in CHAMP+, how comfortable do you feel discussing topics such as sex?
More comfortable   The same   Less comfortable

(6) Since participating in CHAMP+, how confident are you that you can ask medical staff a question re: your/child's HIV?
More confident   The same   Less confident

(7) Since participating in CHAMP+, how confident do you feel that you can initiate a conversation with you caregiver/child if there is something you want to talk about?
More confident   The same   Less confident

(8) Since participating in CHAMP+, how *connected or close* do you feel to your family?
Closer   About the same   Not close

(9) Since participating in CHAMP+, how *connected or close* do you feel to other CHAMP+ participants?
Closer   About the same   Not close

APPENDIX (continued)

(10) Since participating in CHAMP+, how *connected or close* do you feel to CHAMP+ facilitators?
Closer   About the same   Not close

(11) Since participating in CHAMP+, how *connected or close* do you feel to the medical staff at Harlem Hospital?
Closer   About the same   Not close

Index

Page numbers in italics designate figures; page numbers followed by "t" designate tables.